MENTAL ILLNESS AND SOCIAL POLICY

THE AMERICAN EXPERIENCE

MENTAL ILLNESS AND SOCIAL POLICY

THE AMERICAN EXPERIENCE

Advisory Editor
GERALD N. GROB

NEUROSYPHILIS

MODERN SYSTEMATIC DIAGNOSIS AND TREATMENT

PRESENTED IN ONE HUNDRED AND THIRTY-SEVEN CASE HISTORIES

BY

E[lmer] E. Southard
and
H[arry] C. Solomon

ARNO PRESS
A NEW YORK TIMES COMPANY
New York • 1973

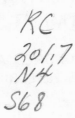

Reprint Edition 1973 by Arno Press Inc.

Reprinted from a copy in
  The Medical Library Center of New York

MENTAL ILLNESS AND SOCIAL POLICY:
  The American Experience
ISBN for complete set: 0-405-05190-5
See last pages of this volume for titles.

Manufactured in the United States of America

——————◆——————

Library of Congress Cataloging in Publication Data

Southard, Elmer Ernest, 1876-1920.
    Neurosyphilis: modern systematic diagnosis and
treatment presented in one hundred and thiry-seven
case histories.

    (Mental illness and social policy: the American
experience)
    Reprint of the ed. published by W. M. Leonard,
Boston, which was issued as Monograph no. 2 of the
Psychopathic Hospital, Boston, and in the Case
history series.
    1. Neurosyphilis. I. Solomon, Harry Caesar,
1889-   joint author. II. Title. III. Series.
IV. Series: Massachusetts. State Hospital,
Boston. Psychopathic Dept. Monographs, no. 2.
V. Series: Case history series. [DNLM: WC165 S726n
1917F]
RC201.7.N4S68 1973   616.8'92'09   73-2418
ISBN 0-405-05228-6

NEUROSYPHILIS

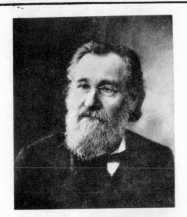
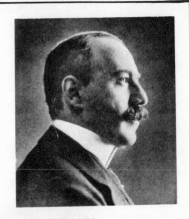

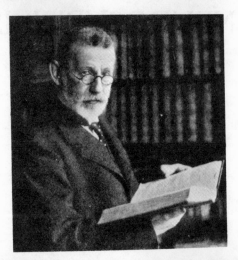

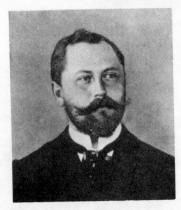
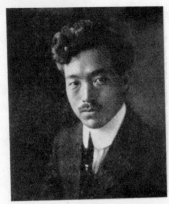

METCHNIKOFF   WASSERMANN

EHRLICH

SCHAUDINN   NOGUCHI

NEUROSYPHILIS

MODERN SYSTEMATIC DIAGNOSIS AND TREATMENT

PRESENTED IN ONE HUNDRED AND THIRTY-SEVEN CASE HISTORIES

BY

E. E. SOUTHARD, M.D., Sc.D.,

Bullard Professor of Neuropathology, Harvard Medical School; Pathologist, Massachusetts
Commission on Mental Diseases; Director, Psychopathic Department,
Boston State Hospital; Vice-President, American
Medico-Psychological Association

AND

H. C. SOLOMON, M.D.,

Instructor in Neuropathology and in Psychiatry, Harvard Medical School; Special Investigator in Brain Syphilis, Massachusetts Commission on Mental Diseases; Acting
Chief-of-Staff, Psychopathic Department, Boston State Hospital

WITH AN INTRODUCTION BY
JAMES JACKSON PUTNAM, M.D.,
Professor Emeritus of Diseases of the Nervous System, Harvard Medical School

BY VOTE OF THE TRUSTEES OF THE BOSTON STATE HOSPITAL
MONOGRAPH NUMBER TWO
OF THE
PSYCHOPATHIC HOSPITAL, BOSTON, MASSACHUSETTS

BOSTON
W. M. LEONARD, PUBLISHER
1917

To

MASSACHUSETTS

A STATE THAT
BOTH TOLERATES AND FOSTERS
RESEARCH

PREFACE

THIS book is written primarily for the general practitioner and secondarily for the syphilographer, the neurologist, and the psychiatrist. Our material is drawn chiefly from a psychopathic hospital, that modern type of institution in which the mental problems of general medical practice come to a diagnostic head weeks, months, or years before the asylum is thought of.

It is this peculiar nature of psychopathic hospital material — a concentrated essence of the most difficult daily problems of general practice — that brings together such an apparent *mélange* of cases as are here described, ranging from mild single-symptom diseases like extraocular palsy up to genuine magazines of symptoms as in general paresis; from feeble-mindedness, apparently simple, up to apparently simple dotage, both feeble-mindedness and dotage really syphilitic; from the mind-clear tabetic to the maniacal or deluded subject who looks physically perfectly fit; from the early secondaries to the late tertiaries or so-called quaternaries; from peracute to the most chronic of known conditions; from the most delicate character changes to the profoundest ruin of the psyche.

Although the bulk of our case-material is drawn from general practice through the thinnest of intermediary membranes, the psychopathic hospital, yet we have tried to depict the whole story by presenting enough autopsied cases from district state hospitals to show exactly what treatment has to face. Nor have we hesitated to insert cases in which treatment has failed.

In addition to (a) the Psychopathic Hospital, Boston, group of incipient, doubtful, obscure, or complicated cases (the early clinical group) and (b) the Danvers State Hospital, Hathorne, group of longer-standing, committed, fatal cases (the finished or autopsied group) we present (c) a miscellaneous group of cases, including many from private neurological or psychiatric practice.   No doubt those familiar with Boston medicine will see traces of the teaching of our former chiefs, notably Professors James Jackson Putnam and Edward Wyllys Taylor.   We are obliged to them for some well-observed cases.

We have dedicated our work to the Commonwealth, but perhaps we should more specifically ascribe to the Massachusetts Commission on Mental Diseases (formerly the State Board of Insanity) the spirit that permitted our special study of neurosyphilis treatment.   To these authorities, who have countenanced and encouraged a somewhat costly piece of special work since 1914, we offer our thanks, hoping that other states will be one by one stimulated to the state-endowment of research.   States doing full duty by research can be counted on one hand.

To our Psychopathic Hospital colleagues and the internes, and especially to Drs. Myrtelle M. Canavan and Douglas A. Thom of the Commission's Pathological Service, we also offer our best thanks.

The Danvers traditions are tangible here: cases of Drs. A. M. Barrett, H. A. Cotton, H. W. Mitchell, H. M. Swift, and others are presented.   We have been especially aided by the more recent work of Dr. Lawson G. Lowrey.

Nor should we have been able to present our samples of brain correlation without drawing on the collection arranged and analyzed by Dr. Annie E. Taft, Custodian, Harvard Department of Neuropathology.   The photographs, part of a collection of brain photographs now numbering over 10,000 representing 700 brains of all sorts, were made by Mr. Herbert W. Taylor.

The Wassermann testing work has been done by Dr. W. A. Hinton of the State Board of Health.   Dr. Hinton himself wrote out the text description of the Wassermann method. The method of his laboratory is held to the standards of control set by previous chiefs, viz. by Professor F. P. Gay, who brought immunological methods direct from the laboratory of Bordet (whose method the Wassermann method essentially is), Prof. W. P. Lucas, and the late Dr. Emma W. D. Mooers, who had assisted Plaut in his first work with the Wassermann method in Kraepelin's Munich Clinic.

The material combed by us to secure this illustrative series amounts to over 2000 cases of syphilis of the nervous system, including over 100 autopsies in all types of case. We have presented these with very varying fulness, chiefly to illustrate the contentions at the heads of the case-descriptions.

In using the book, we suggest early reference to the Summary and Key, where for convenience are placed numerous cross-references permitting extended illustration of almost every proposition from several cases.

We have not made a large feature of the Medicolegal and Social section. This kind of thing well deserves a volume by itself, with all the legal and social-service implications drawn out in their amazing richness and detail. The social service slogan, "A paretic's child is a syphilitic's child" has already accomplished a great deal of good in our local world. Some day we may not be compelled to *drive* the paretic's spouse and offspring to the Wassermann serum test! The general practitioner must help here.

A note on the Treatment section. This is manifestly not the last word or even, we hope, our own last word, since the systematic work of the Massachusetts Commission must be kept up for some years to get a reliable verdict. Some of the results give rise to greater optimism than has prevailed in asylum circles, especially *re* general paresis. We are confident that *no one can now successfully make a differential diagnosis between the paretic and the diffuse non-paretic forms of neurosyphilis in many phases of either disease,* even with all laboratory refinements. If this be so, it is *improper not to give the full benefits of modern treatment to all cases in which the diagnosis remains doubtful* between the paretic and the diffuse non-paretic forms of neurosyphilis. We ourselves advocate modern treatment, not only in the diffuse, but also in early paretic forms of neurosyphilis.

It would have been out of place in a book in this Case History Series to have dealt extensively with the history of our topic. We have compensated inadequately for this lack by a few remarks at the head of the Summary and Key. We are, like all others in the field, under the inevitable obligation to Nonne of Hamburg, whose great work has gone into three editions, the second of which has appeared in English translation (Nonne's Syphilis of the Nervous System, C. R. Ball, translator). Mott's work, embodied in a large volume of the Power-Murphy System of Syphilis, has also been attentively consulted, as well as the various systematic works on neurology and psychiatry. The topic of Neurosyphilis is getting wide and appropriate attention in this country through special journals, both those dealing with nervous and mental diseases, and those dealing with syphilis. Syphilis is in a sense the making of psychiatry and will go far to pushing psychiatry into general practice.

At the last moment we have been led to deviate from our plan of presenting only local cases familiar and accessible to us. In a section on Neurosyphilis and the War, we present excerpts and digests of English, French, and German cases of neurosyphilis that have appeared in association with the war. Our own country has not suffered greatly as yet either from the lighting up of neurosyphilis under martial stress or from the immediate or remote effects of syphilis obtained in the unholy congress of Mars and Venus. Space forbids a large collection of these martial cases, but, as will be seen, a fair sample of problems is presented.

Speaking for the moment as the senior author of this book, I wish to say that, were it not for the energy, industry, and ingenuity of the junior author, Dr. H. C. Solomon, the book would not have been written. Nor, in all probability, would the systematic work of the Commonwealth on neurosyphilis and its treatment ever have been begun. I can also accord the highest praise to Mrs. Maida Herman Solomon for her social-service work in this new field.

Perhaps, in closing, we owe an apology to John Milton for our borrowings from the two Paradises. Had he known much about syphilis, Milton might have written still stronger mottoes for us.

E. E. SOUTHARD

74 FENWOOD ROAD
Boston, Massachusetts

TABLE OF CONTENTS

PAGE

SECTION I. THE NATURE AND FORMS OF SYPHILIS OF THE NERVOUS SYSTEM (NEUROSYPHILIS). CASES 1 TO 8 17

CASE

1. Paradigm: protean symptoms, nervous and mental. Autopsy, with meningeal, parenchymatous, and vascular lesions............... 17
2. Tabes dorsalis (tabetic neurosyphilis). Autopsy.................. 31
3. General paresis (paretic neurosyphilis). Autopsy................. 37
4. Cerebral thrombosis (vascular neurosyphilis). Autopsy........... 42
5. Juvenile paresis (juvenile paretic neurosyphilis). Autopsy......... 45
6. Extraocular palsy (focal meningeal neurosyphilis). Autopsy........ 50
7. Gumma of brain (gummatous neurosyphilis). Autopsy............ 53
8. *Meningitis hypertrophica cervicalis* (gummatous neurosyphilis). Autopsy.. 56

SECTION II. THE SYSTEMATIC DIAGNOSIS OF THE FORMS OF NEUROSYPHILIS. CASES 9 TO 38... 63

CASE

9. Neurasthenia *versus* neurosyphilis............................. 63
10. Paretic neurosyphilis *versus* manic-depressive psychosis............ 68
11. Neurosyphilis *versus* manic-depressive psychosis................... 71
12. Dementia praecox *versus* neurosyphilis. Autopsy................. 74
13. Neurosyphilis: negative Wassermann reaction (W. R.) of serum..... 77
14. Diffuse neurosyphilis: six tests apt to run mild................... 80
15. Paretic neurosyphilis: six tests strong.......................... 85
16. Taboparesis (tabetic neurosyphilis): tests like those of paresis....... 92
17. Paretic *versus* diffuse neurosyphilis: confusion *re* tests.............. 97
18. Vascular neurosyphilis: positive serum, negative fluid W. R......... 101
19. Seizures in diffuse neurosyphilis................................ 103
20. Seizures in paretic neurosyphilis................................ 106
21. Aphasia in paretic neurosyphilis................................ 111
22. Aphasia in paretic neurosyphilis................................ 115
23. Remission in paretic neurosyphilis.............................. 117
24. Remission in diffuse neurosyphilis.............................. 122
25. *Paresis sine paresi*.. 126
26. Paretic neurosyphilis. Autopsy................................ 131
27. Gummatous neurosyphilis. Operation.......................... 137
28. Extraocular palsy (cranial neurosyphilis)....................... 140
29. Tabes dorsalis (tabetic neurosyphilis): six tests apt to run mild....... 141
30. Tabetic neurosyphilis, clinically atypical......................... 143
31. Cervical tabes.. 146
32. Erb's syphilitic spastic paraplegia.............................. 147
33. Syphilitic muscular atrophy.................................... 149

9

CASE   PAGE
34. Neurosyphilis of the secondary period.......................... 151
35. Juvenile paretic neurosyphilis: optic atrophy.................... 154
36. Juvenile paretic neurosyphilis.................................. 157
37. Simple feeblemindedness, syphilitic 159
38. Juvenile tabes... 161

SECTION III. PUZZLES AND ERRORS IN THE DIAGNOSIS OF NEUROSYPHILIS
        (INCLUDING NON-SYPHILITIC CASES). CASES 39–82............. 165

CASE
39. Paretic *versus* diffuse neurosyphilis. Autopsy.................... 165
40. Paretic *versus* vascular neurosyphilis, cerebellar. Autopsy......... 169
41. Paretic *versus* vascular neurosyphilis, cerebellar. Autopsy......... 172
42. Tabetic combined with vascular neurosyphilis. Autopsy........... 175
43. Tabetic neurosyphilis: mental symptoms, non-paretic. Autopsy.... 177
44. Cerebral gliosis. Autopsy..................................... 180
45. Neurasthenia *versus* neurosyphilis.............................. 183
46. Hysteria. Neurosyphilis of the secondary period................. 185
47. Manic-depressive psychosis *versus* paretic neurosyphilis........... 187
48. Cerebral tumor.. 190
49. Early post-infective paretic neurosyphilis....................... 192
50. Atypical paretic neurosyphilis, hemitremor. Autopsy............. 197
51. Paretic neurosyphilis. Autopsy............................... 199
52. Manic-depressive psychosis *versus* paretic neurosyphilis........... 202
53. Syphilitic (?) exophthalmic goitre. Autopsy..................... 205
54. Argyll-Robertson pupils...................................... 209
55. Argyll-Robertson pupils: pineal tumor. Autopsy................. 212
56. Neurosyphilis (?) with negative spinal fluid...................... 216
57. Disseminated syphilitic encephalitis, seven months post-infective.
        Autopsy... 218
58. "Pseudoparesis".. 222
59. Syphilitic paranoia?.. 225
60. Paretic neurosyphilis *versus* alcoholic pseudoparesis.............. 227
61. Alcoholic pseudoparesis *versus* paretic neurosyphilis.............. 231
62. Alcoholic neuritis and paretic neurosyphilis...................... 234
63. Chronic alcoholism *versus* paretic neurosyphilis................... 236
64. Neurosyphilis, diabetic pseudoparesis, or brain tumor.............. 238
65. Neurosyphilis and diabetes.................................... 240
66. Neurosyphilis: hemianopsia................................... 242
67. Paretic neurosyphilis *versus* syphilis and cerebral malaria.......... 245
68. Paretic neurosyphilis: gold sol test "syphilitic." Autopsy.......... 247
69. Lues maligna... 250
70. Neurosyphilis *versus* multiple sclerosis......................... 253
71. Atypical neurosyphilis.. 256
72. Huntington's chorea *versus* neurosyphilis....................... 258
73. Senile arteriosclerotic psychosis *versus* neurosyphilis.............. 262
74. Hysterical fugue *versus* neurosyphilis........................... 264
75. Tabetic neurosyphilis *versus* pernicious anemia................... 267
76. Congenital neurosyphilis...................................... 270
77. Congenital *versus* paretic neurosyphilis......................... 272
78. Juvenile paretic neurosyphilis................................. 275

CASE PAGE

79. Epilepsy *versus* juvenile neurosyphilis................................ 277
80. Addison's disease and juvenile paretic neurosyphilis. Autopsy...... 279
81. Neurosyphilis of the secondary period........................... 283
82. Taboparetic neurosyphilis and typhoid meningitis. Autopsy....... 284

SECTION IV. NEUROSYPHILIS, MEDICOLEGAL AND SOCIAL. CASES 83–98... 289

CASE

83. A public character, neurosyphilitic. Autopsy..................... 289
84. Debts, neurosyphilitic.. 295
85. Suicidal attempt by a neurosyphilitic.......................... 296
86. Neurosyphilis and juvenile delinquency......................... 298
87. Neurosyphilis in a defective delinquent........................ 300
88. *Paresis sine paresi* in a forger............................... 303
89. Trauma: juvenile paretic neurosyphilis......................... 306
90. Trauma: paretic neurosyphilis.................................. 308
91. False claim for trauma: neurosyphilis.......................... 309
92. Traumatic exacerbation? in neurosyphilis 310
93. Trauma: cranial gumma at the site of injury.................... 311
94. Occupation-neurosis *versus* syphilitic neuritis............... 312
95. Character change: neurosyphilis................................ 314
96. A neurosyphilitic family....................................... 316
97. A neurosyphilitic's normal-looking family...................... 318
98. The neurosyphilitic's marriage................................. 319

SECTION V. THE TREATMENT OF NEUROSYPHILIS. CASES 99–123.

(CASES 99–103 SHOW THE VARIETY OF STRUCTURAL LESIONS THAT
    TREATMENT HAS TO FACE)............................... 323

CASE

99. An incurable spastic paresis in paretic neurosyphilis. Autopsy...... 323
100. A theoretically curable case. Autopsy........................... 328
101. A highly meningitic case, theoretically amenable to treatment.
    Autopsy... 332
102. A highly atrophic case, theoretically not amenable to treatment.
    Autopsy... 335
103. Paretic neurosyphilis with markedly focal lesions. Autopsy........ 338

(CASES 104 TO 123 ARE EXAMPLES OF TREATMENT INCLUDING SUC-
    CESSES AND FAILURES.)

104. Diffuse neurosyphilis: treatment successful after nine months...... 342
105. Atypical neurosyphilis: treatment successful..................... 346
106. Argyll-Robertson pupil not necessarily of bad prognosis: treated case
    an insurance risk... 350
107. Spinal fluid cleared: symptoms persistent....................... 355
108. Arteriosclerosis does not contraindicate treatment.............. 359
109. Symptoms of intracranial pressure relieved by treatment.......... 362
110. Therapeutic improvement in tabetic neurosyphilis................. 366
111. W. R. rendered negative in tabetic neurosyphilis................. 367
112. Example of successful treatment of paretic neurosyphilis.......... 370
113. Another example.. 372

CASE   PAGE

114. Clinical recovery but tests persistently positive in treated paretic neurosyphilis... 375
115. Improvement delayed in treated paretic neurosyphilis............. 377
116. Non-neural syphilis in treated paretic neurosyphilis................ 380
117. Partial recovery in treated paretic neurosyphilis.................. 382
118. Laboratory signs improved: clinical situation stationary: treated paretic neurosyphilis.. 384
119. Another example.. 386
120. Failure of treatment.. 388
121. Treatment, at first mild, later intensive.......................... 390
122. Intensive treatment... 392
123. Syphilitic feeblemindedness improved by treatment 395

SECTION VI. NEUROSYPHILIS AND THE WAR.

CASES A TO N FROM BRITISH, FRENCH, AND GERMAN WRITERS (1914–1916)

CASE

A. Tabes "shell-shocked" into paresis? (Donath).................. 401
B. Latent syphilis "shell-shocked" into tabes? (Duco and Blum).... 403
C. Aggravation of neurosyphilis by service? (Weygandt)........... 404
D. Aggravation of neurosyphilis *by* service? (Todd)................ 406
E. Aggravation of neurosyphilis *on* service? (Todd)................ 409
F. Duration of neurosyphilitic process important. (Farrar).......... 411
G. Latent syphilis lighted up to paresis by war stress without shell-shock. (Marie)... 412
H. Paresis lighted up by "gassing"? (de Massary) 414
I. Epilepsy in a neuropath lighted up by syphilis acquired at war. (Bonhoeffer).. 415
J. Syphilitic — after Dixmude epileptic. (Bonhoeffer).............. 417
K. Syphilitic root-sciatica in a fire-works man. (Dejerine, Long) 418
L. Paresis lighted up in civilian by domestic stress of the war. (Percy Smith).. 420
M. Shell-shock pseudoparesis. (Pitres and Marchand).............. 421
N. Shell-shock pseudotabes. (Pitres and Marchand)................ 424

SECTION VII. SUMMARY AND KEY.................................. 427

APPENDICES:

A. The six tests.. 471
B. Common methods of treatment.................................. 486

INTRODUCTION

IT is a privilege to be allowed to write a word of introduction to a textbook which so richly fulfils its function as does this volume on the manifold disorders classified under Neurosyphilis, a subject of which the importance for the welfare of society is found to loom the larger the more deeply its mysteries are probed.

The case-histories with which its pages are so amply stocked are carefully analyzed in accordance with a broadly chosen plan, and the generalizations that precede and follow them are obviously based on a wide and varied personal experience such as alone could render a familiarity with the literature of the subjects treated adequate to its best usefulness. Both writers were indeed well adapted for this task. Dr. Southard, as everyone is aware, has long been a highly conscientious, ardent and productive worker in the department of pathological anatomy, and of late years a careful student of clinical diagnosis and methods, both at the Danvers State Hospital and still more, at the Psychopathic Hospital which he worked so hard to found; while Dr. Solomon's researches, in the special field of neurosyphilis, have been of the highest order.

Undoubted as are the merits of the case-system of instruction that has been so much in vogue in recent years, and excellent as is the modern supplementation of this method by the use of published records, the danger is still real that the student will have presented to him a picture of nature in disease that is too diagrammatic, too concise, with the result that while the task of memory is lightened through simplified formulation, the training of the doubting and inquiring instincts is often given too little stimulus and scope. In this book this danger is deliberately met through the casting of emphasis rather on the pluralistic aspects of the processes at stake than (primarily) on their unitary aspects.

13

The student who utilizes this volume cannot but emerge from his study a more thoughtful person than he was at the period of his entry. He will have seen that clinical rules of thumb cannot be followed to advantage, and that, on the contrary, surprises are to be expected and prepared for. Let the recognition of this fact, if it seems to increase the difficulties in the way of diagnosis, not lead to pessimism in that respect, or to hopelessness in therapeutics. On the contrary the writers' bias is towards the worth-whileness of clinical efforts and an increased respect for accuracy and thoroughness in the utilization of modern methods of research. The chance is indeed held open that even the gaunt spectre of "General Paresis" may prove to be less terrible than it seems, and for this hope good grounds are given.

It is in this way made clear, on the strength of anatomical evidence of much interest, that even if in the treatment of a given patient, the time arrives when a fatal or unfavorable result seems manifestly foreshadowed, it may be still worth while to renew the treatment with fresh zeal, for the sake of combatting some symptom or exacerbation, for which a locally fresh process furnishes the cause.

Another noteworthy principle here emphasized and illustrated is that the relationship between "functional" (hysterical, neurasthenic, migrainoid) symptoms and the signs (or symptoms) of organic processes is clinically important and worthy of much further study. This is a matter which, in a general sense, has interested me for many years. Above and over the "organic" hovers always the "functional," as representing the first indication of the marvelous tendency to repair, or substitution, for which the resources of nature are so vast. Yet this functional tendency also has its laws, of which, in their turn, the organic processes display the action in quasi diagrammatic form. Hysteria, neurasthenia, migraine, etc., do not arise *de novo* in each case, but conform to typical, though not rigid, formulas, susceptible of description. I have recently had the opportunity to study in detail an analogous series of transitions between the movements (and emotions) indicative of apparently purposeless myoclonic movements (on an epileptoid basis) and the movements of surprise, engrossment, purposeful effort, the excitement and joy by which the former were excited and into which they shaded over.

Taken altogether, this book represents work and thought in which, for amount and kind, the neurologists of Boston may take just pride.

JAMES J. PUTNAM.

St. Hubert's, Keene Valley, New York.
August, 1917.

Me miserable! which way shall I fly
Infinite wrath and infinite despair?
Which way I fly is Hell; myself am Hell;
And, in the lowest deep, a lower deep
Still threatening to devour me opens wide,
To which the Hell I suffer seems a Heaven.

Paradise Lost, Book IV, lines 73-78.

I. THE NATURE AND FORMS OF SYPHILIS OF THE NERVOUS SYSTEM (NEUROSYPHILIS)

> **PARADIGM** to show possible abundance and variety of symptoms and lesions in **DIFFUSE NEUROSYPHILIS** ("cerebrospinal syphilis"). **Autopsy.**

Case 1. Mrs. Alice Morton * was in the hands of at least five well-known specialists in different branches of medicine and surgery during the nineteen years of her disease. It appears that she acquired syphilis upon marriage at the age of 23 to a man who later became tabetic and acknowledged syphilitic infection previous to marriage. Mrs. Morton remained without children and there were no miscarriages.

At the age of 27, she developed iritis, paresis of the left eye muscles, and ulceration of the throat, with destruction of the uvula. The syphilitic nature of her disease was at once recognized and the classical treatment was given, although, through numerous shifts in consultants, this treatment was never pushed to the limit. At 28 Mrs. M. began to suffer from severe headaches resembling migraine and accompanied by attacks of paræsthesia; at 35, came severe pains in the back and difficulty in walking.

At 36, the migraine attacks began to be accompanied by blurring of vision and dizziness. The difficulty in walking became extreme, affecting particularly the right foot. The

---

* The cases chosen to illustrate the propositions of the boxed headings always illustrate several other points. See the footnotes of Section VI for lists of cases illustrating special points. The names assigned to the cases are fictitious and chosen to suggest race or descent.

legs became spastic, there were pains and hyperæsthesia of the chest, and severe cramps of the legs. Anti-syphilitic treatment at this time yielded marked improvement.

During her thirty-sixth year, Mrs. M. sustained curious transient losses of vision and of hearing. She was also irritable, and at this time developed her first pronounced mental symptoms, namely, delusions concerning her relatives. There were also a few seizures of an epileptiform nature.

At 38 there was a spell of total deafness, followed by improvement. The eye muscles were also subject to a variable involvement with intervening spells of improvement. The *knee-jerks were lost, but] after a time returned* in less pronounced form. Shortly, an absolute paralysis and extensive decubitus developed, and death occurred at 39.

The autopsy is briefly summarized below, but it is important in the understanding of Mrs. M.'s case (particularly some of the sensory symptoms and the transiency of certain symptoms) to consider the pre-infective history. Although there seems to be no doubt that the patient acquired syphilis at about 23 years of age from a syphilitic husband, who himself later became tabetic, yet it is of note that the patient was the only child of parents, both of whom also suffered from mental disease. Mrs. M.'s father died of what was called softening of the brain (one should avoid terming *all* old cases of *so-called* " softening of the brain " syphilitic, since the older diagnosticians did not always distinguish between non-syphilitic arteriosclerotic effects and syphilitic disease). Mrs. M.'s mother also died insane (confusion and emotional depression). It is clear, then, that we do not need to suppose that every symptom shown by Mrs. M. is directly due to destructive or irritative lesions immediately due to the spirocheta pallida. The case is, in fact, an excellent lesson as to the association of structural and functional effects in neuropathological cases.

Mrs. M. as a child had shown talent, but was somewhat nervous and eccentric. At one time, she had an attack of hysterical dysphasia; at another time, an attack of hysterical dyspnea; during another period, an apparent obsession (kicking the mopboard at regular intervals). Moreover, she had for years suffered from migraine of a severe and unusual type.

Both the hysterical tendency and the migrainous tendency became mingled with the results of the neurosyphilis in later stages of the disease in such wise that it was hard to tell exactly where the structural phenomena left off and the functional phenomena began.

For example, at the age of 32, nine years after infection and four years after the earliest nerve symptoms traceable to syphilis, and at about the time of the onset of spinal cord symptoms, an attack was described as follows:

> The patient had a very severe attack of migraine (?) yesterday, preceded and accompanied by paraphasia, so severe that for three hours she was unable to make herself understood, and indeed felt "as if her ideas were getting away from her." This attack was ushered in by a numbness of the forefinger and thumb of the right hand, which lasted for about three hours, though the earlier attacks had lasted for only about ten minutes. During this period the hand felt as if it had been frozen and the loss of muscular power was so great that she was unable to hold objects in the hand. In some of the attacks this paræsthesia has affected the entire left half of the body, and occasionally the right half. Sometimes the seizures come on with great suddenness, so that once, when she was attacked while in the middle of the street, she had considerable difficulty in reaching the sidewalk. After the worst part of the attack is over a certain amount of paraphasia may persist for some days, together with awkwardness in the use of the right hand and numbness. She has had a great deal of nausea and vomiting, without reference to the taking of food.*

Bearing in mind the mingling of structural with functional symptoms in this case, let us consider the autopsy findings.

Peripheral neurosyphilis: The lesions of the cranial nerves were characteristically asymmetrical. Whereas the left third nerve looked entirely normal, the **right third nerve** had its diameter reduced two-thirds. On the other hand, the fourth nerves were equal and apparently normal. The sensory portion of the left fifth nerve was normal; the right fifth nerve was normal. The **right sixth nerve** agreed with the

---

* Notes of Dr. James J. Putnam.

ANATOMICAL

FORMS OF NEUROSYPHILIS

AUTONOMIC (SYMPATHETIC) NEUROSYPHILIS?

PERIPHERAL NEUROSYPHILIS

CENTRAL NEUROSYPHILIS
    MENINGEAL
    VASCULAR
    PARENCHYMATOUS
    MENINGOVASCULAR
    VASCULOPARENCHYMATOUS
    DIFFUSE (=MENINGOVASCULOPARENCHYMATOUS)

GUMMA

CHART I

CLINICAL FORMS OF NEUROSYPHILIS

HEAD AND FEARNSIDES, 1914

SYPHILIS MENINGOVASCULARIS
  CEREBRAL FORMS
  HEMIPLEGIA
  AFFECTION OF THE CRANIAL NERVES
  MUSCULAR ATROPHY
  LATERAL AND COMBINED DEGENERATIONS
  EPILEPSY

SYPHILIS CENTRALIS
  DEMENTIA PARALYTICA
  TABES DORSALIS
  MUSCULAR ATROPHY
  OPTIC ATROPHY
  GASTRIC CRISES
  EPILEPTIC MANIFESTATIONS

CHART 2

right third nerve in being atrophic, and was in fact reduced to a mere thread without contained nerve fibres at a point 2 mm. from its superficial origin. Although the right third nerve was atrophic, it was the **left seventh and eighth nerves** which had become atrophic; the process had spared the right seventh and eighth nerves. The remainder of the cranial nerves were grossly normal, except that the **optic nerves** had an outer zone of a translucent nature. So far, no spirochetes have been demonstrated in any portion of the nervous system of this case, but such asymmetrical and focal cranial nerve lesions are perhaps due to local spirochetal infection, punctuating (as it were) the diffuse process.

How much of the transient blindness, deafness, and ocular paralysis can be explained on the anatomical findings in these nerves? Possibly a portion of the phenomena can be so explained. Thus, the mechanical conditions of pressure inside and outside these nerves, both in their peripheral course and in their passage through the membranes, can be readily understood to differ during the acute and subacute inflammation, during the process of repair in the pial tissues, and during the process of overgrowth of neuroglia tissue about the superficial origins of the nerves. Of course, the majority of lesions of these nerves were entirely extinct at the time of the autopsy, and their history could be surmised only from the appearances in the *left eighth nerve*. Here occurred a sharply marked focal area of gliosis with apparently total destruction of nerve fibres and related with a *lymphocytosis* of the investing membrane (one of the few areas of lymphocytosis found anywhere in this case).

If it were not for the pre-infective history, the hysterical dysphasia and dypsnea, the youthful obsessions, the migrainous tendency, and the psychopathic inheritance, we might be tempted to try to explain the transient blindness, the deafness, and ocular palsies on the basis of mechanical and toxic variations in the conditions of the peripheral cranial nerves. The existence of a trace of lymphocytosis in the left eighth nerve leads to the hypothesis that treatment might still be effective in this particular region (see below in discussion of spinal symptoms).

Spinal neurosyphilis: Not only the spinal cord but also the posterior and anterior nerve roots exhibited severe lesions. These lesions were both meningeal and parenchymatous. The meningeal process differed in its intensity in different parts of the spinal cord, being severest in the thoracic region. At one point in this region, the dura mater was so firmly attached to the pia mater that the line of demarcation between the two membranes was hard to make out. In fact, it seems clear that there could have been no free intercommunication between the spinal fluid above these adhesions of dura to pia mater and the spinal fluid below the adhesions. Accordingly, it seems that *lumbar puncture*, had it been practised in this case, *would have failed to show features representative of the whole cerebrospinal fluid system.* Moreover, since at no point in this region of adhesions or in the pia mater of the spinal cord below this point, were found any lymphocytes, it seems clear that the ordinary lumbar puncture would have failed to reveal a pleocytosis. Whether this fluid would have yielded a positive globulin and excess albumin test, it is now impossible to say; but it appears that the process in the lower part of the spinal cord was to all intents and purposes extinct.

However, there was one region of more severe inflammatory involvement. The *spinal cord in the cervical region showed a lymphocyte infiltration* of its vessels amounting to a mild myelitis (meaning, thereby, an inflammatory process of the spinal cord remote from the pia mater). Moreover, in this region, there was, besides the perivascular infiltration of the substance, also an infiltration of the overlying membranes themselves, especially in and near the posterior root zones.

The lessons of this finding are several: The inflammatory process in this case does not appear to have been entirely extinct! Can we not suppose that treatment might still have benefited this local inflammation (perivascular infiltration of the cervical spinal cord substance and overlying lymphocytic meningitis)? Can we not also picture the gradual ascent of the inflammatory lesions from lower segments to higher segments and possibly conceive of the gradual elevation of the zone of hyperæsthesia manifested in this case as following the gradual displacement upward of the lymphocytic process? Are there spirochetes in this tissue? So far none have been discovered, possibly through inaccuracies of available technique. To the neuropathologist, however, the lesion looks like a local reaction to organisms.

In addition to the spinal meningitis, chronic and acute, as above described, there were extensive parenchymatous spinal lesions.

In the first place, the meningitis had affected practically all the posterior roots so that the explanation of the posterior column sclerosis of this case is clear. The meningitis had apparently been so marked, also, that all the fibres anywhere near the periphery of the spinal cord had been likewise destroyed. The posterior columns and the posterior root zones were markedly sclerotic; or as we say (having reference to the overgrowth of neuroglia tissue) gliotic. But there was as much sclerosis (gliosis) of the lateral columns (particularly in the posterior two-thirds) as there was in the posterior columns and root zones. In fact, the entire posterior half or two-thirds of the spinal cord markedly outstripped the anterior portions of the cord in the severity of the gliosis (sclerosis) shown.

But although we can explain the posterior column sclerosis, the sclerosis of the posterior root zones and the marginal sclerosis (*Randsklerose*) round the entire periphery of the cord, on the basis of long-standing effects of old meningitis, we cannot thus explain another finding, namely, the destruction of the fibres in the lateral columns. This, in fact, is explained through lesions (mentioned below) that affected the encephalon. The net result of all these lesions of the spinal cord was to leave only the gray matter and a small amount of surrounding fibres (belonging to short tracts uniting near-by segments) intact. Briefly stated, **every long tract in the spinal cord appeared upon examination to be extensively degenerated.** The genesis of this parenchymatous loss was, however, double, being in part due to a local meningeal process (sometimes known as " perimeningitis ") and in part due to a cutting off of the pyramidal tract fibres on both sides by lesions higher up in the nervous system.

Can we offer any explanation of the **partial return of knee-**

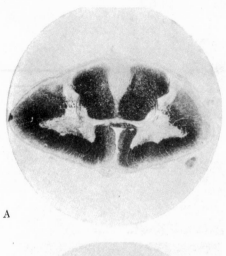

A

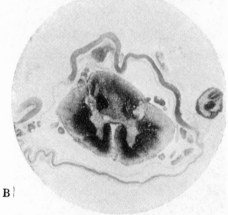

B

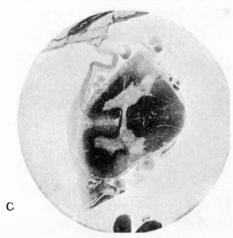

C

CASE 1. SPINAL CORD (THREE LEVELS) SHOWING:

A. Marginal sclerosis — effect of old meningitis now extinct.
B. Posterior column sclerosis — effect of meningitis about posterior roots also now extinct.
C. Bilateral pyramidal tract sclerosis — effect of cerebral thrombotic lesions.

Note distortion of tissues in B and C, partly artificial (tissues in places diffluent).

ANATOMICAL FORMULAE

MENINGOVASCULOPARENCHYMATOUS INVOLVEMENT

M, V, P, or Combinations Applied to the Classification of Head and Fearnsides

I. SYPHILIS MENINGOVASCULARIS

CEREBRAL FORMS	M or V or MV*
HEMIPLEGIA	V
AFFECTION OF THE CRANIAL NERVES	M
MUSCULAR ATROPHY	M
LATERAL AND COMBINED DEGENE-RATIONS	M
EPILEPSY	M or V

II. SYPHILIS CENTRALIS

DEMENTIA PARALYTICA	MVP or VP
TABES DORSALIS	MP
MUSCULAR ATROPHY	P
OPTIC ATROPHY	P
GASTRIC CRISES	(M? or) P?
EPILEPTIC MANIFESTATIONS	P?

* M = meningeal
 V = vascular
 P = parenchymatous

CHART 3

jerks after their temporary total loss at a certain period of the disease? We may assume that the knee-jerks were functionally lost about a year before the death of the patient through the partial or even almost complete destruction of the entering posterior root fibres at that level of the spinal cord which is directly related with the knee-jerk. The later partial return of the knee-jerks apparently requires us to suppose the maintenance of some fibres and collaterals by which a functional connection can be effected between the fibres of the posterior roots and the anterior horn cells which innervate the quadriceps femoris. Let us now suppose that *pari passu* with the actual return of the knee-jerks, the destructive processes that are affecting both pyramidal tracts high up in the nervous system are now advancing. It is clear that, whatever inhibitory influence these pyramidal tracts have been exerting up to this time upon the knee-jerk reflex arc, that influence is now to be decidedly reduced in amount and possibly absolutely lost. Upon the loss of such inhibitory influences exerted from above, the few persisting connections of the posterior roots and anterior horn cells are now permitted to resume their functions.

Encephalic neurosyphilis: The lesions mentioned above as causing destruction of the pyramidal tracts of the spinal cord were symmetrically destructive and atrophic lesions of the gray matter of both corpora striata with atrophy of the anterior segments of the internal capsules. There was a degenerative process of the corpus callosum especially affecting the forceps minor of the tapetum. The ventricles were largely dilated, indicating a considerable destruction and atrophy of the white matter in general.

After the above discussion of the possible effects of pyramidal tract lesion in this case, it is unnecessary further to discuss the paraplegia produced by the cystic lesions of the corpora striata. The theorist might inquire how these cystic lesions are produced: whether by vascular blocking or by toxic effects of the accumulations of spirochetes. Evidence is lacking which would completely sustain either hypothesis. Still, we do know that lesions almost identical in appearance may be produced by the necrosis consequent to the plugging of nutritive vessels in an organ like the brain supplied with end arteries. Therefore, it is probable that most pathologists would believe these lesions of the corpora striata to be produced by vascular plugging of the nature of thrombosis.

It is worth while to note that there was a suggestion of foci of encephalitis made out upon the gross examination. The cortex in general showed strikingly few lesions. However, the convolutions did show in places numerous ill-defined areas of hyperemia and slight swelling. These areas were of irregular distribution and only a few mm. or cm. in diameter. No gross vascular lesions were demonstrable in connection with these focal areas. Microscopically, however, venous plugs of polymorphonuclear leucocytes were found, and the local hyperemias were found to be largely due to venous congestion. However, very few polymorphonuclear leucocytes were found outside the blood vessels.

The white matter of numerous convolutions showed microscopically certain pale spots suggestive of an early atrophic process. Very possibly these represent a general tendency in the cerebrum to the same process of parenchymatous loss which had proceeded to such a marked degree in the spinal cord.

There was a single large so-called cyst of softening in the cerebellum (1.5 mm. across by 0.5-7.5 cm. in depth).

How far can we explain the symptoms of this case on the basis of these encephalic lesions? We can offer no correlation with the cerebellar lesion; and possibly this lack of correlation is to be expected on account of its failure to affect the vermis. As to the cystic lesions of the corpora striata, their effect in producing paraplegia at the close of life is obvious, and their possible relation to the partial return of knee-jerks has been discussed. Literally amazing was the comparative integrity of the cortical gray matter of this case when the spinal cord and the interior structures of the encephalon had been subjected to such severe and numerous lesions. The only mental symptoms noted in the case were sundry delusions directed against the patient's relatives and a certain optimism which led the patient to cling as if with an obsession to the belief that in the end she would get well.

VARIOUS FORMS OF NEUROSYPHILIS COLLECTED FROM SEVERAL SOURCES

MENINGEAL NEUROSYPHILIS (M)

GUMMA OF DURA MATER	M
GUMMATOUS MENINGITIS (Pial)	M
SYPHILITIC MENINGITIS (Pial)	M
SYPHILITIC CRANIAL NERVE PALSIES (Primarily Pial)	M
SYPHILITIC BULBAR PALSY	M
SYPHILITIC ROOT–NEURITIS	M
SYPHILITIC TRANSVERSE MYELITIS	M
SYPHILITIC NEURITIS (Some Cases by Extension)	M
SYPHILITIC EPILEPSY (Some Cases)	M
SYPHILITIC MUSCULAR ATROPHY (Some Cases)	M

VASCULAR NEUROSYPHILIS (V)

SYPHILITIC ARTERIOSCLEROSIS	V
SYPHILITIC CEREBRAL THROMBOSIS	V
SYPHILITIC APOPLEXY	V
ANEURYSM	V
SYPHILITIC EPILEPSY	V

PARENCHYMATOUS NEUROSYPHILIS (P)

GUMMA	P
CEREBROSPINAL SCLEROSIS	P
SYPHILITIC PARANOIA	P?
SYPHILITIC CHOREA	P
SYPHILITIC EPILEPSY	P
TABETIC PSYCHOSIS	P?
SYPHILITIC MUSCULAR ATROPHY	P
SYPHILITIC NEURITIS	P

CHART 4A

MENINGOVASCULAR NEUROSYPHILIS (MV)

CEREBRAL SYPHILIS	MV
CEREBROSPINAL SYPHILIS	MV
SYPHILITIC EPILEPSY	MV

MENINGOPARENCHYMATOUS NEUROSYPHILIS (MP)

CEREBRAL SYPHILIS	MP
CEREBROSPINAL SYPHILIS	MP
TABES DORSALIS	MP
ERB'S SYPHILITIC SPASTIC SPINAL PALSY	MP

VASCULOPARENCHYMATOUS NEUROSYPHILIS (VP)

CEREBRAL SYPHILIS	VP
CEREBROSPINAL SYPHILIS	VP
PARETIC NEUROSYPHILIS (GENERAL PARESIS)	VP
LISSAUER'S GENERAL PARESIS	VP

MENINGOVASCULOPARENCHYMATOUS NEUROSYPHILIS (MVP)

CEREBRAL SYPHILIS	MVP
CEREBROSPINAL SYPHILIS	MVP
PARETIC NEUROSYPHILIS	MVP
TABOPARESIS	MVP

DOUBTFUL (TOXIC?, IRRITATIVE ?) NEUROSYPHILIS (?)

"PARESIS SINE PARESI"
SYPHILITIC NEURASTHENIA
TABETIC PSYCHOSIS
SYPHILITIC PARANOIA
SYPHILITIC POLYURIA, POLYDIPSIA
SYPHILITIC NEURALGIA

CHART 4b

Summary: We have here dealt at length with a long-standing Diffuse Neurosyphilis affecting to some extent the entire **meninges** and producing a destruction of posterior column fibres and numerous other fibres of the spinal cord (**tabetiform** portion of the neurosyphilis **picture**). We have also found central lesions of the corpora striata affecting the destruction of both pyramidal tracts (**paraplegic** portion of the neurosyphilis **picture**). We have found evidences of acute inflammation (**lymphocytosis**) in the cervical region of the spinal cord and in the left eighth nerve (**progressive inflammatory** neurosyphilis **picture**). In short, we have presented a case of **diffuse** (meningovasculoparenchymatous) **neurosyphilis** characterized by an ascending character in a course of at least 16 years; we have indicated a number of possible clinical correlations, not only with the major portion of the clinical course (symptoms of myelitis and pyramidal tract destruction), but we have also mentioned, merely for their suggestive value, a number of finer correlations between histological findings and certain clinical features (notably transient losses of vision and hearing, and a partial return of the lost knee-jerks). Bearing in mind the clinical and anatomical findings of this case, we shall be able to discuss the cases that follow in a briefer and more condensed fashion.

TABETIC NEUROSYPHILIS ("tabes dorsalis," "locomotor ataxia") complicated by vascular neurosyphilis (hemiplegia). Autopsy.

Case 2. Francis Garfield had been a successful lumberman and had enjoyed good health until his forty-fifth year. Suddenly one day, while walking on the street, Garfield lost the use of his legs and for a time was quite unable to walk. However, he recovered locomotion and after a time there was nothing wrong with his leg movements except a slight ataxia.

At the age of 52 Garfield had to give up work. It appears that he had been becoming cranky, sometimes, for example, shouting, whistling and slamming doors, apparently to annoy the family. His intellectual capacity seemed to be maintained, although his memory was slightly impaired.

At 67 years there was an ill-defined seizure, followed a few days later by another seizure with aphasia (wrong words used and lack of understanding of things said).

For years Garfield had been totally deaf in the right ear (following explosion of a gun?). Now, however, the left ear also showed a sensory impairment. Slight slurring of speech had been noticed first in the sixty-sixth year.

Physically there was a slightly enlarged heart with accentuated second aortic sound and irregular rhythm. **Neurologically,** inability to stand or walk; marked ataxia in his leg movements; upper extremities quite well controlled; the pupils were small and unequal, the left being larger than the right; although the reactions were difficult to test, the pupils seemed to react slightly to direct light stimuli; the knee-jerks were absent; tests for sensibility so far as could be determined did not show any abnormalities; there was much complaint of sharp pains in the legs.

There is no doubt that we are here dealing with a case of TABES DORSALIS plus certain complications due to VASCULAR LESIONS. The case went on to death from rupture of **aortic**

MAIN FORMS OF NEUROSYPHILIS

(CLASSIFICATION OF THIS BOOK)

DIFFUSE NEUROSYPHILIS
    (non-vascular forms of " cerebral," " spinal " and " cerebrospinal syphilis ")

VASCULAR NEUROSYPHILIS
    (" cerebral arteriosclerosis," " cerebral thrombosis ")

PARETIC NEUROSYPHILIS
    (" general paresis ")

TABETIC NEUROSYPHILIS
    (" tabes dorsalis ")

GUMMATOUS NEUROSYPHILIS
    (" gumma of membranes, of brain ")

JUVENILE NEUROSYPHILIS
    (paretic, tabetic, diffuse)

CHART 5

POSSIBLE INVOLVEMENT

BRAIN AND CORD SYPHILIS

[M]embranes, [V]essels, [P]arenchyma

[MVP] EARLY, LATENT?, SYMBIOSIS?, ATTENUATION?....

MVP   CEREBRAL, CEREBROSPINAL SYPHILIS, PAR-
          ESIS   MVP

[M]VP PARESIS; SYPHILITIC ARTERIOSCLEROSIS   VP

M[V]P ? SYPHILOTOXIN FROM MENINGITIS   MP

MV[P] SYPHILITIC MENINGITIS; CEREBRAL OR
          CEREBROSPINAL SYPHILIS   MV

[MV]P SYPHILOTOXIC ATROPHY OR SCLEROSIS   P

M[VP] SYPHILITIC MENINGITIS   M

[M]V[P] SYPHILITIC ARTERIOSCLEROSIS   V

      M, V or P in brackets [ ] means not involved.

CHART 6

NEUROSYPHILIS

SIX TESTS

BLOOD WASSERMANN

SPINAL FLUID WASSERMANN

    "   "   CYTOLOGY

    "   "   GLOBULIN

    "   "   ALBUMIN

    "   "   GOLD SOL

CHART 7

aneurysm (also doubtless a syphilitic complication). The death occurred at 71, four years after admission to Danvers Hospital.

This case has been especially worked up and published by Dr. A. M. Barrett on account of the fact that the vascular lesions of the brain had produced a condition of pure word-deafness. Reference is made to the Journal of Nervous and Mental Disease, Vol. 37, 1910, for a complete description of the brain findings and an analysis of the word-deafness, a summary of which is as follows:

> "Reaction to Words and Sounds. — Total deafness to words spoken, but gives attention to sounds; no ability to recognize meaning of sounds heard; no ability to repeat words heard. Spontaneous Speech. — Retained ability to speak spontaneously, with rare paraphasic utterances; occasional inability to speak readily the word desired, but later always giving the correct reaction; calculation fair; spelling good except for occasional paraphasia; spelling good for words pronounced. Reaction to Things Seen. — Objects correctly recognized and named except for an occasional paraphasic reply; mistakes in pronunciation not recognized; correct color recognition. Reaction to Things Felt. — Good for familiar objects; an occasional paraphasic reply. Reaction to Words Seen. — Reads printing and writing understandingly; unimpaired reading except for an occasional paraphasic reply; meaning of familiar signs recognized; slight difficulty in readily understanding meaning of arithmetical signs. Writing. — Spontaneous writing and drawing ability retained; ataxia (tabetic) in writing movements; no ability to write from dictation. Internal language. — No evidence of impairment."

The brain post mortem showed severe atheromatous degeneration of the arteries at the base of the brain. Both middle cerebral arteries showed scattered atheromatous patches. The pia mater was transparent and delicate, except in the regions of both Sylvian fissures. There were residuals of old softening in both temporal lobes. In the fresh brain the regions of the right and left first temporal convolutions were sunken inward, and the pia intimately adherent to the softened areas. The limits and more exact localizing of these softenings were worked out from serial sections.

Barrett found in his serial sections that, although the transverse temporal convolutions of the left hemispheres were intact, these convolutions were undermined throughout their entire extent by degenerations in the fibres of the center of the first temporal convolution. Barrett, accordingly, regarded his case as essentially a case of subcortical tissue destruction. He agrees with various authors that the pure word-deafness of his case is the result of an isolation of the receiving station in the transverse convolutions of the left hemisphere. The tissue destruction produced by the vascular lesion. had cut off the transverse convolutions from the internal geniculate body.

We are here, however, not considering the origin and relations of pure word-deafness but present the case as one of **tabes dorsalis** of 20 years standing, terminated by two characteristic syphilitic complications, first, an extensive destruction of brain tissue through **cerebral thrombosis** and secondly, fatal **aortic aneurysm.**

Summary: We have here dealt briefly with a long-standing case of NEUROSYPHILIS of the TABETIC type: A characteristic but not necessary complication of the case is the LATE CEREBRAL VASCULAR INVOLVEMENT. The **posterior column sclerosis** is virtually the only spinal change. Spinal meningeal changes are absent (although it is to be assumed that chronic inflammatory changes in the posterior roots were at one time present in some quantity and although the spinal fluid characteristically shows lymphocytosis in tabetic neurosyphilis).

Whether the spirochetes produce special toxic components able to cause tabes or whether special kinds of spirochete are the tabes-making kinds is hard to say. Special qualities of individual tissue may be involved.

The **cerebral lesions** of a **cystic** nature are of vascular origin, like the differently localized encephalic lesions of Case I (Alice Morton). Vascular syphilis is not a special property of the vessels of the nervous system. In fact this very case died of **aortic aneurysm.**

PARETIC NEUROSYPHILIS ("general paresis,"
"dementia paralytica," "softening of the brain").
Autopsy.

Case 3. James Dixon, 44, was first seen at the Danvers Hospital, reciting verses in a dramatic and noisy way. He remained good-natured and jolly; nor was there any change in his euphoria until he had become physically weaker and more generally demented. In fact, Dixon appeared to become more and more expansive as he became physically weaker. He was in the habit of describing himself as "O. K., No. 1, Superfine."

Physically the patient was gray and bald on vertex, had a dusky complexion, was very thin (6 ft. in height, weight 155 lbs.); the mucous membranes were pallid; the teeth rather poorly preserved; the heart was somewhat enlarged; the pulse irregular in rhythm, of poor volume and tension.

Neurologically, the patient showed a characteristic Romberg sign and ataxia in walking a straight line. The tremulous tongue was protruded to the left, and there was a coarse tremor of the extended fingers. The knee-jerks were absent, and the Achilles jerks could not be obtained; the plantar reactions were slight; the arm reflexes were present. The pupils were stiff to light. There was a marked vocal tremor. The sensations could not be tested on account of the patient's mental state.

It appears that Dixon had left school at about 16, at about 22 had gone into the provision business, and later had become a hotel clerk. He had married at 28; there had been two miscarriages, at three months and six weeks respectively; one child was stillborn; four children were living.

The patient was not very alcoholic. The patient's wife thought the symptoms had been coming on since his forty-first year when irritability set in, but he was not discharged from work until about a year since. He was taken back again after his wife's pleas, and remained at work about three months; but for ten months before admission to the hospital, Dixon had done practically nothing, had shown a marked memory failure and speech defect, at the same time claiming to be a person capable of doing and accomplishing everything. He had become careless of his personal appearance, collected a drawer-full of stumps of cigars, carried lumps of coal in his pocket, laughed causelessly, and spat on the carpet.

We here deal with a case of unknown duration from the initial infection, but with symptoms lasting about three years and three months. Aside from the cause of death (empyema of left pleural cavity associated with acute hemorrhagic splenitis, acute ileitis, and bronchial lymphnoditis), the body showed a number of other lesions outside the nervous system. There was the usual sclerosis of the aorta, though perhaps less marked than usual. There was a curious acute arteritis with fusiform dilatation of the arteria profunda femoris, with an edema of the thigh muscles and blebs of the overlying skin. There were also multiple chronic caseating lesions of the liver, without evidence of fibrosis. The explanation of these liver lesions is not yet clear. There was a cloudy swelling of the kidney.

The calvarium was dense and the dura mater thick and adherent. There was a chronic leptomeningitis, which, however, was rather unusual in being most marked in the posterior cisterna and along the sulci of the cerebellar hemispheres. There was a general cerebral sclerosis, with a question of atrophy of the superior temporal gyri (suggesting the so-called Lissauer's paresis). There was a marked cerebellar sclerosis with a consequent sclerosis (grossly palpable) of the commissural fibres of the pons. There was a generalized slight spinal sclerosis. As a fair sample of the variety of head findings in paretic neurosyphilis, the details of the **head examination** are presented.

Crown bald, with a slight fuzzy growth of short hairs. Scalp slightly adherent to calvarium; latter of usual thickness but denser than normal. Dura adherent to calvarium in region of vertex; dura not remarkable. Sinuses normal. Arachnoid villi moderately developed. Pia mater a trifle thickened and rather evenly through-

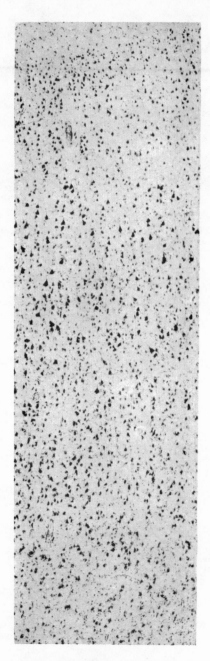

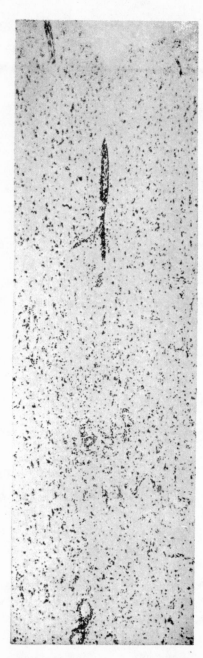

A. Normal postcentral cortex. (Compare B.)

B. Nerve-cell losses. Perivascular deposits of mononuclear cells, amongst which are numerous plasma cells. Note decrease in number of nerve cells. Note irregular disposition of nerve cells. From paretic neurosyphilis.

out the cerebral portion. Linear sulcal markings are remarkable for their absence. The wall of the cerebello-medullary cisterna is thick and opaque. The most prominent pial thickenings are over the cerebellum. These are linear or may show feathery out-growths and are seated over the sulci, particularly in the neighbor-hood of the fissure and about the great cerebellar notch. They correspond fairly well with the focal variation in consistence of under-lying tissues noted below.

Brain weight, 1265 grams. Consistence somewhat increased throughout and somewhat evenly increased. The prefrontal region shows the maximal increase of consistence but the remainder of the frontal region and corresponding occipital region are much firmer than normal. The two superior temporal gyri appear to be firmer than adjacent gyri and are possibly slightly diminished in superficial diameter. The hippocampal gyri are fairly firm. The substance on section is a trifle more moist than normal. The gray and white matter cut quite evenly. Diminution in depth of gray matter, if existent, could not be demonstrated. The ventricles show a moderate sanding throughout, best marked in the fourth ventricle. The basal ganglia are not remarkable except for the development of numerous dilated perivascular spaces about the lenticulostriate vessels. The **pons** is atrophic, but more so on the right side. The pons, like the prefrontal cortex, shows on section a distinct increase of consistence immedi-ately beneath the pia mater. The white bands of the pons on section are distinctly firmer than the interven-ing substance. The olives are of equal consistence. Weight of cerebellum, pons, and medulla, 155 grams. The **cerebellum** shows an obvious atrophic and gliotic process of a symmetrical character. The superior surface, including both vermis and hemispheres, shows a consistence above normal and general reduction of the depth measured from the white matter. The re-duction in depth gives rise to a visible depression as compared with tissue posterior to the postclival sulci. The lobus cacuminis, though slightly raised from the surrounding lobes, is equally firm, if not firmer. The superior and inferior surfaces show practically an equal increase of consistence. The dentate nuclei are not especially increased in consistence. The flocculi are reduced in size about one-third.

There was slight universal increase in consistence of **spinal cord,** best marked in lumbar region.

Microscopic findings are here presented merely in sufficient detail to establish the diagnosis. The left superior frontal gyrus shows extensive and somewhat irregular cellular and fibrillar gliosis of the plexiform layer, together with an increase of thickened vessels having lymphocytes and plasma cells in their sheaths.

The perivascular infiltrations are most extensive in the lower layers of the cortex. The lamination is in places thoroughly obscured, except that representatives of the layer of large external pyramids are almost always demonstrable.

The layer of medium-sized pyramids has undergone more numerical loss of elements than have the other layers.

Gliosis of white matter.

Specimens from the cerebellum show a destructive process of great severity, but a little irregular in extent, affecting chiefly the Purkinje cell belt. The Purkinje cells are often absent throughout one side of a given lamina, and there has ensued a dense accumulation of neuroglia cells along a former Purkinje cell belt, together with a considerable gliosis of the molecular layer. Considerable gliosis of the white matter, both diffuse and perivascular in distribution.

Perivascular plasma cell infiltrations as in cerebrum, but largely meningeal or in the white matter.

Sections from the corpora striata demonstrate a mild and early granular ependymitis, considerable subependymal gliosis of cellular type, considerable perivascular gliosis in the white portions of the tissue, and a moderate infiltration of perivascular sheaths with pigmented cells, lymphocytes, and plasma cells. There is little evidence of alteration in the nerve cells. Some are unevenly pigmented.

Summary: We here present a case with numerous and widespread neurosyphilitic lesions. However, the gross cerebral vascular complications of Case 1 (Alice Morton) and of Case 2 (Francis Garfield) are notably absent in James Dixon. Rather atypical (there seems to be *always something atypical in cases of neurosyphilis!*) are the liver lesions and arteritis of the leg, atypical, that is to say, for PARETIC NEUROSYPHILIS.

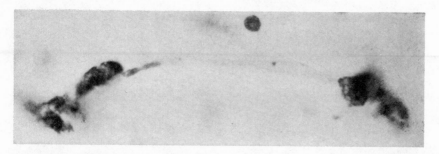

Apparent new formation of small blood vessel.   Photographed by Dr. A. M. Barrett.

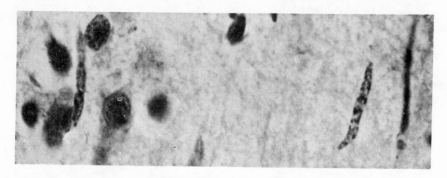

Rod cells (Stäbchenzellen) in paretic neurosyphilis.   Photographed by Dr. A. M. Barrett.

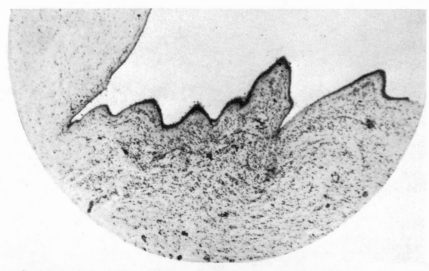

Granular ependymitis — microscopic appearance of a marked example of "sanding" of ventricle.

Highly typical of paretic neurosyphilis and almost constant therein is the aortic sclerosis.

Characteristic and constant in paretic neurosyphilis is the **Plasmocytosis and Lymphocytosis, Perivascular** in distribution about small cortical vessels. There is also a characteristic (though characteristically less prominent) **Plasmocytosis and Lymphocytosis, Meningeal** in distribution. The pleocytosis of the spinal fluid, almost constant though variable in amount in life, is an indicator of the meningeal picture and less directly of the parenchymatous picture.

Granular Ependymitis ("sanding" of ventricle floors) is characteristic and may be regarded as part of the parenchymatous picture. This ependymitis is an indicator how chemical changes could be readily produced at least in the ventricular fluids, since the limiting membranes of the nerve tissue are here subject to multiple breaks. The "sanding" is a neuroglia reaction to these multiple small breaks (Weigert's explanation).

Parenchymatous losses have led to **Atrophy and Sclerosis,** of very varying extent in different parts of the encephalon. The atrophy is characteristic in paretic neurosyphilis, but by no means constant. Numerous cases have come to autopsy without clearly defined gross atrophy. Sclerosis is also characteristic and even more frequent than atrophy, doubtless because sclerosis represents an earlier phase of a process eventuating in gross atrophy.

A **Tabetiform Picture** characterizes the spinal cord, but in this case the tabetic clinical picture did *not* precede the paretic clinical picture. We are consequently to regard the tabetic spinal process as incidental and on all fours with the **Cerebellar and Pontine Atrophy.**

**VASCULAR NEUROSYPHILIS ("syphilitic cere-
bral thrombosis"). Autopsy.**

Case 4. James Pierce was an almshouse transfer to the
Danvers Hospital in his fiftieth year. He died three years
later. The accompanying brain pictures demonstrate so
extensive a lesion of the left hemisphere that it is of great
interest to determine if possible the genesis and course of his
disease. It appears that syphilis had been acquired somewhere about the age of 38 or 40, so that the total duration of
the process was between 13 and 15 years. In Pierce's forty-
third or forty-fourth year, he had a shock while walking in
the streets of his native city, whereupon he was subsequently
transferred to the Danvers Hospital, whose data have been
summed up as follows (we are obliged to Dr. Charles T.
Ryder for these data):

> **Neurological examination:** Neuromuscular condition:
> Barely able to walk or stand without assistance;
> hemiplegia of right side; swings foot out and drags toe
> out and around in attempting to walk. Right hand
> held by side, flexed at right angle; fingers contracted
> and thumb thrown across palm. Can lift arm from
> side; practically no movements of forearms or fingers;
> atrophy of deltoid, arm, forearm, and hand. Mus-
> cular movements of left upper extremities fairly well
> performed; good strength.
> **Cranial nerves:** Refuses to respond to any tests to
> determine hearing or vision, but evidently hears what is
> said to him, and in his movements gives no evidence of
> deafness. Right corner of mouth droops; tongue pro-
> trudes straight.
> **Reflexes:** Pupils dilated; margins irregular; left
> pupil larger; they vary in size but it is impossible to
> determine whether the variation is due to light or ac-
> commodation reflex. Reflexes of right side extremely
> exaggerated throughout; there is little ankle clonus;
> Babinski is not obtained, patient holding his toes in
> flexed position in resisting attempts to elicit reflexes.

Sensations: Reaction to pain stimuli on either side. Evidently some anesthesia on right side, but pressure is apparently very painful. There is considerable spasticity of limbs on right side on passive motion. Too demented to make accurate tests.

The above examination was made on May 6, 1904. On May 20th the record states:

There is almost complete sensory aphasia with word deafness; some paraphasic circumlocution. Many of his words are very well enunciated but have no meaning. Is apparently unable to recognize objects or their uses.

Brother stated that he was always supposed not to be over bright. Physician's certificate states that he is epileptic, averaging two attacks per week. On the 15th of May he had a general convulsion; was unconscious for half an hour, and dull and drowsy for two hours afterwards. On the 19th, he had a similar attack in the afternoon, the convulsion lasting a minute, and he was stuporous for an hour.

On November 8th he had a severe epileptic convulsion. His body was curled up to the right. The convulsive seizure lasted for two minutes and was followed by complete unconsciousness for an hour, when the patient roused and appeared as usual in a few minutes. From that time to December 15th he had five epileptic convulsions; he was much more feeble, and unable to help himself as much as formerly.

Nov. 7, 1905: Patient has had occasional convulsions since last note, but none during the last three months. He is confined to bed, has become very much demented, and shows very marked speech defect, so that he is almost unintelligible. He understands only the simplest directions. Legs are considerably contracted and knees are flexed. Arm and hand on the right are paralyzed and show some atrophic changes; partially flexed. Left elbow-jerk is very lively. On May 23, 1906 he was reported as having Achilles on right side only, and Babinski on right side. He died January 5, 1907.

The autopsy findings were as follows:

Head: Calvarium of moderate thickness; diploë present; dura slightly adherent over bregmatic region. Longitudinal sinus contains cruor clot. Dura is somewhat thickened and slightly more opaque than normal. Pacchionian granulations, small but fairly numerous. Pia contains throughout a considerable excess of clear serous fluid. The convolutions in general are of good breadth and proportion. There is an atrophic area roughly circular in outline and about 2 cm. in diameter in the posterior part of the right third frontal convolution corresponding to Broca's area on the opposite hemisphere. The space thus formed is filled with edema held by the pia. On the left side is a similar subpial collection which covers the site of the posterior portions of all of the third frontal convolutions, parts of the lower end of the precentral convolution, and the whole of the first temporal convolution, which have disappeared entirely. The basal vessels show slight changes.

Cerebellum and basal ganglia are grossly normal.

The spinal membranes are negative. The regions of the pyramidal tracts in the cord are firm, project slightly from surface of section, and are china white.

Summary: Here is a picture made up almost purely of VASCULAR NEUROSYPHILIS, with SECONDARY SPINAL (PYRAMIDAL TRACT) CHANGES. Doubtless the genesis of this picture is allied to that of Case 1 (Alice Morton) and to that of the terminal vascular complications in a tabetic, Case 2 (Francis Garfield).

The absence of meningeal and parenchymatous (i.e., outside the region of necrosis produced by the vascular disease) lesions is characteristic of an important group of neurosyphilitic diseases. It is clear that the case, although one of *extensive* lesions, is *not* one of *diffuse* lesions in the sense of Case 1 (Alice Morton).

The spinal fluid picture in life may nevertheless show (as other cases amply demonstrate) a certain amount of lymphocytosis and possibly plasmocytosis, together with a variety of other changes. Treatment might be expected to keep down these associated changes, although obviously the effects of the necrosis are final and definite. Franz in Washington has succeeded in " reeducating " some of these hemiplegics, employing lower mechanisms of the nervous system.

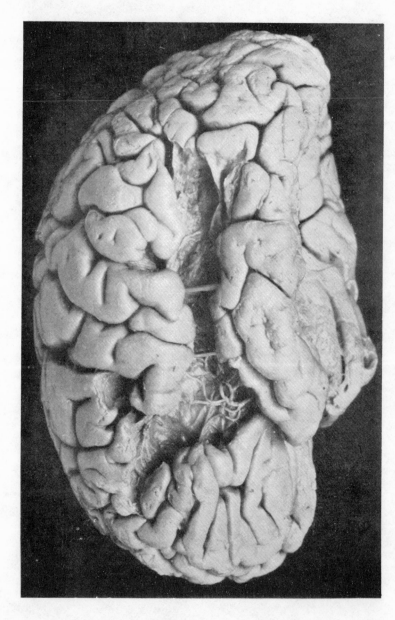

Vascular neurosyphilis — effects of syphilitic thrombosis of Sylvian artery 10 years before death. (Case 4.)

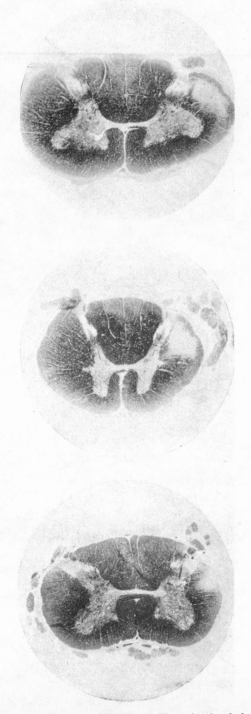

Case 4. (See previous figure for brain lesion.) Three levels of the spinal cord showing unilateral pyramidal tract sclerosis, 10 years after cerebral thrombosis.

JUVENILE PARETIC NEUROSYPHILIS ("juvenile paresis"). Autopsy.

Case 5. John Lawrence was an under-sized negro, who came under hospital observation when he was 23 years of age. There was some evidence that the patient's father was a neurosyphilitic although accurate data were out of the question. At all events, John had Hutchinsonian teeth, a forward bowing of the tibiae, and Argyll-Robertson pupils. These findings together with a history of backwardness at school seem to stamp the diagnosis. It seems that there had been a change for the worse from the age of 18, though the boy had been able to sell newspapers and black shoes up to within a year of his arrival at the hospital. During the last months of his life, he showed a general incoördination, with false movements suggesting those of a drunken person. There were numerous tremors, the glance was shifting, and there was a tendency to nystagmus. Some of these phenomena (taking into account that the Hutchinsonian teeth were not entirely typical and there was even at times some doubt as to whether the pupils were actually stiff) led to a question of the diagnosis multiple sclerosis.

There was, however, little doubt that the case was one of juvenile paresis. Among the symptoms found at various times in this case are the following: disorientation for time, place and persons, confusion, with coarsely irrelevant replies to questions, ill-defined and transitory delusions of persecution, auditory, tactile, and visual hallucinations, and defective memory.

Early in life, the patient had had a habit of falling asleep in school hours, and had experienced a number of falls at various times. During an attack of measles he had had a number of spasms, each of which lasted ten minutes or more.

The **autopsy** showed death to be due to an early bronchial pneumonia. The thymus was persistent, measuring 3×2×.5 cm. The marrow of the femur was red.

There was a moderate degree of **sclerosis of the aorta** confined to a few plaques in the arch (not a characteristic syphilitic scarring of the aorta). The spleen was small and had a thickened capsule.

The majority of the lesions, however, were in the **nervous system,** and the following description is taken from the routine hospital records to exemplify the findings in a fairly characteristic case of JUVENILE PARESIS.

Head: Scalp closely adherent to **calvarium.** Calvarium heavy without diploë. **Dura** adherent to calvarium in bregmatic region. Sinuses contain liquid blood. Arachnoidal villi in considerable quantity. **Pia mater** contains considerable clear fluid and shows diffuse haziness and focal thickenings. The diffuse haziness is almost universal and is best marked over the superior surface of the cerebellum. The focal thickenings are of general distribution over the veins of the sulci on the superior surface of the brim and are heaped up to form considerable linear mounds near the region of the arachnoidal villi. The superior surface of the cerebellum is traversed by similar linear mounds of fibrous tissue running at an angle to the laminæ. There is no notable increase of fibrous tissue at the base.

Brain: Weight 965 grams. The sulcation is roughly symmetrical except in the occipital poles where there is unusually rich and complex but shallow sulcation. The cortical substance is everywhere firmer than normal, but the sulci fail to flare notably. In a few places there is a focal increase of consistence of still greater degree with apparent local hypertrophy (or gliosis with increase of substance). These foci are in the right second temporal gyrus (3 cm. in diameter) and in the left first temporal gyrus (of same size but somewhat less firm) and are of a whitish, waxen appearance, being visible several feet away by reason of their color and apparent encroachment upon the adjacent sulci. The foci are sharply limited by the sulci laterally, but pale out gradually before and behind.

The convolutions of the vertex show another type of lesion. The tissue of the greater part of the vertex resembles that of the flanks and base in being firmer than normal and of a grayish pink color. Behind the fissure of Rolando on the right side and behind the anterior limits of the ascending frontal region on the left side the brain tissue of the vertex becomes suddenly still firmer and of a yellowish gray color. This lesion disappears gradually into the occipital microgyria behind and the gyri gradually lose their yellowish tint. The lesion fades away gradually so that it fails to involve the temporal convolutions.

The cerebral tissue cuts firmly and smoothly. The tissue of the frontal region is a little edematous. The white matter is of a normal appearance. The ependyma of all the ventricles is somewhat sanded. The fourth ventricle is most affected.

The **cerebellum** is not edematous and is as firm as the normal olivary bodies. The cerebellar hemispheres are symmetrical and of a normal appearance, save that the laminæ are slightly narrower than usual and very compactly set. The color, where not obscured by the haziness of the pia mater, is of a grayish pink somewhat suggestive of freshly tanned shoe leather. The substance cuts smoothly and firmly. The dentate nuclei are unusually firm. The **pons** is small, but of the usual color. Lower structures normal except the **cord** which is small and shows curious deviations from the normal markings. The posterior horns and gray commissure are at many levels the only structures to preserve the normal gray appearance, so that the H or butterfly appearance is replaced by a crescent. At these levels traces of gray matter often stand out in the loci of the anterior horns.

The important **anatomical diagnoses** in the nervous system are as follows:

Atrophy of cerebrum, 965 grams (there is of course a question whether we are not dealing with a degree of cerebral hypoplasia).

Focal scleroses of cerebrum, suggesting the tuberous scleroses of Bourneville.

Occipital microgyria.

Cerebral and cerebellar gliosis.

Chronic ependymitis.

Gliosis of the gray matter of the spinal cord.

Chronic diffuse and focal leptomeningitis.

The **microscopic examination** confirmed the diagnosis of **paresis**. The hypertrophic nodules were of special interest.

They were found to be overlain by a characteristic though thin exudate of lymphocytes and plasma cells, together with pigmented cells. The nodules appeared to be supplied with an unusual number of vessels of small calibre, about which were a few lymphocytes. The large vessels and those with well-developed adventitiæ were surrounded by more numerous lymphocytes and by more focal accumulations of pigmented cells. The cortex in the middle of a nodule had almost lost its characteristic cortical layering. The cortex was here reduced (specimen from temporal lobe) to about one-quarter of its normal thickness, and was found to be composed largely of expanded neuroglia cells and vascular tissue, with a few nerve elements, small, shrunken, and dark-staining. The destructive process appeared to have borne hardest on the layer of internal large pyramids and the fusiform layer. There was, however, nowhere any evidence of focal necrosis such as ought to characterize a true gumma. The sections stained by the Marchi method failed to show evidence of fatty degeneration within the focus, although there was a marked diffuse accumulation of fatty granulations along the nerve fibres in the underlying white matter. A special study of the cerebellar material was made by one of the authors.[*] Occasional Purkinje cells showed the characteristic binucleate condition, which has frequently been noted in recent literature.

The cerebellum of this case was perhaps the most markedly diseased of all portions of the nervous system. As noted, the cerebellar tissue was exceedingly firm. How far the notable incoördination of the case (he was observed on staff rounds characteristically curled up in a heap, showing quite an unusual degree of general incoördination) was due to the cerebellar lesions, it is perhaps not possible to say.

Summary: John Lawrence, JUVENILE PARETIC NEUROSYPHILIS, is a foil to Case 3 (James Dixon), paretic neurosyphilis due to acquired syphilis.

Both showed **Cerebral Atrophy,** but Lawrence the more

---

[*] E. E. Southard: Lesions of the granule layer of the human cerebellum; *Journal of Medical Research*, XVI, 1907.

markedly because of hypoplasia incidental to the congenital origin of his condition.

Whereas Dixon gave little or no sign of **stigmata,** Lawrence (besides being undersized, having suspicious teeth, and showing at autopsy a persistent thymus) showed a **Hydromyelia** and curious trefoil shape to the spinal cord. Dixon on the other hand had liver lesions and arterial lesions of the leg.

The suggestion of **Tuberous Sclerosis** in Lawrence is not found in Dixon; but we have not found it elsewhere. Bourneville did not describe tuberous sclerosis as syphilitic.

Binucleate Purkinje cells emphasize the congenital source of the lesions in Lawrence.

Plasmocytosis and Lymphocytosis, Perivascular, and (less marked) **Meningeal,** are found in both the congenital and the acquired cases, as also parenchymatous changes, both **nerve cell losses** and **gliosis.** Both also show granular **ependymitis.**

It is clear that, over and above the factors of destruction evident in both Lawrence and Dixon, the congenital case, Lawrence exhibits also the effects of arrest (in brief not merely atrophy but also hypoplasia). Early treatment is, therefore, theoretically indicated in the juvenile group, which means early diagnosis. Early diagnosis and treatment are still more to be recommended because these juvenile cases progress often very slowly at first.

**FOCAL BASILAR MENINGEAL NEUROSYPH-
ILIS ("syphilitic extraocular palsy," plus other
symptoms). Autopsy.**

Case 6. Flora Black, a housewife of 43 years, had been
tired out for a year but had been apparently in fair health.
She awoke one day with double vision due to a left internal
strabismus. The visual difficulty gradually passed away so
that five months after the sudden seizure she was apparently
quite well again. There was one exception: about three or
four months after the attack of diplopia, Mrs. Black had begun
to feel a kind of weakness in various parts of the face and there
were also fairly definite paresthesiæ. In the sixth month
after the initial attack, the patient began to be unable to
chew and was fain to support the lower jaw with a bandage
to aid in mastication. Deglutition was, however, quite unaffected and there was never any regurgitation of food.
There were pains in the face, the forehead and the back of
the neck.

Upon **physical examination** at entrance to a general hospital, no changes in the body at large were discoverable.
There was a slight edema of the ankles, otherwise no sign
of bodily disease.

Conditions in the **head** were as follows: The facial lines
were (notes by courtesy of Dr. E. W. Taylor) smoothed out;
both upper and lower eyelids and the corners of the mouth
drooped slightly and more markedly on the left side. There
was slight photophobia and considerable lachrymation.
The patient was unable to pucker forehead, nose or mouth.
The unsupported lower jaw fell and the patient was unable
to open the mouth widely. The movements of the tongue
were normally performed. Speech was mumbling. Sensations of touch, heat and cold were preserved all over the
face except that the left cheek below the level of the mouth
yielded a less accurate registration of tactile sensations.
A hot test tube did not feel as hot in the lower left cheek as

elsewhere. Quinine and sugar could not be tasted over the left half of the tongue in front. Smell and hearing were also diminished on the left side. It appeared that there was a complete paralysis of the 5th and 7th nerves and a partial paralysis of the 8th, 11th and 12th, as well as a defect in smell.

The patient died suddenly, three weeks after admission, running a slight temperature during her stay. The autopsy showed (rather surprisingly) a double ovarian carcinoma with metastases into the retroperitoneal glands. Both kidneys were found to be riddled with nodules of carcinoma. The pelvic veins were thrombosed and there was a complete occlusion of the pulmonary artery. There was a riding embolus in the foramen ovale and there was coronary embolism.

The striking nature of these complications and the interest of the case neurologically would warrant its publication in complete detail. We here present the case with utmost brevity as an example of a SYPHILITIC CRANIAL NEURITIS by extension from the meninges.

The **brain** was in general without change but there was a considerable exudate over the entire **pontine region** which had involved several cranial nerves. The 5th nerves, especially the left, showed gross effects of the inflammatory lesion. There seems to be little or no doubt that this neuritis was of syphilitic origin despite the complication of the case with carcinoma of the ovary and despite the fact that the case was observed and came to autopsy before the modern methods of systematic diagnosis could be applied. It is the best case available to us for the demonstration of a focal cranial nerve lesion of the type characteristic of neurosyphilis. We may well suppose that similar conditions would have been found at various stages in the development of Case 1 (Alice Morton). The pontine region of Case 1 was entirely free from lymphocytic exudate at the time of the autopsy. Possibly the clearing up of the pontine pia mater in Case 1 was a therapeutic effect of the thorough treatment therein used. Whether a case like Mrs. Black's could be cured (aside from the ovarian carcinoma and its complications) by the institution of vigorous systematic treatment is a matter of doubt.

Still, in a general way, these cases of focal syphilitic neuritis are among the most favorable cases for treatment.

Summary: We present the case of Flora Black to emphasize how slight in extent and theoretically curable neurosyphilis may be. We fear that Case 1 (Alice Morton) may present too unrelieved and pessimistic a picture. The extensive vascular lesions and complications of Alice Morton, of Case 2 (Francis Garfield), of Case 4 (James Pierce) arrest attention by the incurability of their residual effects (if we omit modern attempts at reeducation of lower arcs). On the other hand the unrelenting progress to destruction of important parenchymatous structures, as shown in the paretic James Dixon (Case 3) and his juvenile replica John Lawrence (Case 5), as well as in Alice Morton (Case 1) and the tabetic Francis Garfield (Case 2), lead to a certain justifiable pessimism. For it is only the meningeal and fine vascular infiltrations of these cases that we can theoretically hope to combat, probably by destroying the spirochetes in these meningeal and perivascular loci. We seem theoretically less able to stop the progress of the often highly systemic and symmetrical, parenchymatous lesions of the tabetic and paretic group.

The condition in Flora Black is clearly much more hopeful, both being more focal and being almost purely meningeal and therefore accessible to therapy.

The two cases which conclude our general survey of neurosyphilis are also focal cases, one of gumma (Lecompte) and one of focal dural lesion (Wyman).

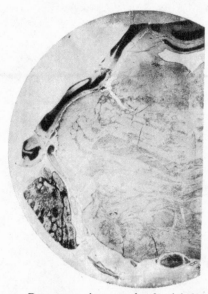 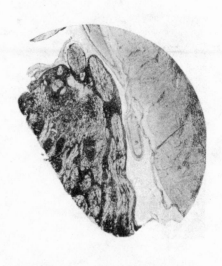

1. Pons, normal except for focal infiltration of left fifth nerve.

2. Higher power view of infiltrated left fifth nerve.

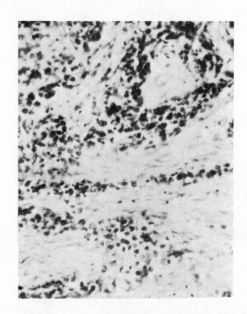

3. Detail of infiltrated left fifth nerve, showing: 1, diffuse infiltration with mononuclear cells; 2, perivascular infiltration; 3, strands of relatively unaffected nerve fibers.

Microscopic appearances in Case 6. Extraocular palsy (focal meningeal syphilis, especially of left fifth nerve). Illustrates exquisite focality of the syphilitic process sometimes found, as well as its unilaterality (giving rise to asymmetrical symptoms and signs). Process in itself probably curable.

GUMMATOUS NEUROSYPHILIS (" gumma of brain "). Autopsy.

Case 7. Mrs. Lecompte was a woman of middle age, who, according to the history given by her son, had been entirely well until her final illness, which began approximately two years before admission to Danvers Hospital. The beginning of her trouble seemed to be chiefly headaches, which would last continuously for several days, or more than a week at a time. These headaches lasted throughout the course of the disease. In the morning, on arising, she would feel very dizzy, but this would pass away during the day. She had had a number of spells of unconsciousness, lasting about fifteen minutes. In these attacks she would breathe heavily, there was frothing at the mouth, twitching of the hands, and the eyes would roll about. Her memory failed gradually, her disposition changed and she became very irritable. Vomiting occurred almost every day, and at times was of a projectile character. She became hallucinated; the hallucinations were chiefly of a visual nature.

About four months before admission to the hospital, after one of her seizures, the entire right side was found to be completely paralyzed, and she complained that it was numb. At this time, she had difficulty with her speech. In a few days, however, she was able to talk correctly again, and in a week she was back at work, although the right side was weak and awkward. She continued to grow worse, and then began to have spells lasting several days, so that it became necessary to have her placed in a hospital.

On admission to the hospital, aside from obesity, the general viscera showed no points of special interest, and there was no evidence of any new growth outside of the nervous system. She was unsteady on her feet, standing with them wide apart. The gait was quite ataxic; the whole right side was weaker than the left and used more awkwardly. There was a paralysis of the right side of the face; the right angle of the mouth drooped; the right eyelid could not be closed but remained continuously open; nor could the right side of the forehead be wrinkled. Vision and hearing were not affected. She miscalled tastes and smells; whether this was due to aphasic difficulties or to cranial nerve involvement could not be divined. There seemed to be some difficulty in deglutition. The knee-jerks were markedly exaggerated; slight clonus was obtained but was not always present. Both pupils reacted well to light and distance and consensually. Sensation could not be readily tested. There was marked ataxia, especially with the eyes closed. The speech was thick and mumbling. The patient was unable to write or copy. Mentally the patient was quite dull; at times, stuporous; when aroused, was found to be entirely disoriented. Memory almost entirely absent. In general she showed herself to be very much confused.

She remained practically in this condition, even gaining in weight, for the following two years, when suddenly one morning, she had an epileptic seizure, vomited, coughed a great deal, with bleeding from the mouth and ears, and died in a few hours.

The symptoms in this case pointed to brain tumor. The only inconsistent thing was the long-continued life, — four years, — after the symptoms were observed. As she lived before the W. R. and spinal fluid tests were known, no light was gained in these ways. The post-mortem examination showed the patient had a GUMMA OF THE BRAIN.

The **summary of the anatomical diagnoses** at autopsy was:
Decubitus.
Lymphadenitis of the mesenteric nodes.
Chronic fibrous peritonitis.
Chronic fibrous myocarditis.
Pulmonary hypostasis.
Thrombosis of vein in right adrenal, with hemorrhage.
Syphilitic leptomeningitis.
Gumma of left hemisphere.
Focal softenings in the pons.

The **anatomical description of the head** (Dr. A. M. Barrett) is as follows:

The sutures in the **calvarium** are well outlined; diploë large in amount. The **dura** is diffusely but lightly adherent to the calvarium; it is very dense, especially over the left hemisphere. The meningeal arteries are thickened but not atheromatous. The sinuses contain a small amount of fluid blood and post-mortem clot. The inner surface shows nothing abnormal. There is a great flattening of the convolutions of the left hemisphere, which is not the case on the right side. Over the convexity, the **pia** is thin and not abnormal except for some slight adhesions between the frontal lobes and the two lips of the Sylvian fissures. The pia at the base over the cisterna, pons, and medulla is thick, cloudy, and of a grayish gelatinous appearance. It is so thick that it is easily removable in a large piece.

The surface of the left hemisphere is dry, and the whole brain is flabby and bulges as if from internal pressure. A section through the hemispheres at the region of the optic chiasm shows a hard, firm area in the left hemisphere deep down in the white substance. It is about $2\frac{1}{2}$ cm. in diameter, with a wavy border. The central part is of a silver-gray gelatinous-like appearance, with red spots and whitish streaks radiating from the centre. In the pons on the right side, in a plane passing through the posterior corpora quadrigemina, are two pinhead size softenings among the pyramidal fibres. The ependyma of the fourth ventricle is granular.

Microscopic examination of the tumor: The area evidently contains several central necrotic foci surrounded by zones of infiltration and proliferation, with bordering areas of nervous tissue showing secondary reactions. The necrotic area stains poorly. From the edge there are projections of reddish homogeneous bands, some intermixed with well-differentiated fibrillæ, probably glia fibrils. The bordering zone is densely infiltrated with lymphoid, plasma, and a few epithelial cells. The nerve tissue outside of this zone is spongy and infiltrated with lymphoid and plasma cells. There are a few scattered, shrunken nerve cells. In this zone and in the zone of infiltration near the necrotic area, there are scattered cells resembling giant cells. There are many obliterated vessels in the area, and other vessels show many infiltrating lymphoid and plasma cells in the walls. The examination of the specimen stained by the methods for bacilli of tuberculosis are negative. The growth is a classical gumma.

GUMMATOUS NEUROSYPHILIS (gumma of
spinal meninges, "meningitis hypertrophica cervicalis of Charcot?"). Autopsy.

Case 8. John Wyman was first seen in his thirty-sixth
year by Dr. James J. Putnam. He denied syphilitic infection
and stated that the first symptoms had come four months
before. He had begun to notice a numbness of the fingers, at
first of the right hand and shortly thereafter of the left hand.
After a few weeks there had been difficulty in walking, and a
few weeks later headaches, especially on the right side, developed. Two weeks before he was first seen medically, he
had begun to have a feeling of tightness or constriction in
his arms.

It appears that micturition had been impaired early,
that is to say, a few weeks after the initial sensory disorder
had begun. A catheter was used for a time and improvement
followed. Shortly before consultation retention of urine
developed again, this time associated with rectal incontinence. The feet began to feel heavy and dead. Then
the legs began to be increasingly weak so that the patient
was almost bed-ridden. Vision appeared to be normal except that reading was followed by fatigue. The speech
was also slow but the slowness could be attributed to fatigue.

Notes of Dr. Putnam's **physical examination** are as follows:
The patient lay in bed on the left side, without motion, and
almost incapable of motion. The tongue was protruded,
and there was no paralysis of facial muscles, or of the eye
muscles (the right pupil had been reported to be slightly
larger than the left). There seemed to be a disinclination to
move the head, but with some effort it could be moved, and
without pain. The arms and hands were held rigidly in
median positions; many movements were possible, but all
were imperfect and of slight amplitude. The fingers were
flexed to a moderate degree, and could not easily be straight-
ened, and there was, in fact, a general rigidity of most of the

muscles of the body below the neck, and even, in some degree, of the neck. The immobility was so great that the general impression made was almost that of a patient with fracture of the spine in the cervical region. Even the breath, and especially the inspiration, was imperfect. The legs were more freely movable than the arms, but still the motions were very stiff and awkward, and of slight amplitude; with effort the whole leg could be lifted from the bed, and flexed or extended with moderate force. The right leg was rather stronger than the left, but the left hand and arm were stronger than the right. The sensibility was almost absent over the hands and lower part of the arms, and was impaired over the entire head and neck, except the forehead, the middle part of the face, and the nose. It is interesting to compare the conditions of the sensibility here present with those seen in cervical syringomyelia. The sensibility of the upper part of the forehead was less good than of the lower part, and there was slight impairment even over portions of the lower jaw. The sensibility of the left (stronger) arm was rather more impaired than that of the right arm, while on the contrary the sensibility of the left leg was better than that of the right leg, though the difference between them was not great. These statements apply to sensory tests by contact, heat, cold, and pricking. Knee-jerks were highly exaggerated, and likewise the wrist-jerks. All forced attempts at movements were attended by a high degree of muscular tremor, especially when the patient was fatigued or under emotional strain. The fingers especially were the seat of coarse tremor.

The remainder of this clinical description (courteously supplied us by Dr. Putnam) may be quoted. A second examination which included also a few facts not given in the first examination was made on the following March 28, 1905. This report says " the ends of the fingers became numb about June 1, 1904. Work was given up on July 3, and at that time the patient was walking very badly. No treatment was used and no satisfactory diagnosis made. In the course of July he improved somewhat, and during August he was able to ride out a little (these spontaneous improvements are of interest for the diagnosis). He went away from home for a short time, but from the time of his return, about the last of September, he grew worse rapidly, and fell into the condition above described, in which he was wholly unable to help himself, even to turning in bed. At times he had a great deal of pain in the neck and forehead. Antisyphilitic treatment was recommended, and for a time potassium iodid and other iodid preparations were given, but at first in relatively small doses (grs. 75 daily). Under this treatment the excretion of urine rose to four quarts daily as a maximum though sometimes the quantity was not so great."

Under this treatment the patient began soon to improve, and continued doing somewhat better till about five months later. He became able to walk downstairs and out of doors, and regained considerable use of his hands. The quantity of urine passed became greatly increased by the use of the iodid.

About the middle of March he became worse again. A careful examination of the sensibility showed that in general the condition was much the same as that previously reported. The iodid treatment, with perhaps some mercurial, was resumed; the potassium iodid was given in doses which were increased up to 850 grains daily, although this maximum dose was taken only for about one week. This large quantity gradually impaired the sense of taste for the time being, and blurred his vision, but otherwise did him no harm. Under this he improved, so that he became able to run more or less, and went about freely, and attended to his business, though still retaining some stiffness in his movements.

This improvement continued until about two years later, when he again had a relapse, and was seen medically once more. His condition at this time was still a pretty good one, but the movements were stiff and awkward. The bin-iodid of mercury was advised, which was taken in doses of $\frac{9}{25}$ grain daily. It will be remembered that this was long before the days of salvarsan treatment.

This was toward the end of June, 1907. Contrary to expectation, there was no material gain from this treatment, and the patient died early in October, without being seen again.

The **autopsy** was limited to the **nervous system** and the findings were as follows (Dr. A. R. Robertson):

Head: Hair abundant, fair, of fine texture and rather curly. Scalp of medium thickness and strips readily from calvarium. The latter appears normal and upon removal is of about the normal thickness. It lifts readily from the dura mater, except for the numerous attachments of Pacchionian granulations.

Meninges: The dura is smooth, moderately injected and shows no areas of thickening; it lifts readily from the pia-arachnoid. The pia-arachnoid shows discrete and in many places diffuse areas of opacity. There is a moderate amount of subpial clear fluid and the vessels are moderately injected. Over the anterior surface of the medulla and lower portion of the pons and largely confined to the right side there is a very marked thickening of the pia-arachnoid to which the dura is densely adherent. This thickening extends down anteriorly and laterally on the right side over the upper part of the cervical cord. The thickened meninges over the upper part of the medulla completely surround the right vertebral artery, shortly before it joins its fellow of the opposite side to form the basilar. Dissection of the arteries shows them to be patent and thin walled. Over the **cerebrum** and cerebellum the pia-arachnoid strips readily leaving a smooth surface. Section of the cerebral cortex, basal nuclei, pons and cerebellum show no gross lesions. The ventricles are moderately distended with fluid. The ependyma contains numerous small cysts. Section of the **pons** shows no lesions of the nervous tissue, but very marked thickening of the surrounding meninges as noted above.

Cord: Throughout the cervical and dorsal region the dura is quite tensely distended with an abundance of clear, light, straw-colored fluid. Upon snipping the dura this fluid escapes with a small spurt, as if under considerable pressure. The cord within, for the most part, lies free, but over the upper three or four centimeters of the cervical portion it is densely adherent to the dura anteriorly and laterally on the right side. Cross sections were made through the upper three or four centimeters of the cord, and over this area the cord is constricted by very marked thickening of all the meninges. The meninges here average from one to three millimeters in thickness. On the right side **and**

somewhat anteriorly opposite the junction of the atlas and axis there is a single nodular, firm mass which on section shows a yellowish, firm center surrounded by very dense, pearl-gray tissue. The demarcation between the homogeneous yellowish centre and its surrounding gray tissue is very sharp. This nodule measures about 0.75 to 1 cm. in diameter. The adjacent cord is deeply indented by it. Below this nodule there is a translucent, grayish appearance of both posterior sensory columns which extends downwards and diminishes in intensity until it finally disappears in the upper dorsal region. This same appearance is well marked on the right outer margin of the upper cervical cord corresponding to the crossed pyramidal tract, and extends downwards diminishing in intensity until it disappears about the mid-dorsal region. The left pyramidal tract appears to be similarly but very slightly involved; section of the lower dorsal cord entirely negative. **Microscopically,** characteristic GUMMA.

It is a question whether this case is one of the group described in 1871 by Charcot under the name of *pachymeningitis cervicalis hypertrophica.* Charcot did not regard his new disease as syphilitic, and it is very probable that syphilis is not responsible for all cases. Charcot, however, noted that his new disease was not incurable: he noted that the resulting paraplegia, although it might be very marked and accompanied by flexion of the leg on the thigh and although the paraplegia might have lasted a very long time, might end in recovery. Charcot thought that surgical intervention was necessary. He described three periods in the disease, the first or neuralgic (pseudo-neuralgic) was characterized by sharp pains in the neck and by the sensation of constriction in the upper part of the thorax. The second phase of the disease was, according to Charcot, the paralytic phase, in which a cervical paraplegia accompanied by muscular atrophy developed. Sometimes cases were found to remain in this paralytic phase and even to end spontaneously in cure. If the muscular atrophy was degenerative, then the atrophy was never replaced; but, according to Charcot, some cases of atrophy were simple and accordingly curable. If, however, the spinal cord itself became involved in the meningeal inflammation, then phenomena of transverse myelitis set in with a spastic paraplegia and involvement of the bladder and rectum. Muscular atrophy never developed in the legs, at least in typical cases.

Among the causes of this condition the following have been mentioned: cold, overexertion, alcoholism, tuberculosis and syphilis. Syphilis undoubtedly plays the major part. Even before the days of the W. R., observers, among whom may be mentioned Dejerine-Tinel and Pforringer, discovered syphilis in nearly all sufferers from *pachymeningitis cervicalis hypertrophica*.

It should be differentiated from caries of the spine and cord and meningeal tumors. The spinal fluid examination makes this somewhat easy.

Antisyphilitic remedies are indicated, and should be tried even when the etiology is obscure, if only as a therapeutic test.

But what have been thy answers?   What but dark,
Ambiguous, and with double sense deluding,
Which they who asked have seldom understood,
And, not well understood, as well not known?

Paradise Regained, Book I, lines 434-437.

II. THE SYSTEMATIC DIAGNOSIS OF THE MAIN FORMS OF NEUROSYPHILIS

PARETIC NEUROSYPHILIS ("general paresis") sometimes persistently receives the diagnosis **NEURASTHENIA** simply through omission to apply approved diagnostic methods.

Case 9. Greeley Harrison, a man of 46, certainly looked like a neurasthenic. He wanted aid for nervous indigestion of years' standing, headache, insomnia, nervousness, failing memory, and deafness. He volunteered, in fact, that he had neurasthenia, and that he had been treated for this by hypophosphites.

During the practically negative **physical examination,** Harrison complained of headache and throbbing in the head, and during examination of the abdomen felt much nauseated and proceeded to vomit rather persistently. There were hemorrhoids.

Neurological examination showed that the left pupil was smaller than the right, was irregular, failed to react consensually, and reacted very slowly to direct light. For the rest, however, the neurological examination was negative. On account of the nausea and vomiting, special examination of the gastric contents was made, but nothing abnormal was found.

Mentally, it was rather striking that the patient's memory was quite inaccurate both for remote and for recent events. His school knowledge was very meagre. As for delusions, the only approximation thereto was the patient's continually dwelling upon his bodily symptoms. Emotionally, he varied between depression and a sanguine attitude.

Although there was no symptom directly suggesting syphilis in the Harrison case, the slightly abnormal pupillary reactions and the amnesia warranted the suspicion of syphilis. The blood and spinal fluid both proved positive to the W. R.; the gold sol reaction was of the " paretic " type; there were 18 cells per cmm.; there was considerable globulin, and an excess of albumin. On the whole, therefore, we felt entitled to make the diagnosis GENERAL PARESIS. Why should not a careful observer have considered syphilis seriously? Yet in our experience such cases are frequently diagnosticated neurasthenia, thus entailing dangerous delay in treatment (in this case, five years' delay).

Going over the history of the case with still greater detail, we learned that for a number of years past, there had been symptoms of a neurological nature. For instance, five years before, at the age of 41, the patient had been apparently overcome when working near a stove, and went upstairs talking incoherently, but recovered shortly. Thereafter, such spells occurred almost every month; later, more frequently; still later, the attacks were associated with unconsciousness and amnesia. Occasionally preceding the attack there would be twitching of the mouth, jerking of the arms, and incoherent talk. Throughout these last five years, in point of fact, the patient had been unable to do regular work, had been given to much complaining, and had been far less efficient than formerly. In short, it would seem that, with the improved technique now in the possession of medical science for the diagnosis of general paresis, cases like that of Harrison will be diagnosticated earlier and earlier.

1. How typical is the insidious onset of symptoms in the case of Harrison? The onset of symptoms in neurosyphilis is ordinarily considered to be sudden, and this statement is generally true despite the fact that after the diagnosis is established a number of mild prodromal symptoms can be remembered by the relatives. However, some cases, of which Harrison is an example, have an exceedingly insidious onset without sudden access of striking symptoms. Joffroy and Mignot remark that with the improvement of clinical methods, the course of paretic neurosyphilis must now be stated

to take some six or seven years for completion. In point of fact, there were early episodic symptoms (seizures almost monthly) which should not have escaped medical attention. They did escape medical attention, however, and Harrison was wont to say " Why wasn't I told that my disease was syphilis five years ago?"

2. Is there such a disease as syphilitic neurasthenia? According to Kraepelin, syphilitic neurasthenia has been described as occurring shortly after infection and in the first stages of syphilis. There are milder and severer forms; the milder forms show discomfort, difficulty in thinking, irritability, insomnia, cephalic pressure, indefinite variable, uncomfortable sensations, and pains. The severer cases acquire anxiety, more pronounced emotional disorder, dizziness, disorder of consciousness, difficulty in finding the right word, transient palsies, pronounced sensory disorders, nausea, and increase of temperature. Kraepelin is in doubt whether there is any definite clinical picture of this sort, and whether there is any causal relation between the syphilitic infection and such symptoms as those described. If the effect of knowledge concerning infection is a merely psychic effect, then it is improper to term the neurasthenia in question a syphilitic neurasthenia. For the relation of hysteria to the acquisition of syphilis, see below the case of Alice Caperson (46). In point of fact, modern work has shown even in the primary and secondary stages of general syphilis more or less pronounced neurosyphilitic phenomena in the shape of the so-called meningitic irritation of French authors. (Besides the case of Caperson (46), see the case of Fitzgerald and the discussions under these cases.)

3. What is the relation of the early symptoms of this case to the so-called preparesis of Dana? The case might well have been an example of Dana's preparesis. For a discussion of this, see Case of William Twist (13).

4. What is the classical differential diagnosis between paretic neurosyphilis and neurasthenia? The testing of the blood by the W. R. is unconditionally necessary. If the W. R. is negative, the diagnosis of paretic neurosyphilis is extremely improbable. (It must be borne in mind that a number of cases of paretic neurosyphilis have been shown to have a negative W. R. in the serum, and receive a proper diagnosis only after spinal fluid examination.) Next to the serum W. R. stand the

pupillary and aphasic symptoms. In the presence of Argyll-Robertson pupil or even a slight speech defect, the diagnosis of neurasthenia must certainly be made with caution if at all. Kraepelin remarks: The sudden occurrence of neurasthenic disorders in a male of middle age without any evident cause therefor is always suspicious. Yet it must be emphasized that a complaint of occasional dizziness, slight speech defect, tremor of tongue, and a moderate increase of tendon reflexes do not possess any marked diagnostic significance. Clear insight and understanding of the nature of the disease phenomena, a persistent search for recovery, reasonableness in conversation, progressive improvement under appropriate treatment, speak for neurasthenia.

Joffroy and Mignot differentiate what they call preparetic neurasthenia from other neurasthenic states, not only on the basis of its etiology but on the basis of its symptoms. They also call attention to the fact that neurasthenia, being a pure neurosis, develops either on a manifestly hereditary basis or upon some physical injury, weakening disease, or moral shock. The pure neurotic suffers a great deal more than the patient who is destined to become a victim of paresis. The character change in neurasthenia does not amount to that entire transformation of personality (even to the performance of criminal acts) that we find in paretic neurosyphilis; at the most, the neurasthenic shows minor emotional disturbances and a certain pathological egoism. The psychotherapeutic test also rather readily dissipates many of the neurotic, hypochondriacal fears and feelings. Although both pure neurasthenia and the paretic pseudoneurasthenia are characterized by sexual weakness, the sexual anæsthesia of the preparetic is practically always preceded by a stage of sexual over-excitement. These finer clinical indications, however, fade into insignificance beside the data that can and should be obtained from laboratory tests.

5. How exceptional is such a case as that of Harrison? We have in our experience seen many patients with a similar course and configuration of symptoms, although the majority of these cases in a community advanced enough to provide easy access to a Wassermann laboratory are now diagnosticated far earlier than was the case of Harrison.

6. What attitude shall we take toward so-called syphilophobia? It seems to us that resort to a serum W. R. is indicated, both from the standpoint of the community and still more importantly from the standpoint of the patient. We are even inclined to suggest for a case of persistent syphilophobia, when the serum W. R. has proved negative, a lumbar puncture. Syphilophobia must be considered, not as a syphilitic psychosis, but as a phobia to be classified among the psychoneuroses. It becomes a difficult question to decide at times whether a patient who has had syphilis, has had a considerable course of treatment and shows the symptoms of a syphilophobiac should be further treated for syphilis or merely for his phobia. We have seen recently such a patient who gave a certain history of syphilis and who was greatly disturbed lest he should be developing paresis. This fear bothered him greatly. Examination showed irregular pupils, but no other signs of syphilis. The W. R. in blood and spinal fluid was negative as were the other spinal fluid tests. It was considered wise to treat him only for his phobia and under this treatment he was given some relief.

PARETIC NEUROSYPHILIS (" general paresis ")
may look precisely like MANIC-DEPRESSIVE
PSYCHOSIS.

Case 10. The mental picture in Lyman Agnew, an architect, 58 years of age, was wholly characteristic of manic-
depressive psychosis. In the first place, there had been (at
55) a previous attack of depression, lasting a few months,
from which Agnew had completely recovered. He had
remained entirely well up to four months before consultation.
(Manic-depressive psychosis is, at least in a majority of
cases, hereditary. There had been mental disorder in one
maternal cousin, and mental impairment in the patient's
mother some time before her death from cerebral hemorrhage.
There was no other report of mental disease in the family.)

It appears that in the interval between attacks, Agnew
had been working very hard and had been fairly successful
in paying off a mortgage on his house. A marked elation,
somewhat natural, followed this success and continued to an
abnormal degree. Agnew labored under considerable excitement, was over-fussy, and at times showed a flight of
ideas. His mania or hypomania gradually diminished and
depression set in, in which depression he arrived for consultation. He had marked ideas of self-accusation, was emotionally unstable, wept much, and showed a characteristic
retardation of activities and unrest.

Physically, there was no neurological disorder. The patient
appeared rather under-nourished. The heart borders lay
2 cm. to the right and at $11\frac{1}{2}$ cm. to the left of the mid-
sternal line. The aortic second sound was very loud. There
was a moderate radial arteriosclerosis. Systolic blood pressure was 210, diastolic 155.

The high blood pressure suggested nephritis, possibly of
arteriosclerotic origin, but urine examination and blood-
nitrogen tests yielded no evidence of kidney disease. Moreover, it is our experience that a manic-depressive psychosis

in persons past middle life is not infrequently complicated by high blood pressure. In point of fact, some authors insist upon a relation between manic-depressive psychosis and the arteriosclerosis which rather frequently sets in in this disease.

Routine examination of the blood serum, however, yielded a positive W. R. Following the approved rule of making an examination of the spinal fluid in all mental cases having a positive serum W. R., we proceeded to lumbar puncture. The fluid was clear and contained 35 cells per cmm., the albumin was in excess, and there was a positive globulin reaction. The gold sol reaction was of the " paretic " type; the W. R. was strongly positive.

On this basis, it seems worth while to consider the diagnosis of GENERAL PARESIS or that of some form of non-paretic neurosyphilis. The former is the diagnosis which we prefer.

1. What is the classical differential diagnosis between manic-depressive psychosis and neurosyphilis? The laboratory tests have naturally supplanted the older purely clinical methods of differential diagnosis. The difficulties lodge, in the first instance, in depressive states. It would appear to be impossible on purely clinical grounds in certain cases to tell the depression of neurosyphilis from the depression of manic-depressive psychosis, since the slightly greater interest in the outer world taken by manic-depressive patients and their greater responsiveness to diagnostic threats (suggestion that patient is to be pinched or cut) are of no special value in the individual case. Identical considerations hold for the maniacal phases of manic-depressive psychosis, for these maniacal phases may even develop delusions (Kraepelin) of precisely the same nature as the characteristic expansive delusions of the excited paretic.

2. If the clinical symptoms are insufficient in differential diagnosis, are not the pupillary signs and the speech defect of greater value? They are of value if present, but as in the case of Agnew, the victim of neurosyphilis may show no pupillary or speech disorder. Instances are familiar, also, in which the pupillary and speech signs are absent in very advanced cases of non-paretic or even of paretic neurosyphilis.

3. Would not a circular course or recurrence of attacks be decisive for manic-depressive psychosis? Paretic neurosyphilis sometimes exhibits the same circular or recurrent course. We conclude that neither the clinical symptoms, the classical pupillary and speech signs, nor the ups and downs of a particular disease, are at all decisive as between manic-depressive psychosis and paretic neurosyphilis. Resort must be had to laboratory tests.

4. What is the significance of the high blood pressure in paretic neurosyphilis? Work from our laboratory (Southard and Canavan) has shown plasma cells in the kidneys in 17 out of 30 paretics (56%), and in 16 of these 17 paretics with renal plasmocytosis, the plasma cells were found in the periglomerular region. What the relation of these findings may be to heightened blood pressure is as yet unknown. The severe syphilitic involvement of the aorta so characteristic in paretic neurosyphilis, as in other forms, may possibly have a bearing on blood pressure.

A POSITIVE SERUM WASSERMANN REAC-
TION associated with mental symptoms (even
with grandiosity) does NOT prove the EXIST-
ENCE OF PARETIC NEUROSYPHILIS ("general paresis").

Case 11. Juliette Lachine came to a general hospital with pain in the right upper quadrant of the abdomen, wherein was found an enlarged liver. This liver was regarded as syphilitic on the ground that the patient had a positive serum W. R. and that her two elder children were clearly suffering from congenital syphilis. The liver mass was promptly reduced by antisyphilitic treatment of the classical sort. When, however, the patient was given an injection of salvarsan, she shortly began to develop marked mental symptoms, whereupon she was removed to the Psychopathic Hospital.

The **mental picture** at the Psychopathic Hospital was as follows: Lack of orientation for time, marked distractibility of attention, with a certain jumping from one subject to another, delusions of a religious nature, claims of wonderful powers possessed by the patient, moods variable, though as a rule of a euphoric and elated nature, with laughing and singing. The activity seemed to be of a mental rather than a peripheral nature. The patient did not regard herself as mentally abnormal. The liver was still 4 cm. below the costal margin in the nipple line. We found the W. R. to be positive in the serum but negative in the spinal fluid. In fact, the spinal fluid was entirely negative.

So far as we are aware the picture presented by this case is one of MANIC–DEPRESSIVE PSYCHOSIS. We regard the disease as merely complicating the syphilis, although it is entirely possible that some visceral condition incidental to the syphilis might be proved (in a higher stage of psychiatric science) to have produced the mania.

In any event, the patient quite recovered from her mental symptoms in a month. She was then able to tell us of a previous attack of depression some 12 years previously, namely, at the age of 26. It apears that she had at that time been committed to a hospital for the insane.

1. In this case, in which the diagnosis of manic-depressive pyschosis and not paretic neurosyphilis was made, are we sure that the symptoms that we term manic-depressive psychosis were not actually produced by syphilotoxins? In other words, in the absence of spinal fluid signs of inflammation or chemical change, might it not be possible for generalized syphilis outside the nervous system to produce manic-depressive symptoms? There is so far in the literature no experimental or other evidence of syphilotoxins. The existence of products and substances permitting the W. R. and the gold sol reaction is not of course evidence of syphilotoxins. Although there is no evidence of soluble syphilotoxins, it is thought that in the so-called Järisch-Herxheimer reaction (the intensification of clinical symptoms after salvarsan injection) effects may be due to the liberation of products from the killed bodies of spirochetes. Such endotoxins are not here in question.

2. Is visceral syphilis, such as gumma of the liver, able to produce characteristic syphilitic reactions in the spinal fluid? We have had an autopsied case in which there was a " paretic " gold sol reaction of the fluid (though without other signs). The autopsy showed gummata of the liver. However, the finer anatomy of the nervous system showed a mild but definite meningo-encephalitic process, which was doubtless responsible for the gold sol reaction.

3. What is the value of grandiose ideas? Ballet distinguishes two groups of grandiose ideas: (a) ideas of self-satisfaction, including ideas concerning extraordinary capacity, strength, power, and wealth on the part of the patient; and (b) ideas of ambition; the latter being of a more exact, constant, uniform and systematizing nature. The more vague and less systematized ideas of self-satisfaction rest in a phase of contentedness and optimism; the more definite ideas of pride and ambition are responsible for striking transformations of personality. General paresis shows, according to Ballet, these ideas of self-satisfaction in their most developed form. A certain variability, absurdity, in-

coherence, and contradictoriness characterize these ideas and the patient has little or no insight into their nature. When such ideas occur at the outset of the disease, they naturally may be of medico-legal interest. Cotard explains these ideas of megalomania on the part of paretics on the ground that they are essentially motor or will disorders and rest upon a sort of hyperbulia, exhibiting itself in exuberant activity. Régis has thought that the delusional generosity and liberality of the paretic, and his willingness to lend his wealth and talents to social progress, is helpful for diagnosis when contrasted with the more personal egoism of the victim of manic-depressive psychosis. The self-satisfaction of the manic-depressive patient often does not reach a delusional stage, but remains a mere feeling of pathological well-being or euphoria. The maniacal patient may compare himself with some great man but he does not identify himself with him. It must be remembered that these ideas of self-satisfaction occur also in alcoholism, but according to Ballet they occur only in the dementing phase of chronic alcoholism, and have no special diagnostic value. They may be a clinical stumbling-block for a time in the cases of alcoholic pseudoparesis. As for the ideas of ambition in which the patients believe themselves to be princes, emperors, divine messengers, and the like, these are less characteristic of paretic neurosyphilis than of delusional psychoses of a non-syphilitic nature. At all events, such ideas if definite, of long standing, and systematized by the patient to form a thoroughgoing portion of his life, are not characteristic of neurosyphilis. The victim of paretic neurosyphilis can as a rule be persuaded out of his delusions, at least for the time being. These distinctions, it must be added, are hardly of value in the early cases of any of the psychoses in question, and cannot be made as a rule in either private or psychopathic hospital practice. Typical examples of grandiosity, although not so frequent as might be thought from textbooks, are always on display in institutions for the chronic insane.

PARETIC NEUROSYPHILIS ("general paresis") may look precisely like DEMENTIA
PRAECOX. Autopsy.

Case 12. Henry Phillips remains a striking case in the
memory of those who knew him and his medical findings.
Phillips came to the hospital voluntarily at 42 years of age
from the bank where he worked as a clerk; he came at the
suggestion of his employer. It seems that he had been
annoying his associates because he had fallen into a habit of
continually scratching himself. Phillips was entirely sure
that he was the victim of what he called the "Scotch itch,"
and explained off-hand that this itch had been put upon him
by the Free Masons as a matter of revenge because he would
not join their order. He said once, for example: "At
times I feel like raising Hell; then I get a psychic intimation;
and then I get to using a foot-rule on my back and to slapping
my face." He explained this psychic intimation as coming
from the order of Scottish Rites. Another example of talk is
as follows: "My father is a fighting man; that is part of it.
They mean to throw me down. I am through now trying
for membership in the Free Masons. They have good cause,
they must fight. They do not want me for some personal
matters. I can go just so far in agreeing and seconding their
advances, but in the end it fails. I have no strength nor
endurance."

Aside from these delusions, there was little abnormality
to be found, though his recollection for minor events of the
immediate present was inaccurate. He was rather abnor-
mally impulsive, gesticulating a good deal while talking,
and was of the appearance that the laity call "nervous."
It appears that he had always been peculiar, subject to
violent fits of temper, in which fits he might throw things at
other members of the family. He always had pronounced
likes and dislikes which he never concealed. He had never
had friends, had always been secretive; and he was often

termed a great student. For some five years he had been studying Japanese from time to time, associating himself with a Japanese.

It never does to jump at the diagnosis dementia praecox. However, the picture seemed characteristic enough for the paranoid form of this disease. Physically, Phillips had no particular abnormality; the knee-jerks were a little lively, and the pupils reacted a little sluggishly. However, the routine W. R. of the serum proved to be positive. Examination of the spinal fluid was resorted to, — as in all cases with a positive serum W. R. — and it also proved to be positive and strongly so; the globulin and albumin were increased, and there was a pleocytosis. A diagnosis of neurosyphilis was hardly avoidable. Phillips later admitted a chancre, which he claimed was located on the mucous membrane of the cheek and acquired by using the same utensils as his Japanese friend, which friend, he stated, had active syphilis.

Antisyphilitic treatment of considerable intensiveness was begun, with intravenous injections of salvarsan and intraspinous injections of salvarsanized serum, but the patient grew steadily worse. His mental symptoms became more marked, although not especially characteristic of general paresis. **Neurologically,** he did develop signs more suggestive of general paresis, and 18 months later died.

The **autopsy** showed features of GENERAL PARESIS. It is not necessary to enter into the question of the details of histological correlation at this time.

1. What conclusion can be drawn from lively knee-jerks? Lively knee-jerks are of very little significance. Not only certain neurosyphilitics but also a variety of neurotic persons, victims of dementia praecox and hysteria, are very prone to have active tendon reflexes. Of course, extreme degrees of exaggeration are of importance, and especially an association of the hyperreflexia with the Babinski reaction, the Gordon, or Oppenheim reflexes, ankle clonus, and the like.

2. Is there any special or differentiating factor in an extragenital chancre as against a genital chancre? Prob-

ably this question should be answered in the negative. Some have claimed that chancres draining by lymphatic channels of the head are more likely to lead to cerebral syphilis. This idea cannot be said to be established.

3. Is there any significance in the story, if true, that Phillips acquired his syphilis from a Mongolian? It seems to be fairly well established that syphilis of the nervous system is extremely rare in China and Japan, whereas bone syphilis is very frequent there. It has been held that this has to do (a) with strains of spirochetes, (b) with the state of civilization, or (c) with the degree of " syphilization." Apparently when a race is first infected with syphilis the lesions are chiefly of the cutaneous and osseous systems; only in later generations the vascular and nervous systems suffer. However, involvement of the nervous systems of Mongolians resident in this country is no rarity, a point possibly in favor of the theory of special strains affecting the nervous system as prevalent in western countries. Little or nothing is known as to the effect of transmission from one race to another, as from Mongolian to Caucasian in Phillips' story.

NEUROSYPHILIS is NOT to be entirely ruled out by a negative serum Wassermann Reaction; for the fluid Wassermann Reaction may be positive.

Case 13. William Twist is a case of note in the matter of the so-called preparetic period (the idea of Charles L. Dana which was scoffed at when first proposed by him in 1910). The patient, a very successful traveling salesman, 35 years of age, was admitted to the Psychopathic Hospital showing a typical picture of general paresis.

Thus, **mentally,** the patient showed elation, grandiosity (millions of dollars to give away), intellectual weakness, disorder of memory, lack of judgment, rambling talk, speech defect, omission of letters in writing and spelling.

Neurologically, there was tremor of the lips, slight irregularity of the pupils, which however reacted well, and lively knee-jerks.

Mr. Twist had sought advice at our out-patient department in his thirty-third year. The records show that at that time he was somewhat depressed, and his speech was even then, according to his own statement, stammering. However, we found the W. R. at that time to be negative in the blood serum. It appeared that his mother had died of consumption; his father was said to have committed suicide. A brother had once recovered from an attack of depression, presumably an attack of manic-depressive psychosis. Accordingly, we thought at the time that the case was probably one of manic-depressive psychosis. Moreover, our routine serum W. R. failed to indicate any syphilitic process. As for the so-called stammering of speech, this appeared to be a matter of the patient's own recollection rather than of our observation. In any event, the patient had gone into the country and appears to have entirely recovered; falling, again, however, into mental difficulties after a short period, and finally arriving at the hospital in the above-mentioned classical condition.

The W. R. in the blood serum proved again negative. The test was repeated a number of times; also, after salvarsan had been given. The salvarsan did not act provocatively, and the blood serum has remained consistently negative.

In cases of syphilis the W. R. is at times negative. Swift claims that in such cases an injection of salvarsan will often produce a positive W. R. if the blood is tested on several days following the injection.

The spinal fluid, however, did show a positive W. R. as well as a gold sol reaction of a " paretic " type. There were at the first examination 194 cells per cmm., there was a moderate excess of albumin, and a positive globulin test. In short, there was no question of any other diagnosis than GENERAL PARESIS.

1. How can the negative W. R. of the blood serum be explained? It is difficult or impossible to explain this. Figures differ as to the percentage of cases of general paresis with negative blood serum; perhaps 3 to 5% of these cases yield a negative serum W. R.

    It is important to note the long preparetic period: at least a year and a half. Could our diagnostic methods be sharpened a trifle, such cases as these could be obtained early in this preparetic period and it might then be safe to promise good therapeutic results.

2. What is the nature of the preparesis of Dana? When Dana's brief paper on preparesis was written, there was of course hardly any idea that cases of paretic neurosyphilis could be cured or would recover, except possibly vanishingly few *curiosa* about which there would always rage a diagnostic question. Accordingly, Dana, having found certain cases that seemed to him to have early signs of paresis but had apparently been cured by treatment, proposed to call them cases of preparesis. His idea was that he would thereby not offend those who held that general paresis was theoretically a fatal disease. With modern work and the display of more and more atypical cases of neurosyphilis, and the observation of relatively numerous cures or remissions under treatment, the designation of preparesis for a separate entity, or even for a subform of neurosyphilis, becomes superfluous.

3. What is the percentage of cases of paretic neurosyphilis that show a negative serum W. R.? Among the best figures are those of Müller, who found that of 386 examples of paretic neurosyphilis, 379 showed all reactions positive, or 98.5%.

4. What is the meaning and value of the so-called provocative salvarsan injection? In practice, there may be a series of negative W. R.'s in the blood serum before a positive reaction is finally obtained, owing to technical difficulties or biological peculiarities. Where intensive work is being done upon the neurosyphilis problem, it is beyond question desirable to make the W. R. test upon at least three separate samples of blood drawn at intervals, for the second or third test may prove positive. This situation makes the interpretation of the so-called provocative salvarsan injection exceedingly doubtful; that is, the reaction might have been positive on repetition without the injection of salvarsan. The present case, as above stated, failed to yield a serum W. R. even after repeated tests and the " provocative."

5. What is the significance of the irregular pupils in this group? Paretic neurosyphilis shows inequality of the pupils in a high per cent of cases. Irregularity of outline of the pupils is commonly thought to be an important sign and to suggest neurosyphilis. It is true that many cases of pupillary irregularity are syphilitic, but the sign is of little or no differential value since congenital malformations and relics of old injuries and adhesions may produce effects identical with those of neurosyphilis.

DIFFUSE (that is, meningovasculoparenchymatous*) NEUROSYPHILIS is typically associated
with six positive tests (serum Wassermann reaction,
fluid Wassermann reaction, spinal fluid gold sol
reaction, pleocytosis, positive globulin, excessive
albumin); but one or more, and frequently several, of these tests are likely to run mild as
compared with the tests in PARETIC NEURO-
SYPHILIS ("general paresis"). The clinical course
of the diffuse (and especially the meningovascular)
cases is likely to be protracted, with a good prognosis as to life (barring fatal vascular insults).

Case 14. We shall present the case of John Jackson, a
surveyor, 31 years of age, suffering from a left hemiplegia,
with this in mind: To exhibit difficulties in diagnosis in the
presence of an embarrassment of symptomatic riches.

The patient arrived at the hospital, in the first place, because he had been threatening a woman who lived next door
to him. He believed that this neighbor had been talking
about him and circulating reports against him. Excited by
these ideas, he had threatened to cut her throat.

Now the occurrence of hemiplegia in adult life before the
approach of senium is always suspicious of syphilis, and this
suspicion we naturally entertained from the beginning.
However, there was upon the scalp a crooked linear furrow
about six inches long, running from the vertex to the right
parietal eminence. Another furrow about an inch long
was present upon the forehead. These furrows appeared to
be of a bony nature and were not tender. There was evidence of an old decompression operation on the right side of
the head; there were also large scars on both sides of the

---

* Proof of marked parenchymatous lesions must hang on
post-mortem data; the inference here as to the presence of
parenchymatous lesions is a clinical inference.

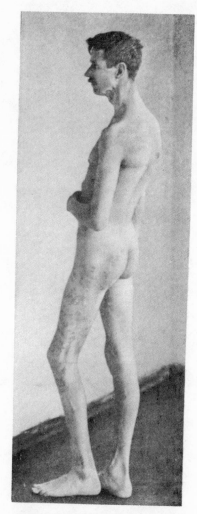

Station in syphilitic hemiplegia.
Syphilitic pigmentation of skin.

neck, evidently the result of old operations; and there were numerous palpable glands — the largest about the size of a lima bean — all firm and not tender.

It seems that at the age of eight, according to the patient's mother, Jackson had received a head injury and had remained unconscious for three weeks. Upon recovery, he had to relearn both to walk and to talk; however, he was able to begin school where he left off. He became more nervous and irritable after the accident than previously. Nothing further had developed until, at about 25 years of age, a tubercle was discovered in his eye (the right pupil was smaller than the left, reacting more slowly; right iris bound down by adhesions, with white opacity of anterior chamber). For two years, 25 to 27, the patient was under medical treatment for tuberculosis, and at the conclusion of this period numerous glands were removed from the neck and diagnosticated tuberculous. However, the neck did not heal and he carried bandages upon it for two years.

At 28, the patient's mother described the occurrence of a slight shock, with head retraction, for a minute or two, and inability to speak. Thereafter there had been five or six similar attacks, less severe, and without loss of speech. The attacks were never accompanied by convulsive movements. Then occurred a paralytic stroke, leaving the patient with a left hemiplegia, which had somewhat improved. Mentally, the patient had gone down hill, becoming less alert and more apathetic, and to some extent amnestic. One had to consider, accordingly, the somewhat doubtful possibility of post-traumatic and post-operative conditions, and the question of tuberculosis (possibly errors in diagnosis; the lungs showed no evidence of tuberculosis).

Physically, the signs of a left hemiplegia were appropriate. Spasticity on the left side was found; there were Babinski, Gordon, Oppenheim reflexes and ankle clonus on the left side (all absent on the right). Speech defect was present. **Mentally,** aside from the delusions noted at the beginning of our analysis, a striking feature was the patient's childishness. While reciting delusions, the patient was overactive and evinced a somewhat childish interest. Arithmetically, Jack-

TYPICAL LABORATORY FINDINGS IN NEUROSYPHILIS (NONNE, 1915)

DIAGNOSIS	W. R., BLOOD SERUM	W. R., 0.22 CC. BLOOD SERUM	SPINAL FLUID, 1.0 CC.	PHASE I, GLOBULIN	PLEOCYTOSIS
PARESIS OR TABOPARESIS	POSITIVE IN ALMOST 100%	POSITIVE, 85-90%	POSITIVE, 100%	POSITIVE, 95-100%	POSITIVE, ABOUT 95%
TABES (not combined with paresis)	POSITIVE, 60-70%	POSITIVE, 20%	POSITIVE, 100%	POSITIVE, 90-95%	POSITIVE, 90%
CEREBRO-SPINAL SYPHILIS	POSITIVE, 70-80%	POSITIVE, 20-30%	POSITIVE ALMOST ALWAYS	POSITIVE almost always; NEGATIVE only EXCEPTIONALLY	POSITIVE ALMOST ALWAYS

CHART 8

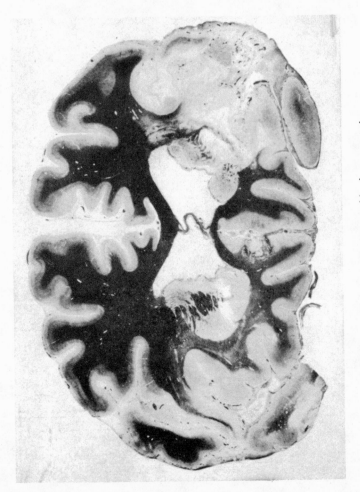

Syphilitic thrombosis.   Contours of brain preserved.

son had preserved a fair ability but his apathy and lack of interest interfered with tests, and possibly also with the exercise of memory. As above noted, we were compelled to maintain the suspicion of syphilis throughout despite the attractive hypotheses of traumatic and post-decompressive effects and cerebral tuberculosis. A history of the acquisition of syphilis an unknown number of years before admission entered to strengthen the suspicion of the syphilitic nature of the mental symptoms.

The W. R. proved positive in blood and spinal fluid. The gold sol reaction was of the syphilitic type; 37 cells were found per cmm.; there was a slight amount of globulin and a slight excess of albumin.

We made a diagnosis of CEREBROSPINAL SYPHILIS rather than general paresis on account of, first, the slow course of the disease; second, the vascular type of the cerebral insult, hardly typical of paresis; and third, the mild spinal fluid reaction. Treatment will hardly cure the hemiplegia, at least so far as restoration of cerebral tissues lost in the insult is concerned. We were perhaps entitled to consider that, as in the cases of Petrofski (17), O'Neil (19), Robinson (45), the meningitic process could be arrested. Unfortunately, our treatment of 20 injections of salvarsan over a period of 10 weeks, followed by a number of months of bi-weekly injections of mercury salicylate, proved incapable of making any change in the mental and physical picture or in the laboratory findings.

1. Can we explain the apparently poor reaction to treatment of the cerebrospinal syphilis in the case of Jackson by supposing a more deep-seated involvement than the meningovascular involvement indicated by the hemiplegia and the signs in the fluid? Autopsied cases in our experience show focal parenchymatous involvements that have not caused obvious clinical symptoms at any time during the course of the disease. These symptomatically silent lesions may have been present.

2. What is the comparative prognostic value of seizures in paretic neurosyphilis and in such a meningovascular case as that of Jackson? Paretic seizures are often and indeed characteristically recovered from. More-

over, autopsies in paretic neurosyphilis characteristically show no gross focal destructive lesions to correspond with the seizures. The paretic seizures are apparently more irritative than paralytic. However, the seizures of the meningovascular group of neurosyphilis are also, though less commonly, recovered from, so that the differential diagnosis on the basis of the outcome of seizures is not safe. Rarely paretic neurosyphilis itself also develops seizures from which no recovery is made.

3. What is the relation of neuropathic heredity to neurosyphilis? The family history of John Jackson is undoubtedly poor, since his father died of diabetes and a paternal uncle was insane; and on the mother's side, the grandmother died of tuberculosis and an aunt died insane. This general question was more interesting in the days before the syphilitic nature of general paresis and of allied diseases was known. However, we may still hold perhaps that not only syphilis but also various intoxications, especially alcoholism, do flourish upon a neuropathic soil. This question, like that of Krafft-Ebing's celebrated claim of the relation between syphilization and civilization, needs revision in the light of more extensive applications of the W. R. in larger and larger groups of persons under various community conditions.

The SIX TESTS (serum Wassermann reaction, fluid Wassermann reaction, pleocytosis, gold sol reaction, globulin, excess albumin) are likely to run STRONGER in PARETIC NEUROSYPHILIS (" general paresis ") than in DIFFUSE (especially meningovascular) NEUROSYPHILIS; in particular, the gold sol reaction is likely to prove " paretic " rather than " syphilitic." The clinical course of paretic neurosyphilis (" general paresis ") is likely to terminate in death within a few years.

Case 15. Pietro Martiro was a well-developed and nourished man, 30 years of age, who had been doing erratic things and acting peculiarly for a few weeks before entering the hospital. In the hospital, Martiro proved to be very excitable and given to violence. He had marked delusions of grandeur, saying he was worth many millions of dollars, was the greatest singer in the world, the greatest athlete in the world, and the like.

Physically, there was no disorder except overactivity of some reflexes. The diagnosis of GENERAL PARESIS offered no difficulties, and it was confirmed by the laboratory tests (positive serum and fluid W. R., " paretic " gold sol reaction, 42 cells per cmm., an excess of albumin, and a positive globulin test).

Treatment: The perfect physique of this case and the extremely brief clinical duration (a few weeks) would naturally suggest a probably favorable outcome. However, cases with marked delusions of grandeur have very frequently proved to be cases with extensive brain tissue loss as shown in certain studies with Danvers material.

In any event, the treatment in this case proved unavailing. Enormous doses of salvarsan, twice a week, aided by mercury and potassium iodid, were given. Although other cases had been helped by such intensive treatment, Martiro went

PARETIC NEUROSYPHILIS (GENERAL PARESIS)

PHYSICAL SYMPTOMS

EARLY HEADACHE

VISUAL DISORDER

HYPALGESIA

ADIADOCHOKINESIS

ATAXIA

NASOLABIAL FLATTENING

VOCAL CHANGE

SPEECH DISORDER

WRITING DISORDER

LOSS OF MANUAL DEXTERITY

PUPILLARY CHANGES

REFLEX CHANGES

SEIZURES

LATE: PARALYSIS, CONTRACTURE

CHART 9

PARETIC NEUROSYPHILIS (GENERAL PARESIS)

MENTAL SYMPTOMS

INTAKE IMPAIRED

CONSCIOUSNESS CLOUDED

FATIGUABILITY INCREASED

HALLUCINOSIS RARE

AMNESIA — RECENT! CHRONOLOGY AND STORAGE
    IMPAIRED. FABULATION

OVERSUGGESTIBILITY

JUDGMENT IMPAIRED

FANTASTIC DELUSIONS

INSIGHT INTO ILLNESS NIL

EARLY IRRITABILITY OR HEBETUDE

QUICK SHIFTING EMOTION

CHARACTER CHANGE

CONDUCT SLUMP

CHART 10

steadily downhill, nor was there the slightest diminution in the intensity of any of the spinal fluid reactions. After 50 injections of salvarsan over a period of 30 weeks without improvement, treatment was discontinued. A few months later, the patient died.

1. What is the duration of paretic neurosyphilis ("general paresis")? If we omit the doubtful, early, and prodromal stages and count the beginning of the disease with the occurrence of definite symptoms, we find (Kraepelin) that almost half the patients with pronounced paretic signs die within the first two years of their disease. Kraepelin's observations upon 244 cases are as follows:

Year:	1	2	3	4	5	6	7	8	9	10	14
Cases:	51	63	52	41	22	4	5	2	2	1	1

The average duration of the disease in months has been calculated as varying from 24 to 32 months. Juvenile paresis runs a slower and more insidious course. The duration of paresis, according to many observers, diminishes with the increasing age of the patient. It is now held that a combination of tabes with paresis does not prolong the duration of the paresis. As noted above in the discussion of Case Harrison (9), our conceptions of the characteristic duration of paretic neurosyphilis must alter with the increase of our knowledge due to the early application of laboratory tests.

2. What is the significance of the term *general paresis?* The case of Martiro is, of course, a good instance to show that the term is sometimes a misnomer. The characteristic generalized motor incapacity denoted by the term *general paresis* is shown in patients in the institutions for the chronic insane in their last few months of life. The term *paresis* is perhaps to be preferred to the term *paralysis* because the paralysis is not complete but partial; but perhaps the best reason is that the word *paresis* is a shorter word. When the mental side is to be emphasized, the term *paralytic dementia* is employed. In this book we have used the term *paretic neurosyphilis* to mean a more precise statement of the etiology of general paresis (general paralysis, paralytic dementia). The lay term, *softening*

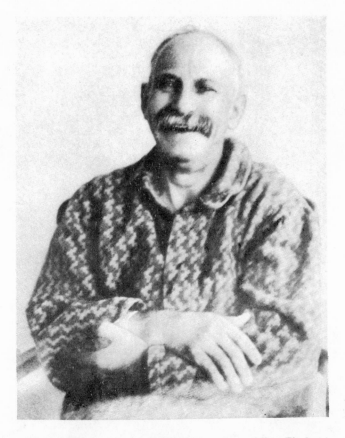

Euphoria in paretic neurosyphilis ("general paresis"). The head, arms and trunk were shaking with mirth; hence, the indistinct outlines of the photograph.

of the brain, like the terms *metasyphilis* and *parasyphilis* is in the present phase of our knowledge to be eschewed.

3. If this fatal case be typical of general paresis (for more favorable results, see Part V), what is the toll of deaths from this disease in the community at large? A striking statement may be quoted from Dr. Thomas W. Salmon's "Analysis of General Paralysis as a Public Health Problem:"

"With the information in our possession at the present time, we are able to state that not fewer than 1000 persons in whom general paralysis is recognized die in New York State every year. Let us compare this with the lives lost from some other important preventable diseases. It means that *one in nine* of the 6909 men who died between the ages of 40 and 60 in New York last year died from recognized general paralysis and that *one in thirty* of the 5299 women who died in the same age-period died from this disease.

"The number of deaths from general paralysis in New York last year about equalled the number of deaths from typhoid fever. The following table gives the number of deaths due to the ten most important specific infectious diseases. Of course, deaths in measles, typhoid fever and scarlet fever will be found also under the names of some of the complications of these diseases, but it should be remembered that these primary diseases are not invariably fatal as general paralysis is. Many of the patients with measles who died from bronchopneumonia would have recovered but for this complication, while the paretics with bronchopneumonia would have died even if this complication had not arisen. No attempt is being made to compare the *prevalence* of general paralysis with that of other diseases — we are trying only to estimate its share in the *mortality*.

" 1. Tuberculosis (all forms) 16,133
    2. Pneumonia 9,302
    3. Bronchopneumonia 7,217
    4. Diphtheria and croup 1,854
    5. Influenza 1,381
    6. Measles 1,071
    7. Typhoid Fever 1,018
       General paralysis (recognized) . . 1,000
    8. Scarlet fever   837
    9. Whooping cough   818
   10. Syphilis . . . .   782"

PARETIC NEUROSYPHILIS (GENERAL PARESIS)

CHARACTERISTICS

AMNESIA

QUICK SHIFTING EMOTIONS

CHARACTER CHANGE

CONDUCT SLUMP

NERVOUS DISORDERS

SPEECH DISORDERS

PUPILLARY CHANGES

REFLEX CHANGES

SEIZURES

CEREBROSPINAL FLUID PICTURE

CHART 11

SYPHILITIC PSYCHOSES

SYPHILITIC NEURASTHENIA

GUMMA

SYPHILITIC PSEUDOPARESIS

APOPLECTIC CEREBRAL SYPHILIS

SYPHILITIC EPILEPSY

SYPHILITIC PARANOIA

TABETIC PSYCHOSIS

HEREDITARY

PARESIS

KRAEPELIN, 1910

CHART 12

TABOPARETIC NEUROSYPHILIS (" taboparesis ") is CLINICALLY a combination of the
symptoms of TABES DORSALIS and those of
GENERAL PARESIS. The COURSE of TABO-
PARESIS is likely to be from a characteristic
tabes dorsalis (often of years' standing) to a characteristic general paresis; the ultimate paretic
picture is likely to retain various characteristics
of tabes. The LABORATORY TESTS in the
paretic phase are characteristic of ordinary (non-
tabetic) general paresis. The PROGNOSIS,
after the paretic phase has arrived, is apt to be
that of general paresis.

Case 16.   Joseph Sullivan, a waiter, 50 years of age, sought
assistance at the Psychopathic Hospital voluntarily.   His
complaint of severe and lancinating pains in the legs, difficulty
with his gait, and a feeling of constriction about the waist,
was forthwith suggestive of tabes dorsalis.   He was a rather
poorly nourished, white-haired man, with a drooping of the
left side of the face.   The pupils reacted sluggishly to light,
the right somewhat better than the left.   A marked Romberg
reaction could be demonstrated.   Ataxia in walking was
marked.   There was some incoördination of the hands, considerable tremor, and writing was poorly performed.   The
ankle-jerks and knee-jerks were absent.   On the whole,
the diagnosis of TABES DORSALIS was clear enough.
    The most appealing situation was **mental.**   Sullivan was
exceedingly apprehensive about his condition on the ground
that it was growing progressively worse; if it was to get
worse, Sullivan feared he would commit suicide.   From his
own account, he had become irritable, quick-tempered, and
often unreasonable.   As usual in these cases, the question
arose whether the depression was psychopathic or natural.
    While in the hospital things shortly came to a crisis.   In
the midst of a fit of depression, Sullivan attempted suicide

TABETIC SYMPTOMS AND SIGNS IN ORDER OF THEIR FREQUENCY

ANALYSIS OF 250 CASES

		PER CENT
1.	ROMBERG SIGN	96.4
2.	ABSENT KNEE-JERKS	90.0
3.	LANCINATING PAINS	88.4
4.	STAGGERING GAIT	87.2
5.	ARGYLL-ROBERTSON PUPIL	80.0
6.	ATAXIA IN UPPER EXTREMITIES	68.2
7.	SPHINCTER DISTURBANCES	67.6
8.	SENSORY DISTURBANCES	58.2
9.	VISUAL DISTURBANCES	43.6
10.	PARESTHESIA AND NUMBNESS OF FEET AND LOWER EXTREMITIES	42.8
11.	GIRDLE SENSE	31.2
12.	PTOSIS OF EYE-LIDS	23.2
13.	PARESTHESIA OR NUMBNESS IN HANDS OR UPPER EXTREMITIES	13.6
14.	STRABISMUS	12.0
15.	VISCERAL CRISES	12.0
16.	LOSS OF SEXUAL DESIRE	11.5
17.	CHARCOT JOINTS	9.2
18.	VERTIGO	4.0
19.	MAL PERFORANS	3.2
20.	PAIN IN JOINTS	2.8
21.	RECTAL TENESMUS	2.8
22.	MENTAL DEGENERATION (other than paresis)	2.4
23.	HEMIPLEGIA	2.4
24.	VESICAL TENESMUS	2.0
25.	DIFFICULTY IN ARTICULATION	2.0
26.	DEAFNESS	1.2
27.	ANOSMIA	0.8

BALDWIN LUCKE.

CHART 13

by beating his head against the wall. Whether this attempt could be regarded psychopathic, however, remained in question. Sullivan had been drinking very heavily although he had stopped about six weeks before admission, fearing that the alcohol was causing a development of symptoms. The remedy was almost worse than the disease because he then became more nervous, lost his appetite, and had a marked insomnia.

According to the patient's own history, he had had several attacks of gonorrhœa and a syphilitic infection at the age of 19; that is, some 31 years before admission to the hospital. However, the first *neurological* symptoms of which the patient was aware came about 27 or 28 years after infection, namely, 3 or 4 years before admission, when facial paralysis developed. At that time, he had suddenly felt a peculiar sensation in the throat and became unable to swallow for a time. His voice remained hoarse and low for some time, and his face began to droop. The lancinating pains and the ataxia also dated back several years.

1. How shall we evaluate the mental symptoms? The prognosis of tabes dorsalis is relatively good so far as life is concerned, and it might even be possible for Sullivan by training to remain capable of being a waiter. The manual incoördination was not marked, and possibly the manual tremor was in part due to alcohol. Accordingly, the mental symptoms, such as emotional lability and memory defect, were in the foreground of attention. In point of fact, the laboratory examinations showed positive W. R. in the serum and the spinal fluid, which latter also contained 60 cells per cmm., positive globulin, and an excess of albumin. THE DIAGNOSIS MADE WAS THAT OF TABOPARESIS, meaning thereby a tabes associated with appropriate symptoms of a mental nature.

2. How shall the term *taboparesis* be used? Some use the term, as we feel erroneously, for instances of general paresis which happen to show crural areflexia (absence of knee-jerks). We feel that the best usage of the term is for instances in which well-defined symptoms of tabes (as well as of paresis) are present, namely, characteristic ataxia, lightning pains, and the like. If the

term is used more loosely, as above mentioned, then practically every case of general paresis might perhaps be termed *taboparesis*, since almost every case of paresis does show involvement of the cord as well as of the cerebrum. Such involvement may lead to hyperreflexia, hyporeflexia, or areflexia according to the localization of the process. In true taboparesis, in which there is a commingling of the features of tabes with those of paresis, we should find the posterior roots of the spinal cord affected. The spinal lesions of paresis itself are more apt to be intraspinal; that is, confined to the nervous system within the pial investment.

3. Bearing in mind that Sullivan was a waiter, what shall be said about the infectivity of these cases? It is counted as a rule as negative, since there are no open spirochete-bearing lesions. The longer the period since infection the less, as a rule, is the chance of contagion in syphilis; and as tabes and paresis occur fairly late in the disease, the infectiousness at this stage is practically negligible.

4. Of what differential value is the insight shown by Sullivan into the nature of his symptoms? Kraepelin remarks that a genuine insight into the nature of the disease does not as a rule occur in paresis. At the beginning of the disease, there may sometimes be a correct understanding of the nature of the disease and of its probable outcome; but the presence or absence of insight into the fact of mental disease is by no means a differential sign of practical value.

5. What is to be said of the occurrence of depression and excited states in paretic neurosyphilis? A variety of classifications of sub-forms of paretic neurosyphilis have been propounded. Kraepelin, for example, deals with four: the demented, depressive, expansive, and agitated forms, but remarks that the division is merely convenient for exposition. The institutional intake does not accurately represent the distribution of cases. Under psychopathic hospital conditions with the relatively easy resort to such institutions, the number of quiet cases increases; under the less advanced conditions in Heidelberg, Kraepelin took in 53% demented paretics as against 56% at Munich (73% women) under the easier conditions of admission. The admissions of demented paretics varied from 37 to 56%. The variations depend much upon the facility with which the cases can be brought to institutions. Where admission

is beset with various legal restrictions, the quiet and demented cases are more apt to be treated for long periods at home. The depressive type of paretic neurosyphilis forms a much smaller group, according to Kraepelin, as only about 12% of his Heidelberg admissions were of this type, and still fewer of his Munich admissions. Other authors give percentages as high as 16 and 19. The so-called expansive group is larger, Kraepelin finding 30% of his Heidelberg cases to be of this group, and 21 to 22% of his Munich cases. The rarest sub-form of paretic neurosyphilis is the agitated form: 6% of Kraepelin's Heidelberg admissions; 14% among males and 5% among females in his Munich admissions, where the diagnosis of agitated paresis was entered on somewhat broader lines. French authors (Sérieux and Ducaste) have enlarged the number of sub-forms of paretic neurosyphilis as follows: Expansive 27%; sensory 24%; demented 24%; persecutory 3%; depressive 2%; circular 7%; hypochondriacal 7%; and maniacal 6%.

DIFFUSE (meningovasculoparenchymatous) NEU-
ROSYPHILIS may look precisely like PARETIC
NEUROSYPHILIS ("general paresis") at certain
periods of clinical and laboratory examination.

Case 17. The police found Gregorian Petrofski crouching
on his knees on a Boston sidewalk, attempting to take
pickets off a fence. Petrofski knew little English; he said
that he had slept in Poland the night before. He did not
appear to be alcoholic.

When he was examined, through an interpreter, he told
how he had been in America two days, and in Boston two
years; that he was at the present time in Poland, and that
his brother had brought him to the hospital and left him
there.

The **physical examination** showed Petrofski to be well
developed and nourished. His pupils were somewhat dilated
and reacted somewhat slowly to light and accommodation.
Neurologically, there was nothing else abnormal found upon
systematic examination although, through lack of coöperation,
sensory and coördination tests proved difficult if not impossible. There was a large ulcer on the under surface of the
glans penis, with several small smooth scars on the upper
surface. There was a purulent discharge from the external
meatus. There were exostoses of both tibiæ.

The initial diagnosis had to consider uremia and diabetes,
which could be easily excluded on examination. Alcoholism
was excluded through absence of alcohol on the breath.
There remained such diagnoses as epilepsy, some post-traumatic condition, or meningitis, to say nothing of the hypothesis of syphilis raised by the tibial exostoses and the lesions
of the penis. The hypothesis of trauma was given up, as
well as epilepsy and meningitis upon the data of the lumbar
puncture. The spinal fluid proved to be clear but with
enormous amounts of globulin and albumin, 80 cells per cmm.,
a "paretic" gold sol reaction, and a positive spinal fluid

W. R. (the serum W. R. was also positive). Accordingly, it was clear that the case was one of neurosyphilis.

Treatment was instituted with injections of mercury salicylate, a grain and a half twice a week, and potassium iodid. After some weeks, diarrhœa and salivation with marked symptoms of mercury poisoning set in; the treatment was suspended, but later re-instituted. In a few weeks Petrofski was apparently quite well, the spinal fluid tests had all become negative, as had the serum W. R.

Petrofski now began to pick up a good deal of English, and gave a consistent narrative of his past life, although the period just prior to and during his early stay in the hospital has remained blank. Without further treatment Petrofski has remained well for over a year.

1. Does the " paretic " gold sol reaction mean general paresis? In connection with this general question, a brief summary of the significance of the gold sol reaction in this group may be made. (1) Fluids from cases of general paresis in the vast majority of cases will give a strong and fairly characteristic reaction, especially if more than one sample is tested. (2) Very rarely general paresis fluid will give a reaction weaker than the characteristic one. (3) Fluids from cases of syphilitic involvement of the central nervous system other than general paresis often give a weaker reaction than the paretic, but in a fairly high percentage of cases give the same reaction as the paretics. (4) Non-syphilitic cases may give the same reaction as the paretics; these cases are usually chronic inflammatory conditions of the central nervous system. (5) When a syphilitic fluid does not give the strong " paretic reaction " it is presumptive evidence that the case is not general paresis, and this test offers a very valuable differential diagnostic aid between general paresis, tabes, and cerebrospinal syphilis. (6) The term " syphilitic zone " is a misnomer, as non-syphilitic as well as syphilitic cases give reactions in this zone, but no fluid of a case with syphilitic central nervous system disease has given a reaction out of this zone, so that the finding may be used negatively; and any fluid giving a reaction outside of this zone may be considered non-syphilitic. (7) Mild reactions may occur without any evident significance,

FREQUENT SYMPTOMS IN DIFFUSE AND VASCULAR NEUROSYPHILIS

("CEREBRAL" AND "CEREBROSPINAL SYPHILIS")

PUPILLARY DISORDER

HEADACHE

VERTIGO

INSOMNIA

DROWSINESS

CHANGE IN DISPOSITION
    Irritability   Slow thinking

SEIZURES

PARALYSES
    Permanent   Transient

APHASIA

HEMIANOPSIA

SENSORY DISTURBANCES

GASTRIC CRISES

SPHINCTER DISTURBANCES

INTRACRANIAL PRESSURE SYMPTOMS

POLYURIA, POLYDYPSIA, GLYCOSURIA

MENIERE'S SYNDROME

NYSTAGMUS

CHART 14

while a reaction of no greater strength may mean marked inflammatory reaction. (8) Tuberculous meningitis, brain tumor, and purulent meningitis fluids characteristically, though not invariably, give reactions in higher dilutions than syphilitic fluids. (9) The unsupplemented gold sol test is insufficient evidence on which to make any diagnosis, but used in conjunction with the W. R., chemical and cytological examinations, it offers much information, aiding in the differential diagnosis of general paresis, cerebrospinal syphilis, tabes dorsalis, brain tumor, tuberculous meningitis, and purulent meningitis. (10) We believe that no cerebrospinal fluid examination is complete for clinical purposes without the gold sol test.

See Appendix B for technical details.

2. What is the relation of the tibial exostosis to neurosyphilis? The syphilographers have always stressed the tibial lesions in the diagnosis of syphilis. Although not so much attention has been paid to these and kindred osseous lesions in neurosyphilis, yet we have frequently found such lesions and they afford an important auxiliary means of diagnosis.

> A POSITIVE SERUM Wassermann reaction with
> a NEGATIVE FLUID Wassermann Reaction may
> be found in NEUROSYPHILIS, particularly in
> VASCULAR NEUROSYPHILIS: the remaining
> signs in the fluid, although frequently positive, may
> even be negative.

Case 18. Frederick Wescott was a promoter, an elderly looking man of 60 years. His health had been failing for 18 months. There had been shortness of breath, dizziness, a tired feeling, inability to " get the words he wanted," and forgetfulness of names. About eight weeks before examination, Wescott had had a convulsion, following which he had been unable to express himself at all well. This convulsion was not accompanied by loss of consciousness. Besides a marked motor aphasia, there was agraphia.

Physically, Wescott showed arteriosclerosis and a blood pressure of 135 systolic, but, except very lively knee-jerks, no other reflex disorders or anomalies were discovered. In particular, the pupils reacted fairly well.

There was, perhaps, no special reason to implicate syphilis in the case, yet Wescott gave a history of syphilis at 35 years. The W. R. of the blood serum proved positive; that of the spinal fluid was negative, and the albumin was but slightly increased; there was a very slight amount of globulin, and there were 16 cells per cmm. in the fluid. The gold sol reaction suggested syphilis.

We felt entitled to make a diagnosis of SYPHILITIC CEREBRAL ARTERIOSCLEROSIS, regarding the convulsion or seizure eight weeks before as due to a vascular insult. The laboratory picture in the spinal fluid in Wescott's case seems to be rather characteristic of this group of syphilitic arteriosclerotics.

1. What is the reason for the negative spinal fluid W. R.? The theory would be that the syphilitic lesion is localized in the vascular system and that the parenchyma

is only secondarily, if at all, involved. The W. R. producing bodies are accordingly not found in the fluid.

2. How frequently are several of the spinal fluid tests negative, while others are positive? Whereas, clinically speaking, the five tests in the spinal fluid (W. R., globulin reaction, excess albumin, pleocytosis, and gold sol reaction) are each indicative of a pathological condition in the central nervous system, yet a specially intensive study of the distribution of these tests has shown that they are prone to occur independently. Consequently, we must concede that they do not all represent the same inflammatory products and chemical conditions. The W. R. producing bodies, the gold sol reaction producing bodies, as well as the globulins and albumins, have been proved to be separate. Special work has also shown that *these tests disappear under treatment at different rates*. There is, unfortunately, no doubt that the rate and intensity, presence or absence, and the order of disappearance of these tests in either treated or untreated cases, do not at all parallel the clinical conditions of the patients.

3. What is the prognosis in vascular neurosyphilis, such as in the case of Wescott? The prognosis is identical with that of cerebral arteriosclerosis in general, that is to say, bad, but with frequent periods of improvement. In the neurosyphilitic type of arterial disease thromboid formation is frequent. Where the lesion is chiefly pervascular infiltration, rather than disintegration of the vessel wall, improvement may very well occur as a result of treatment. Wescott showed slight improvement under treatment. He has already lived two years since his first convulsion, and three and a half years since the onset of symptoms

---

DIFFUSE NEUROSYPHILIS (so-called "cerebrospinal syphilis ") is often marked by **SEIZURES.**

Case 19. Agnes O'Neil, an unmarried woman of 28 years, was first examined five weeks after the initial symptoms. It appears that she had had certain seizures, with unconsciousness and twitching of the limbs (otherwise not well described), followed by confusion of mind and sometimes by a weakness of the left side and a difficulty in speaking. Headache had been almost constant, as well as pains in the arms and legs.

Physically, both in general and **neurologically,** there were no signs or symptoms; mentally, we could discover no symptoms. Syphilis was denied, although possible exposure to syphilis was admitted.

The **diagnosis** of some form of organic brain disease was clear with the picture of convulsions followed by slight aphasia with headaches and limb pains. With onset at 28, the most frequent cause for such epileptiform seizures is certainly syphilis. Examination of the blood and spinal fluid showed a positive W. R., in both. The albumin was also somewhat increased. The clinical picture suggested a fairly generalized meningitic involvement.

The **prognosis** in such cases of generalized meningitic involvement is in general good, and this principle was illustrated in the O'Neil case, in which the symptoms soon disappeared under intensive antisyphilitic treatment. In fact the spinal fluid W. R. became negative in the course of four weeks. The blood serum W. R., however, has remained positive despite eight months of active treatment.

1. Are certain cases of syphilitic epilepsy really cases of Jacksonian epilepsy? As a matter of nomenclature, Jacksonian cortical epilepsy is usually the result of a focal and circumscribed irritative lesion in the cortex. Gumma, local syphilitic meningitis, and syphilitic vascular lesions, as well as scars consequent upon the latter, are among the causes of Jacksonian epilepsy,

CONDITIONS IN WHICH CONVULSIONS OCCUR

NEUROSYPHILIS

HYSTERIA

EPILEPSY MAJOR (GRAND MAL)

EPILEPSY MINOR (PETIT MAL)

DEMENTIA PRAECOX

TOXIC CONDITIONS:
   Asphyxia, Uremia, Alcohol, Absinthe, Lead, Mercury, etc.

ORGANIC BRAIN LESIONS
   Apoplexy, Meningitis, Intracranial Growths

STOKES-ADAMS DISEASE

MALINGERING

DISSEMINATED SCLEROSIS

CHART 15

along with such other focal lesions as trauma, tumor abscess, tubercle, and the like. Even non-syphilitic Jacksonian epilepsy has been observed from time to time in cases of diffuse intracranial pressure. Jacksonian attacks also have been found in so-called genuine epilepsy. Accordingly, we must not conclude from the occurrence of Jacksonian convulsions, even though in a proved syphilitic case, that the convulsions in question are surely due to a focal lesion, for they may be due to diffuse syphilitic lesions.

2. What is the significance of aphasia in Agnes O'Neil? Aphasia is not a characteristic symptom in ordinary Jacksonian epilepsy, but the aphasia is another sign of focal lesion and forms an added argument against the diagnosis of genuine or idiopathic epilepsy. See also discussion of aphasia in paretic neurosyphilis under Case Levenson (22).

2. What is the behavior of the serum W. R. and the spinal fluid W. R. under systematic treatment? Sometimes, as in this case, the serum W. R. remains positive and the fluid W. R. becomes negative; but in other equally well-defined cases, the reverse holds true, and the serum W. R. reaction becomes negative whereas the spinal fluid reaction remains positive. The obvious conclusion is that we cannot always be sure even by faithful tests of either the serum or the fluid alone, whether the treatment has succeeded in abolishing the laboratory signs.

4. Can this case be regarded as one of cure? Not by the definition adopted in this book or by the syphilographers who take into account not only the nervous system but the body which contains it. To be sure, the spinal fluid of Agnes O'Neil is now entirely negative and she is clinically free from symptoms; yet from the broad standpoint of syphilis therapy in general, this patient is not cured, as is evidenced by the positive serum W. R.

PARETIC NEUROSYPHILIS ("general paresis ") is often marked by SEIZURES.

Case 20. Lester Crane, a plumber, 37 years of age, came to the hospital with a slow and defective speech. Moreover, there seemed to be some mental disorder since his answers to questions were not always relevant. It appeared that he was seeing bugs on the wall.

Physically, Crane was a well-developed and nourished man, with overactive knee-jerks and a Babinski reaction on the left side.

It developed that there was an impairment in hearing. The pupils reacted well both to light and to distance. The patient was very restless and smiled in a silly fashion. His memory was decidedly defective in all spheres, and he was very slow in the intake of ideas.

The plumber's wife said that, at about the age of 23 or 24, he had a spell of confusion lasting two or three days, with peculiar conduct, unintelligible talk, and a good deal of weeping. The medical diagnosis at that time took into account the fact that Crane was a plumber and was " lead encephalopathy."

However, according to his wife, Crane had acquired chancre at about 26 years, was treated mercurially for about three years and declared well. He had remained well up to about 18 months before entrance, when, without previous warning, the patient had a convulsion with the continuous movements for about half an hour. He was semi-conscious for about 18 hours and vomited continuously. There was amnesia for the whole affair on regaining consciousness. In a week's time, Crane was entirely well. But six weeks later there was another convulsion. Upon removal to a hospital, the diagnosis of general paresis was made, and the patient was given the Swift-Ellis intraspinous treatment. This seemed to be very successful, and the patient discontinued treatment after 14 weeks (during which time there had been seven treatments) on the ground that he was entirely well.

However, after discontinuing treatment, there was another convulsion in about a month, and further convulsions occurred once a month. For six months, however, the patient took no treatment, but finally returned to the hospital and was given mercury. This treatment appeared to suspend convulsions again for three months, but at the expiration of six months, the patient had three convulsions in one day, and several more during the following days. After the last of these convulsions, there had been numbness on the right side of the body and considerable headache.

The diagnosis of PARETIC NEUROSYPHILIS ("general paresis") is borne out by the laboratory tests. The W. R. of the blood serum was, to be sure, negative, but the W. R. of the spinal fluid was positive, and there was a "paretic" type of gold reaction, together with other laboratory signs.

The case well demonstrates that group of paretic cases in which convulsions periodically occur, leaving the patient worse after each convulsion. Treatment with salvarsan was instituted, and mercury and iodid was given by mouth. During the period of eight months which have now elapsed since the beginning of this treatment, there have been no convulsions; there has been a great improvement in the memory, the hearing has improved, the W. R. in the spinal fluid is much less intense, the gold sol test has become negative, and the other tests are all less intense.

The patient, however, has not been entirely well, for in place of the generalized convulsions, he has had minor seizures, beginning as a rule with a tingling sensation in the right hand, extending up the arm, down the trunk and leg, and through the right side of the face, with a bitter sensation on the right half of the tongue. The patient maintains that this sensation is absolutely confined to the right half of the body (in this connection we may recall case Morton (1), in which there was also a hemiplegia together with other apparently hysterical symptoms at several times during the long course of a disease with abundant structural correlations). During these minor seizures, the patient is unable

LOSS OF DEEP REFLEXES

NEUROSYPHILIS

NEURITIS
  (alcohol, diabetes, diphtheria, lead, arsenic, tubercle, cachexia, etc.)
    Peripheral nerves sensory or motor

PERIPHERAL NERVE PALSIES

TEMPORARILY FROM COMPRESSION BY TURNIQUET

FRIEDREICH'S ATAXIA

SUBACUTE COMBINED DEGENERATION OF POSTERIOR
  AND LATERAL COLUMNS
    Posterior column disease

FOCAL LESION IN GRAY MATTER OF CORD

INFANTILE PARALYSIS (ACUTE ANTERIOR POLIOMYELITIS)

PROGRESSIVE MUSCULAR ATROPHY
  (chronic anterior poliomyelitis)
    Anterior cornua of cord

AMYOTROPHIC LATERAL SCLEROSIS

SYRINGOMYELIA

THROMBOSIS OF ANTERIOR SPINAL ARTERY

LANDRY'S PARALYSIS
    Anterior cornua and peripheral motor nerves

MYOPATHIES
  (pseudohypertrophic and atrophic types)
    Muscle itself

AMYOTONIA CONGENITA

FAMILY PERIODIC PARALYSIS
  (during attacks)

INCREASED INTRACRANIAL PRESSURE
  (especially hydrocephalus and tumors of posterior fossa)

PNEUMONIA

IMMEDIATELY AFTER ATTACK OF MAJOR EPILEPSY
  (post-epileptic coma)

TOXIC COMA
  (uremia, morphine, etc.)

DURING SPINAL ANESTHESIA

COMPLETE TRANSVERSE LESION OF CORD

PURVES STUART

CHART 16

to talk, although he does not lose consciousness and is entirely aware of everything going on about him. These attacks have of late been growing somewhat less frequent.

1. What is the cause of the negative serum W. R.? It is claimed that 3 to 5% of all cases of general paresis yield a negative blood serum. In this particular case, there had been considerable treatment, including some Swift-Ellis treatment, so that it may be that this treatment had reduced a formerly positive blood serum W. R. to a negative one.

2. What is the nature of the typical seizures of general paresis? The most frequent seizures are epileptiform and bear a general resemblance to cortical epilepsy; but more rarely these seizures resemble the ordinary epileptic attack or consist of a violent general shaking of the whole body. A variety of initial minor disorders usher in the attacks: the temperature is often increased. The attacks are over after one or at most after a few hours. Kraepelin speaks of one that lasted 14 days. Sometimes a *status paralyticus* develops, suggestive of the *status epilepticus*. Another rarer form of characteristic seizure is the apoplectiform, which can hardly be told from an ordinary stroke, and may be followed by the usual post-apoplectic phenomena. A good many of the strokes leading to sudden death in middle life are probably cases of neurosyphilis although often set down as early arteriosclerosis of a non-syphilitic nature. Besides the epileptiform and apoplectiform seizures, there are certain seizures of a less definite and complete nature, ranging from simple fainting spells, dizzy spells and petit mal attacks, to various special forms of irritative muscular contractions and temporary speech disorders. Sometimes these attacks occur with complete preservation of consciousness. Transient paresthesias, visual field defects, and especially attacks of vomiting, which, according to Kraepelin, may precede paresis by years (of course in this connection gastric crises of tabes must be thought of), may be counted as sensory seizures.

3. What is the proportion of paretic cases developing seizures? Figures vary from 30 to 90%. According to Kraepelin, seizures occurred in 30 to 40% of his cases at Heidelberg; he was of the impression that treatment in bed had reduced the number of seizures. 65% of

paretics admitted to Munich (under very free conditions of admission) were determined to have shown seizures before their admission to the hospital. Seizures are said to be somewhat more frequent in men than in women. These paretic seizures are not due to either hemorrhages or vascular plugging — at least in the vast majority of cases — and must be ascribed to the effects of microscopic injuries.

4. What is the effect of seizures upon the future course of paretic neurosyphilis? The current idea as expressed, for example, by Mercier, is that " immediately after each crisis the patient is much worse than he was before it, and thereafter there is some improvement, but he never improves up to the point at which he was before the occurrence of the crisis." That is, " The course of the disease is one of sudden plunges, each deeper than the last, each followed by a gradual recovery that is less complete than the recovery from the previous plunge."

5. During what period of the disease are seizures most common? Late in the disease many cases have convulsions, even though there were none for the first year or two. In other cases the convulsion is the first indication of paresis.

DIFFUSE (non-paretic) NEUROSYPHILIS (" cerebrospinal syphilis ") is often marked by APHASIA.

Case 21. Martha Bartlett, a woman of 40 years, was brought to the Psychopathic Hospital aphasic, or at least unable to talk distinctly enough to be understood, or even to give name and address. The police had found her wandering aimlessly about the streets. Although she was well-dressed, she was mud-bespattered and apparently had not changed her garments for several days. It shortly developed that the patient, although unable to express herself either in words or by writing, could understand everything that was said to her and could indicate by the monosyllables *yes* or *no* whether she agreed or disagreed with statements made. It was thus determined that she was pretty well oriented. She was able to understand both speech and printed words. Although she approximated more than is at all common a pure type of *motor aphasia*, it appeared that there was a slight involvement on the sensory side, especially in the sphere of visual imagery.

Neurologically, the patient showed moderate strabismus, slight deviation of the tongue to the right, and considerable tremor on protrusion of the tongue. The right side of the palate hung lower than the left. The ankle and arm reflexes were possibly more active on the left side, and the left grasp was somewhat better than the right. Both knee-jerks were active, but again the reflex on the left side was more active than the right. No other abnormalities of reflex were determined. There was no Rombergism but the gait was somewhat ataxic. For the rest, the physical examination was normal. The blood pressure was 120 systolic, 85 diastolic.

The ready suspicion was that the case was one of apoplexy of slight degree with post-apoplectic phenomena. Upon investigation, this suspicion was confirmed since it appeared that Mrs. B. had been apparently quite well until about six months before admission, when without particular warning

CONDITIONS IN WHICH SPEECH DEFECT IS FOUND

NEUROSYPHILIS

HYPOGLOSSAL PARALYSIS

FACIAL PALSY

PARALYSIS OF PALATE (Post Diphtheritic)

BULBAR PALSY

PSEUDOBULBAR PALSY

MYOPATHY—FACIO–SCAPULO–HUMERAL TYPE OF LAN-
DOUZY AND DEJERINE

MYASTHENIA GRAVIS

FRIEDREICH'S ATAXIA

LARYNGEAL TABES

ALCOHOLIC INTOXICATION

POST HEMIPLEGIC

LENTICULAR DISEASE

BILATERAL ATHETOSIS

MULTIPLE SCLEROSIS

DEAF MUTISM

PARALYSIS AGITANS

CHOREA

STAMMERING

TICS

HYSTERICAL APHONIA

CHART 17

she began to act strangely and promptly fell into a series of convulsions. These convulsions would begin with twitchings of the face, and then spread throughout the body. There would be a period of unconsciousness for two or three hours. It is not certain how many of these convulsive seizures the patient had. At all events she is reported to have recovered therefrom completely, remaining well for three months; whereupon, suddenly, while visiting a friend, she suffered a paralysis of the left side of the body. She remained dazed and had hospital treatment for about a week. Ever since this left-sided paralysis, the aphasic condition above described has persisted.

Such a phenomenon has often been dismissed in the past as due to an early arteriosclerosis, but most neurologists and internists of today would look beyond the diagnosis of mere arteriosclerosis and consider syphilis. The only suggestive feature in the case, aside from the post-apoplectic reflex disorder and spastic phenomena, is the irregularity and diminished light reaction of the pupils. Our suspicions were confirmed by the positive serum W. R. The W. R. of the spinal fluid proved, however, to be negative. There was a moderately strong gold sol reaction of the syphilitic type. There was a slight excess of albumin, and there was an exceedingly slight amount of globulin. There was but one cell per cmm.

On the whole, it would seem best to consider the case of Mrs. Bartlett to be one of CEREBRAL ARTERIOSCLEROSIS OF SYPHILITIC ORIGIN, and a case in which there is no evidence of meningitis or meningo-encephalitis.

1. What is the explanation of the negative spinal fluid W. R.? It may be that none of the W. R. producing bodies have gone over into the spinal fluid. It has been shown by the work of Weston that the W. R. producing body is not identical with the bodies responsible for the other tests in cerebrospinal syphilis. Moreover, it has been clearly shown that these several tests of the spinal fluid do not run at all parallel with one another. Especially is it true that the chemical tests do not correspond at all with the degree or nature of the pleocytosis. On the whole, when involvement of the nervous

system is entirely vascular, it is not only theoretically proper but also practically common, to find a spinal fluid negative to several tests.

2. Omitting consideration of the syphilitic gold sol of this case, what conclusion could be drawn from the albumin and globulin findings? It would not be warrantable to assume syphilis since it is a common finding after cerebral hemorrhage due to non-syphilitic arteriosclerosis to find excess albumin and also globulin in the spinal fluid. Occasionally, also, pleocytosis occurs in cases of cerebral hemorrhage even when the hypothesis of an active meningitis can be excluded. We may recall in this connection the pleocytosis in so-called meningitis sympathica of certain brain tumors. (See also the case of Milton Safsky (48), a case of brain tumor in which there was an excess of albumin, a large quantity of globulin, and a pleocytosis of 146 cells per cmm.)

3. What can be expected from treatment in these cases of vascular cerebral syphilis? The condition offers very little opportunity for therapeutic results. However, antisyphilitic therapy is indicated to prevent if possible further progress of the lesions. Since the lesions are, however, vascular, and since it must remain a question how far these vascular lesions are due directly to spirochetal action, and since in any event it may be difficult to reach the spirochetes thus active, perhaps it is best to place most reliance on potassium iodid. In any event, potassium iodid should be given. Salvarsan and mercury are also indicated. It is common to warn against administration of large doses of salvarsan in this type of case on the ground that further vascular ruptures may be produced. (See Friedberg, 108.)

4. If we conclude that the aphasia of the Bartlett case is due to vascular disease, can we conclude a relation between this vascular disease and vascular tension? It is not safe to draw such a conclusion. The Bartlett case itself showed low blood pressure. To be sure, some cases of neurosyphilis show high blood pressure from which one draws the à la mode clinical conclusion to the effect that the kidneys are probably involved in the arteriosclerosis; but other cases do not show a high blood pressure but may in fact show a low blood pressure. The vascular disease doubtless responsible for the aphasia in the Bartlett case is probably not at all an effect of blood pressure conditions, but is, on the contrary, an effect of local syphilitic vascular lesions.

**PARETIC NEUROSYPHILIS (" general paresis ")
is often marked by APHASIA.**

Case 22. Meyer Levenson, a traveling salesman of 36 years, had for the last two or three years been undergoing a change of disposition, quite interfering with his work. He had begun to take unreasonable aversions to people, had become irritable and emotionally depressed, and often fell to weeping without cause.

About nine months before hospital observation, it seems that a trunk-cover had fallen on Levenson's head, and there is some question as to whether he did not have a convulsion at that time. However, a month later he had a definite seizure, followed by speech disorder, a slight paralysis, and a staggering gait. Four weeks later, however, he had gotten over these post-convulsive difficulties and had gone back to work.

At his work, he became tired easily, his gait and speech did not seem entirely normal, and there was a considerable memory disorder. After five more months, another attack of a convulsive nature, with twitching of hands and face and tongue-biting occurred, and the attending unconsciousness remained for two days. Again improvement followed, though without ability to return to work. Four (?) months later there were several severe convulsions and Levenson would remain unconscious for a day or two at a time. Restlessness, irritability, and irrational talking followed.

Physically, the patient was fairly well developed and nourished; blood pressure 168 systolic, 68 diastolic; pupils reacted very sluggishly to light. There was a marked motor aphasia, which the patient recognized as a speech difficulty. On the whole, however, Levenson was very euphoric and was entirely sure that he was improving and would surely get well.

Shortly after entrance, Levenson had a severe convulsion, with unconsciousness. The movements were mainly on the right side of the body, and there was a post-convulsive weakness of the right side for several days, followed by a slow recovery of strength.

The course of the disease — convulsions followed by improvement — is very characteristic of a paretic onset. The **laboratory findings** were in all respects confirmatory. It was rather striking that a permanent *motor aphasia* followed the convulsions in this case, since the seizures of paresis do not in the vast majority of cases leave permanent paralyses. The course of the disease continued to show convulsions, which would in each instance leave him at a lower terrace of capacity than had been before shown. The patient died four years after the onset of symptoms of a general asthenia. With the exception of the permanent motor aphasia, this case might be regarded as a fairly typical one of general paresis.

1.   What is the general nature of speech disorder in paretic neurosyphilis? Speech disorder is, along with the pupillary changes, one of the most important clinical symptoms in paretic neurosyphilis.   There are aphasic and articulatory disturbances.   The aphasia that accompanies paretic seizures is of a transient nature as a rule.   A case with such long-standing motor aphasia as shown by Levenson is not common.   Paraphasia, with incorrect naming of objects, may last longer.   The so-called " sticking " phenomenon is often observed.

Word deafness is said to be rarer but is difficult to test on account of the patient's dementia.   Agrammatism (incapacity to form correct sentences) is sometimes observed.   But the most characteristic disorder is in the syllabic composition of words.   Syllables are left out (" medaltricity " for medical electricity), or fused (" exity "), or doubled (" electricicity ").   Besides the central speech disorders of which the above are examples, there are disorders in articulation, which at first occur as a consequence of paretic seizures or in states of excitement, but later become permanent. These are divided into paretic and ataxic disturbances.

2.   What is the structural basis of these forms of aphasia? It is believed that they are due to microscopic changes, not to coarse destructive lesions.

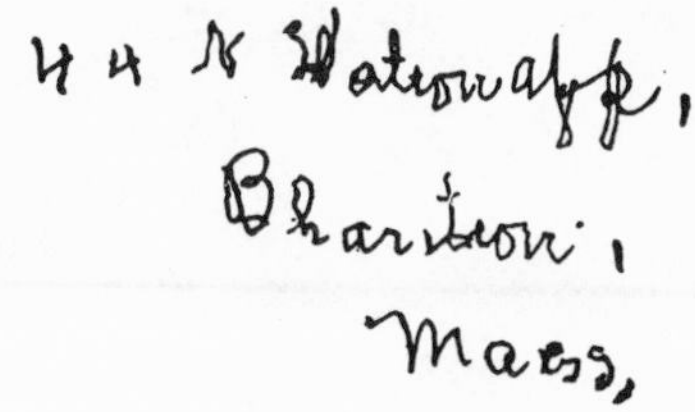

[handwritten] [BROOKLINE,

MASS.]

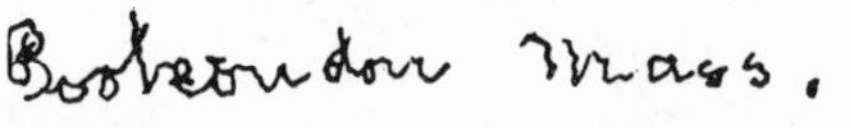

[handwritten] [BROOKLINE, MASS.]

Mss. of Levenson, case 22. Paretic neurosyphilis. Tremor, misspelling.
Metathesis of letters (Bk, not Br) omission of letters (Book).

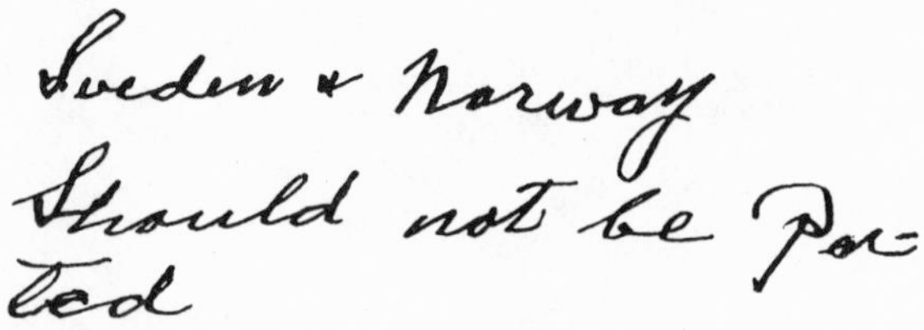

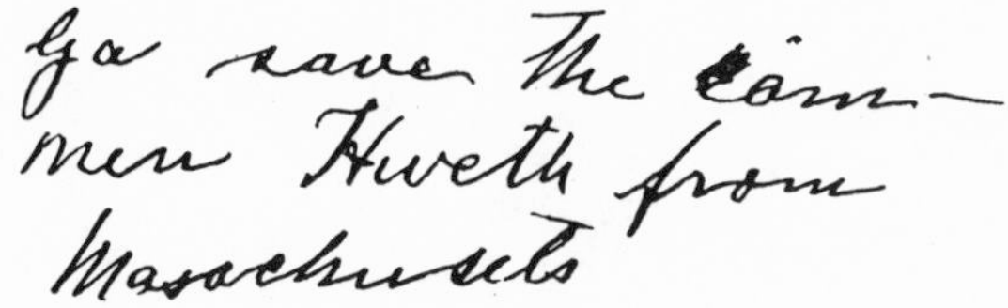

Λ

[handwritten]

[handwritten] [God save the Commonwealth

of Massachusetts]

Mss. of Safsky, case 48, brain tumor. Tremor not marked. Misspelling, omission
of letters. Wrong letters (h in hweth).

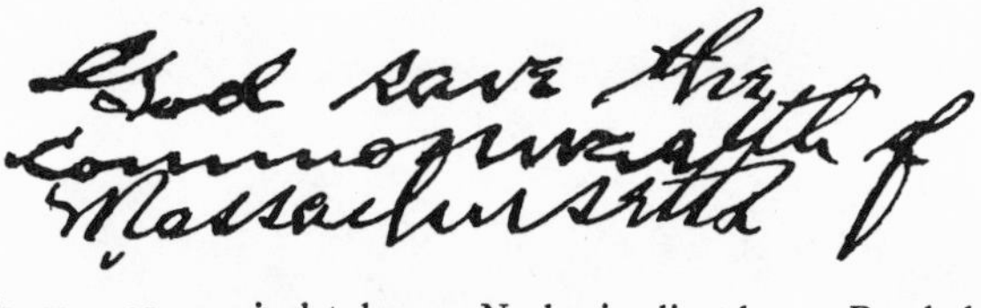

[handwritten]

Mss. of Halleck, case 31, cervical tabes. No brain disorder. Pen-holding and bearing-
on difficulties. Crowding of phrases result of ataxia.

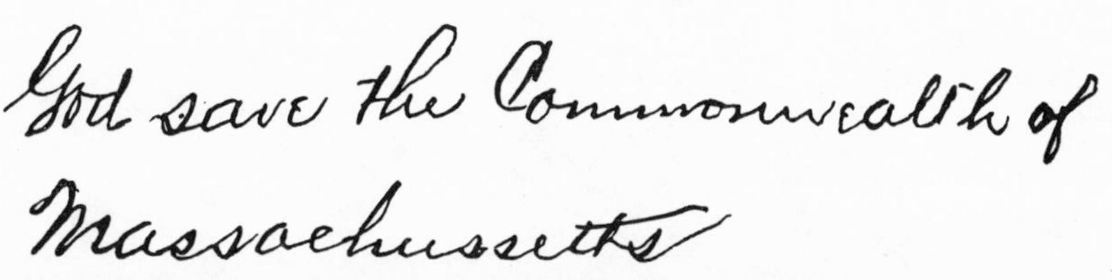

[handwritten]

Mss. of Collins, case 61, paretic neurosyphilis. One misspelling (-chussetts); not psychopathic? Characteristic tremor.

REMISSIONS of identical appearance occur in PARETIC and in DIFFUSE (non-paretic meningo-vascular) NEUROSYPHILIS.

Case 23. Thomas Donovan, a merchant 44 years of age, acquired syphilis according to his own story at the age of 31, and he was at that time treated at a well-known watering-place with mercurial injections. Later he continued treatment under his family physician, and at 34 was pronounced cured. However, four years later — that is seven years after his initial infection and in his 38th year — he had his blood examined and it proved positive. He was accordingly treated by salvarsan and his W. R. became negative. The story did not end there, however, for at 43, mental symptoms appeared of the nature of depression and a diagnosis of paresis was made. He was released from the institution against advice at that time, and without treatment, made a partial recovery.

A sudden outburst of violence brought Mr. Donovan to the Psychopathic Hospital; he was very surly, combative, and difficult to manage, standing 6' 2", and weighing 210 pounds. He was oriented only fairly well and his surliness was streaked with humor. He facetiously said that the Psychopathic Hospital was the largest hospital in the country, and that it was, in fact, a horse hospital; that he had come because he liked the surroundings, not to make money; that he was the healthiest man in the world, never having been sick; that the Psychopathic Hospital was a club, for which you have to get somebody to propose your name. There was amnesia and no knowledge of current events. He regarded the food as poisoned, refused to eat, and was very irritable and untidy.

Physically, there were few abnormalities, but the pupils failed to react either to light or accommodation, and the knee-jerks and ankle-jerks were absent. There was a slight Rombergism. There was a marked speech defect to test

ATAXIA OR INCOÖRDINATION

NEUROSYPHILIS

LESION OF PERIPHERAL SENSORY NERVES

DIVISION OF POSTERIOR ROOTS

TUMORS OR CHRONIC SCLEROSIS OF POSTERIOR COL-
UMNS

SUBACUTE COMBINED DEGENERATION

VESTIBULAR ATAXIA

FRIEDREICH'S ATAXIA

FAMILY PROGRESSIVE HYPERTROPHIC NEURITIS

THROMBOSIS POSTERIOR INFERIOR CEREBELLAR ARTERY

MARIE'S HEREDITARY CEREBELLAR ATAXIA

LESIONS OF CEREBELLUM, TUMORS, ETC.

WRITERS' CRAMP

PREHEMIPLEGIA

MULTIPLE SCLEROSIS

PSEUDO-SCLEROSIS

HYSTERIA

CHART 18

CONDITIONS IN WHICH VERTIGO IS FOUND

NEUROSYPHILIS

HEAD TRAUMA

CEREBRAL ANEMIA AND HYPEREMIA

MENOPAUSE

ARTERIOSCLEROSIS

RENAL DISEASE

CEREBRAL HEMORRHAGE AND THROMBOSIS

INTRACRANIAL TUMORS

MULTIPLE SCLEROSIS

EPILEPSY (Aura)

TOXIC CONDITIONS:
    alcohol, tobacco, constipation

PSYCHONEUROSIS

OCULAR DISTURBANCES

EAR DISEASE

MÉNIÈRE'S DISEASE

MIGRAINE

CHART 19

phrases.   Both serum and spinal fluid W. R.'s were positive; the fluid showed 41 cells per cmm., there were large amounts of globulin and albumin, and the gold sol reaction was of the " paretic " type.

Salvarsanized serum was injected intraventricularly through a trephine opening in the right frontal region.   Injections were made through the corpus callosum into the third ventricle.   There was progressive symptomatic improvement after each of four injections.   In fact, after the fourth injection the patient was allowed to leave the hospital despite the fact that there was only a slight improvement in the spinal fluid findings.   The speech defect had entirely disappeared.   (Speech defect, according to many authorities, including Kraepelin, is of very grave diagnostic significance.) His memory returned.   Mr. Donovan is now able to handle figures rather extraordinarily well.   He now has a good insight into his delusions and tells stories about them with great humor.

1.   What is the definition of a remission in general paresis? Remissions form a foil to seizures; just as seizures mark a sudden advance in the severity of the disease or may even lead to death; so remissions may cause a sudden cessation of both mental and nervous phenomena in the disease.   Whereas the seizures occur most often, according to Kraepelin, in the demented types of paresis, the remissions occur in all cases except in the terminal phase.   Kraepelin quotes Hoppe as observing pronounced remissions of long duration in 17% of male and 15% of female paretics.   Gaupp observed marked improvement in less than 10%, and very marked improvement indeed in only 1% of his cases.   Kraepelin states that such improvements are most frequent in agitated and especially in expansive forms of paresis, and that they are rarer and less complete in the depressive and demented forms.   Sometimes the improvement occurs over night, although the full extent of the remission becomes complete only gradually, perhaps in the course of months.   The sensorium clears, the disorientation disappears, the delusions retreat, and the former delusions are treated as dreams and imaginations.   There is often a good deal of persistent uncertainty as to events during the height of the disease.

The nervous disorders are far more obstinate than the mental. Still, both speech and writing may often greatly improve.

Cotton in New Jersey found, among 127 cases of paresis diagnosticated by modern methods during seven years, that remissions occurred in but five, or about 4%, lasting from a half to three years.

2. Does a remission ever amount to a cure? The classical case quoted in this connection is one observed by Tuczek. This case developed a picture of paresis in 1876, at the age of 36; and a remission, or cessation, of symptoms, occurred in 1878; but in 1883, at 43 years, the patient developed a tabes without any trace of mental disorder, which tabes gradually advanced. By the middle of 1898, when the patient was 58, certain symptoms of excitement and confusion occurred, which led to death with dementia, 22 years after the beginning of the disease. Nissl pronounced the cortex to be undoubtedly the characteristic cortex of a paretic. This observation seems to indicate that a clinical remission tantamount to a clinical recovery may occur without the death of the spirochetes engaged. This observation is to be held in mind in connection with all therapeutic work with neurosyphilis.

Nonne states that during his clinical experience of 19 years he had followed 10 cases of paresis with apparent recovery; but of these ten cases, four had to be thrown out by Nonne because the apparent recoveries turned out to be only long and almost complete remissions, finally issuing in characteristic dementia. Of the remaining six cases, perhaps two should hardly be counted as paretic and Nonne rather preferred to term them cases of syphilitic dementia in the sense of a non-paretic cerebral syphilis. At the end, therefore, of his review of observations, Nonne found himself with four cases of true recovery from paresis.

Spielmeyer holds that there is no theoretical reason why paresis might not be cured, since all the different changes that have been described in the disease can be halted, and many of them can be repaired. In particular, he reminds us that the acute infiltrative process, the neuroglia reaction, and the phagocytic action of the large mononuclear cells are distinctly removable processes. (See discussion below under Section V, for apparent cures and remissions occasionally secured under treatment.)

REMISSIONS of identical appearance occur in
PARETIC (" general paresis ") and in DIFFUSE
(non-paretic) NEUROSYPHILIS.

Case 24.   Michael O'Donnell, a laborer of 48 years, came
home, one day, at 5:30, complaining of severe headache.   His
wife told him he should lie down and, taking him by the arm,
tried to help him to the bed.   At this moment, O'Donnell
lost control of both left arm and left leg, and fell, unable to
move but with consciousness preserved.   The wife noted
that the left side of his face was drawn up and that he drooled.
He was at once carried to a general hospital, remaining there
for about three weeks, talking at random in a delirious manner
and tied in bed.   Two intraspinous injections of salvarsan
were given, and O'Donnell showed considerable improvement
and went home.

However, upon his return from the hospital, he became
very wilful, would not remain in bed, and on one occasion
actually took the mattress from the bed, carried it to another
room, and then returned to his own room and slept upon the
springs.   He became irritable and emotional, insisted upon
going to the hospital, did not go there but upon returning
home insisted that he had been there.   That night, O'Donnell
left the house only partly dressed.

It appears that O'Donnell had been excessively alcoholic,
but that before August 15, when he sustained the left-sided
hemiplegia above mentioned, there had been no symptoms
except that in February he had once been very dizzy.   It
appears that there had been another dizzy spell, three nights
before the paralysis, accompanied by a fall and unconsciousness for about 15 minutes.

O'Donnell was brought to the Psychopathic Hospital some
six weeks after the paralysis, complaining merely of a slight
headache and desirous of treatment.   There were no mental
symptoms of any sort.   **Physically,** O'Donnell was in general
not abnormal (there was a slight pre-systolic murmur and

TRANSIENT OR FLEETING PARALYSES

NEUROSYPHILIS

MYASTHENIA GRAVIS

MYOTONIA CONGENITA (THOMSEN'S DISEASE)

PARAMYOTONIA CONGENITA

MYOTONIA ATROPHICA

INTERMITTENT CLAUDICATION

OCCUPATION NEUROSES

FAMILY PERIODIC PARALYSES

TETANY

EPILEPSY MINOR

HYSTERIA

MULTIPLE SCLEROSIS

APOPLEXY

CEREBRAL THROMBOSIS

CHART 20

a blood pressure of 190 mm. systolic). The pupils were slightly irregular, the left larger than the right; both reacted sluggishly. Both ears were moderately deaf; the tendon reflexes of the left arm and leg were somewhat more lively than those on the right. The systematic **neurological** examination otherwise revealed no abnormalities. The urine was negative. The serum W. R. was positive but the spinal fluid reaction was negative. There were but 2 cells per cmm., and there was a very slight trace of albumin.

1. How shall we account for O'Donnell's transient paralysis? We might invoke brain tumor, alcoholic pseudoparesis, or some form of neurosyphilis. The diagnosis of brain tumor seems quite untenable in view of the absence of premonitory symptoms and in the absence of intracranial pressure. As for alcoholic pseudoparesis it is true that the patient was excessively alcoholic.

   However, against these two diagnoses and in favor of the diagnosis of NEUROSYPHILIS, are the positive serum W. R. and the pupillary reactions (although these are short of the true Argyll-Robertson phenomenon). Dizziness with retention of consciousness and associated with the paralyses mentioned suggests rather a subcortical than a cortical lesion. We are inclined to regard this lesion as probably THROMBOTIC, and to place it possibly in the region of the internal capsule. We are inclined to regard the phenomenon as purely vascular and as not in this case associated with an encephalitis. We are, however, not entirely satisfied with the diagnosis.

2. What shall be said as to treatment? A full-blown left-sided hemiplegia may be produced even when the thrombotic lesion is itself exceedingly small. It is common to explain this on the basis that there is an area of collateral edema about the small necrotic, thrombotic, or hemorrhagic area responsible for the lesion. In short, numerous neurones are functionally rather than structurally affected, or at all events capable of early restitution of function.

3. What is the prognosis in such cases? It appears that now and again patients run for several years without further trouble, both with and without treatment. We are inclined, however, to advocate treatment rather than absence of treatment for a variety of reasons.

In the first place, vascular lesions may at any time become associated with meningitic lesions, and treatment by salvarsan may perhaps be counted on to head off this process; secondly, the treatment with iodids may possibly aid in the resolution of a local thrombotic process.

4. What are the prodromal symptoms of cerebrospinal syphilis? According to Nonne, headache, dizziness, sleeplessness, mental symptoms of the irritability group, loss of capacity as to mental work, whether severe or not, and loss of capacity for difficult thinking; also impairment of memory. Nonne does not regard these phenomena as characteristic of syphilitic vascular disease, and calls attention to the fact that in every organic disease the same subjective symptoms occur. The triad — headache, dizziness, and impairment of memory — is for example now counted as a prodromal symptom complex for arteriosclerotic apoplexy (Cramer). Of course, apoplectic attacks occur without such preliminary symptoms: particularly, according to Nonne, the nocturnal attacks.

5. Can the fleeting paralysis be of service in differentiating the diffuse from the paretic form of neurosyphilis? Probably not. In both forms transient paralyses occur as well as the permanent ones. In general, however, the transient paralyses are more frequent in paretic neurosyphilis, whereas the permanent ones occur more often in diffuse neurosyphilis.

There are cases of NEUROSYPHILIS in which the laboratory signs are positive but in which there are no clinical signs or symptoms (PARESIS SINE PARESI ?).

Case 25. Richard Lawlor* was admitted to the Psychopathic Hospital, October 29, 1914, being sent there from a general hospital where he had gone on account of a self-inflicted wound of the wrist, apparently made in a period of depression with suicidal intent. Routine notes follow.

Family History. Paternal grandparents both died of heart disease. Maternal grandfather died at seventy-two of dropsy. Moderately alcoholic. Maternal grandmother died of shock at fifty-six. Father died at age of forty, after an illness of eight years, from heart disease. Father all his life was subject to fainting spells and headaches. The only paternal cousin died at thirteen months of brain fever. Mother, aged forty-seven, is, to say the least, eccentric. Says "she has several times been given up from tuberculosis." Two maternal uncles died of tuberculosis, one from rupture, one from heart disease. One uncle who " doesn't know anything after he has a teaspoonful of liquor." Several other uncles and aunts whose history is not obtained. Patient is mother's only child. Mother was twice married. There were several miscarriages by both husbands; patient child by first marriage.

Past History. Patient born thirty-two years ago, full term, normal delivery and development. Measles, mumps, and chickenpox in childhood. Subject to headaches since seven or eight years old. Kicked in the face by horse at seventeen or eighteen, not considered serious. Hit by a baseball three or four years ago, leaving him hard of hearing

---

* Reprinted from an article by Southard & Solomon: " Latent neurosyphilis and the question of *Paresis sine paresi.*" Boston Medical & Surgical Journal, XXIV, 1.

on left side. Married ten years ago; no children because he says his wife needed an operation. He denies venereal disease by name and symptoms. For past ten years has had attacks of depression lasting but a short time, but quite severe. Never caused him to quit work as a barber and he felt better when working. His married life he says was fairly happy except for his wife's extravagances, and on this account he left her a little over a year ago, and she has applied for a divorce, which he is willing that she should have, but does not wish to give her alimony. He admits moderate alcoholism.

Present Trouble. Patient states that since he left his wife a year ago he has felt sorry a number of times. He has wished he had her back. He has felt lonely. He has had six or eight periods of depression in that time similar to those he has had for many years, lasting two or three days, and sometimes a week. These were always precipitated by some cause for worry. In these attacks he feels nervous, sleeps poorly, has little or no appetite, sweats during his work and everything looks black. Several times in these attacks he has had suicidal ideas. Ten months ago he considered taking corrosive sublimate. For a little over a week before entrance to hospital he had been out of work and had been " sporting." The day before entrance he had a telephone message from his lawyer which upset him somewhat and he walked the floor all night. He had just been shaving when the idea of suicide came to him. He sat down a minute when suddenly the thought " to hell with the world " came to him; he took the razor and slashed his wrist. He does not remember drawing the razor across his wrist. As soon as he saw the blood he felt sorry, called his mother, and was taken to an emergency hospital and then sent to the Psychopathic Hospital.

Physical Examination. Patient is a well-developed and nourished man thirty-two years of age. Head is normal as to size and shape; there are no scars or marks of injury. Hair and skin not remarkable in any way. Ears negative to external examination. Teeth well kept; two missing, several gold fillings. Tongue very slightly coated. Throat negative. Tonsils easily visible without evidence of inflammation or exudation. Neck, no thyroid enlargement, no abnormal pulsations, no adenopathy. Chest, symmetrical, expansion good, resonant throughout. Breath sounds transmitted normally. No râles or rubs heard. Heart, no enlargement or cardiac dulness. Sounds of good quality, no murmurs heard. Rate regular. Pulses equal, regular and synchronous, and of good volume and tension. Systolic blood pressure 130, diastolic 65. Abdomen, flat, soft and tympanitic throughout; no masses; no tenderness. Liver edge not felt, below costal margin. Spleen not palpable. Extremities negative, except for incised wound on left wrist.

Neuromuscular Examination. Pupils are large, round, regular, equal and react readily to light and accommodation. No nystagmus, strabismus or ptosis. No weaknesses or paresis of facial muscles. The tongue projects medially and shows no tremor. The triceps and biceps reflexes are readily elicited, and are quite active, as are the knee-jerks and ankle-jerks. On one occasion it was thought that the tendon reflexes were slightly more active on the left than on the right. This was never confirmed; always afterwards found equal. There was no tremor of extended hands. Abdominal reflexes not elicited. Cremasteric present on both sides. The plantar response is flexor. There is no Babinski, Gordon or Oppenheim. No Romberg. Coördination tests well performed. No speech defect. No sensory disturbances. Urine examination negative.

Wassermann reaction in the serum: Positive, with cholesterinized antigen; negative, with syphilitic fetal liver antigen.

Wassermann reaction in fluid positive on two occasions. Examination of spinal fluid, November 4: globulin +++, albumin ++, 100 cells per cubic millimeter; large lymphocytes, 8 per cent; small lymphocytes, 90 per cent; plasma cells, 0.7 per cent; endothelial cells, 1.3 per cent. November 11, globulin +++, albumin +++, cells 18 per cubic millimeter. November 26, globulin ++, albumin ++, cells 92 per cubic millimeter; large lymphocytes, 13.1 per cent; small lymphocytes, 82.1 per cent; plasma, 1.2 per cent; endothelial, 3.6 per cent.

Gold sol, November 4, 5555432100.
Gold sol, November 26, 3332100000.

Mental Examination. On entrance to hospital patient seemed slightly depressed and a bit irritable. This condition lasted two days, after which he was agreeable and apparently entirely over his depression. Even during his mild depression, however, he talked freely. There was no evidence of retardation. He told his story readily. Orientation was intact. Memory excellent. Educational knowledge well retained. There was no evidence of any hallucinations or delusions.

1. Was Richard Lawlor insane?
   There was, then, on the mental and physical examination nothing to make a definite suggestion of a psychosis, and the most one could think of was a psychoneurosis or a cyclothymia of at least ten years' duration. The findings in the cerebrospinal fluid and the Wassermann reactions, however, give us material for thought. Certainly one cannot call the man insane; all who saw him agreed on this point.
2. If Richard Lawlor should some day develop mental symptoms, what would be the genesis of the new psychosis? Though writers such as Fildes and McIntosh, and Swift, have suggested an anaphylactic or hyperallergic explanation for the development of symptoms after a normal interval; such a hypothesis could hardly obtain in the present case. The hyperallergic hypothesis for the development of tertiary neurosyphilis would run to the effect that in the secondary stages there had been a definite disease of the nervous system, which, however, absolutely cleared up, leaving no inflammatory vascular or parenchymatous relics of its existence. Nothing would on this hypothesis remain except a hypersensitisation of the tissues. In some later period of the now clinically normal person, one or more spirochetes from a lesion outside the nervous system are carried into the nerve tissues and there set up an anaphylactic or hyperallergic reaction. It is obviously difficult to prove the correctness or incorrectness of the hyperallergic theory without numerous examinations of the spinal fluid, in clinically normal persons after the secondaries have passed. The present case, so far from demonstrating a normal fluid, demonstrates a highly pathological fluid, even though there are absolutely no clinical symptoms which could be regarded as of

nervous origin. The burden of proof at the present time would seem to lie with those who claim hyper-allergy in neurosyphilis. We prefer on present evidence to think that at the conclusion of the secondaries a disease process often remains in the nerve tissues despite clinical quiescence.

3. What is the prognosis in the case of Richard Lawlor? The prognosis *re* neurosyphilis is doubtful. We have, however, boldly termed the condition *PARESIS SINE PARESI*, meaning thereby to suggest that the patient is in considerable danger of the efflorescence of a true diffuse or paretic neurosyphilis. We have no means of telling, however, whether the positive symptoms would be those of a paretic or a non-paretic neurosyphilis. As data accumulate regarding these cases of *paresis sine paresi*, we may be able finally to come upon some case in which trauma shall bring out the clinical symptoms of neurosyphilis. For discussion of this matter, see the case of Bessie Vogel (52) in Part III of this book.

4. Should Lawlor have been brought to a psychopathic hospital? It is a safe working rule to have any person who attempts suicide observed. A large percentage of suicides occur in psychotic individuals and a suicidal attempt is not infrequently the first recognized abnormality. Immediate observation is a necessary safeguard against another more successful attempt.

> **Demonstrates SYMPTOMS and LESIONS of PARETIC NEUROSYPHILIS (" general paresis "). Autopsy.**

Case 26. John Morrill, 49, an operative in a mill town in Essex County, Mass., was described as a " Saturday night and Sunday drinker," with a history of very serious long sprees at the age of 43. It seems that he had had what was called " sciatica " at 35, and was treated in hospital for seven weeks at that time. The nature of this sciatica is in doubt, but there was a history of syphilitic infection at 36 years (scar of glans).

Morrill had been married twice, and two of the children were dead; one daughter was described as " very nervous," but there were four children under ten years of age, all regarded as perfectly healthy.

Morrill had been a mill operative of average capacity, was industrious, and had supported his family despite alcoholism. The syphilis had been treated with reasonable thoroughness.

Aside from alcoholism, there had been no symptoms up to two months before admission to Danvers Hospital. Then there had been insomnia, fatigue, agitation, eruption on foot, loss of ten pounds in weight, hypochondriacal fears, apprehensiveness for the future of the children, incoherent talk; and just before admission, his talk was described as foolish. He had taken to running away and hiding in bushes by a pond and in the cellars of other people's houses.

The patient was of medium height and weight, with thin grayish hair and grayish irides; musculature was slender. The face was blank in expression, the teeth poorly preserved with atrophy of gums, the tongue coated, and the breath foul. There was a gummy secretion of the eyelids, an area of brownish branny eruption over both clavicles, a number of depressed scars over the limbs and back, and another area of scaly eruption on the right heel and the sole of the foot. The heart area was increased, and the sounds were faint at the base, with the first sound accentuated at the apex. The urine showed a trace of albumin.

Neurologically, the Romberg position was maintained with a general tremor and fluttering of the eyelids. In complicated movements, the patient was slightly ataxic. The pupils were irregular, the left being much larger than the right. There were no light reactions to be obtained in window light. The reaction to accommodation was present, though slight. Vision was poor, $\frac{1}{4}$-inch capitals could not be read by left eye at reading distance. The knee-jerks were diminished equally; the Achilles jerks were absent; the other reflexes were normal. Upon the sensory side, the patient gave a history of pains in the legs at irregular intervals for several years. These pains he described as of a darting character. There was little or no sensory disorder, although the outer surface of the right leg required a deeper pressure to elicit sensation. There were no disorders of muscle sense.

If Morrill was to be trusted, he had been born in Ireland, and had come to the United States at the age of 17. He married at 18; there had been seven pregnancies by the first wife, with one stillborn child; one child had died at five weeks. The four children by the second wife were healthy. The first signs of neuritis had occurred at 45 and had received the diagnosis neuritis, although no connection between the neuritis and the syphilis had been noted.

The patient entered the hospital July 26, 1904, and was discharged, improved, January 5, 1905. He returned a little more than a year later, January 15, 1906, and died March 21, 1906. The total duration of the disease from the onset of mental symptoms may therefore be stated as somewhat under two years. When the patient appeared at the hospital the second time, he showed a positive Romberg sign, an unsteady gait, an ataxia that still was moderate, and somewhat more marked tremors, involving fingers, tongue, and face. He was now unable to read $\frac{1}{2}$-inch type with the left eye. The knee-jerks, formerly diminished, were both exaggerated, the left slightly more so. The Achilles reaction, not obtained formerly, now appeared on the right side. The pupils reacted as before. The sensory loss had become more marked, since sharp and dull points could hardly be distinguished. Deep pinpricks were not felt in the leg, and heat could not be told from cold.

The speech in 1904 had been somewhat defective ("truly rural" rendered as "tooly lualal," "sifted soft thistles" as "thoft thsistles"), and there had been little further development of the speech defect. The handwriting had lost appreciably in legibility and had become much more tremulous. During the first period of hospital observation Morrill had what might possibly have been visual hallucinations, but it was impossible to tell whether his story of seeing his wife and children trying to get in through the window was hallucinatory or a matter of fabrication. Memory was decidedly imperfect and few details of recent events could be produced. The association of ideas was almost a so-called "flight" of apprehensive, fearful ideas, loosely connected, incoherently expressed, and dealing chiefly with his work and his children. Judgment was imperfect; the height of the room was estimated as 24 feet, but the height and weight of persons were estimated with fair accuracy, and also the length of small objects, whose lengths were doubtless remembered rather than estimated. The estimate of time elapsing during a medical examination was accurate, but the estimate of longer durations involving over-night memories was hopelessly imperfect. Emotionally, there was a dulling of sensibility, an appearance of suspicion and apprehensiveness; the patient fancied himself to be in a hopeless condition as a result of syphilis, but at the same time accompanied his statement of his hopelessness with laughter. A sample of his hypochondriacal ideas: "I am all gone; I am good for nothing; I am all gone now; I can't drink now; can't write or talk at all; worse than when you saw me first; nothing in my inside; all wrong through me again; I aint got no swallow* now; I can't die even; my heart aint much good; I can't hear it beat; I don't think it flutters; no life in these hands; they are all cold and dead " (pointing to his arms and moving them about). During such a portrayal the patient laughed in a silly way.

During the second hospital stay, Morrill was at first restless, sleepless, profane, imperfectly oriented for time, possibly for place, and also for the attendants. A few weeks later he became stuporous and confused, and his feebleness and physical exhaustion were finally ended by death, March 21, 1906. Death was preceded by a semi-comatose condition; a left otitis media had developed.

At the **autopsy**, it appeared that death was due to an early bronchopneumonia associated with acute splenitis and doubtless related to the otitis media of the left side. The body at large showed, aside from these acute lesions, a few chronic lesions, including slight scars of the left apex, and chronic adhesive pleuritis, chronic diffuse nephritis, and aortic and coronary syphilis. The aorta showed slight linear and nodular markings, with a single small dark ulcer in the upper thoracic region, but the aorta did not show the characteristic scarring which syphilitic aortas often show. The femoral marrow was of a dark red chocolate color. The thyroid appeared to be smaller than normal. A slight sacral decubitus had developed.

The description of the head (E.E.S.) is given in full on account of the encephalitic lesions shown. These encephalitic lesions may be summed up as follows:

Local cerebral **atrophy** and **sclerosis** of the frontal, orbital, and central regions, especially of the left operculum and left supramarginal gyrus.

Extension of sclerosis to hippocampal gyri with effacement of substantia reticularis alba.

Slight chronic internal **hydrocephalus.**

Granular **ependymitis** (especially of floor of 4th ventricle).

Compensatory edema of frontal and central pia mater.

Cerebellar sclerosis (culmen monticuli, lobus culminis, lobus cacuminis).

Spinal sclerosis (grossly evident in the posterior columns of the upper thoracic region and of the lumbar enlargement).

The details are as follows:

Head: — Bald on top. Hair gray. Scalp normal. Calvarium thin, deeply excavated by arachnoidal villi to right of vertex. Diploë absent. Dura closely adherent in bregmatic region. Dura of usual thickness.

Sinuses contain cruor clot. Arachnoidal villi slight. Pia mater hazy and over sulcal veins porcelain white over all of vertex except occipital poles and over flanks (notably left). Thickened also around circle of Willis, over culmen monticuli and in posterior cerebellar notch. Edema of pia corresponding to atrophy of frontal and central regions. Cerebral atrophy most marked in orbital surfaces of both frontal lobes, in left area of Broca, and in left supramarginal region. The ascending branch and the ascending ramus of the posterior limb of the left Sylvian fossæ both readily admit the thumb by reason of atrophy of adjacent substance. Induration corresponds closely with atrophy, but is not more marked about the left Sylvian fossa. There is sclerosis of both hippocampal gyri, with loss of the substantia reticularis alba. The culmen monticuli and lobus culminis are firmer than the clival regions, and the lobus cacuminis is again slightly firmer than the clival region. Cerebellum a little softer than usual. Pia strips with usual readiness from all regions. The subpial region of the frontal lobes is a trifle grayer than that of the rest of cerebrum. Ventricles slightly dilated. Surfaces evenly sanded. Floor of fourth ventricle shows numerous coarse, closely set granules. Brain wt. 1200 grms. Cord shows a slight increase of consistence over one or two upper thoracic segments and in lumbar enlargement corresponding with a slight graying out of posterior columns. In places there is a suggestion of graying out also in lateral columns. A few calcified plaques in posterior lumbar pia.

Analysis of these details shows a number of lesions that characterize paretic neurosyphilis (among others, granular ependymitis, frontal atrophy, chronic leptomeningitis), but the lesions are more than merely frontal, extending as they do back as far as the postcentral regions on both sides, and even as far as the left supramarginal gyrus. The cerebellar involvement although frequent, can hardly be said to be characteristic in paretic neurosyphilis. The spinal involvement is characteristic of a case which is probably to be regarded as one of taboparesis; that is, of paretic neurosyphilis following a number of years after the establishment of tabetic neurosyphilis. The aorta is almost constantly affected by sclerosis in paretic neurosyphilis. The absence of diploë in the skull is not infrequent and the adherent dura mater is often found.

Microscopically, the tissues showed the characteristic lesions of PARETIC NEUROSYPHILIS; nerve cell destruction, fibrillar and cellular gliosis, lymphocytic and plasma cell deposits about the small vessels.

1. What are the clinical evidences of syphilis outside the nervous system? The brownish branny eruptions of the skin, the depressed scars and the scaly eruption on right heel and sole are very suggestive of syphilis. Such clinical evidences of syphilis are very important in systematic examination. Although the laboratory tests are of the utmost assistance in the diagnosis of syphilis, the clinical signs should not be neglected, and no physician should rest satisfied with laboratory signs alone. X-ray diagnosis of bone conditions sometimes succeeds when all other methods have failed.

GUMMA of cerebral cortex verified by operation; death.

Case 27. The presenting picture in the case of David Tannenbaum was that of deep dementia, in which condition the patient was brought to the hospital. There was a meagre history to the effect that about four months before admission, he had lost his job in a hotel through lack of further work. We heard that at this time he had begun to suffer with excruciating pains in the head; at first, worse at night, later, worse by day. It appeared that this pain, though it came and went, was chiefly localized on the left side of the head. For a fortnight, Tannenbaum had been dragging his legs, until finally he had become unable to walk at all.

Pari passu with these developments, Tannenbaum had become mentally confused and irritable, and his memory had become untrustworthy. For several days before admission, an appearance of marked dementia was presented, with slow incoherent, or at all events, irrelevant words, and a complete disorientation for person. However, his vison had become so poor that it would have been hard for him to have recognized any one.

It appeared that the family history was entirely negative; that the patient was without education but had been physically very strong, and had been fairly successful at first in the junk business, and later in the clothing business; but latterly he had been less fortunate in the clothing business, and finally had to resort to work as a laborer around a hotel.

His wife had had eleven pregnancies with but one miscarriage. Nevertheless, out of the eleven pregnancies, there were now but four living children.

Physically, Tannenbaum was a rather small man; he was flabby and looked as if he had recently lost weight. The skin showed areas of pigmentation on the face and sides of the neck, and some dark copper-colored circular areas, marble-size, in the neck (syphilitic?). There was a slight radial arteriosclerosis. The heart was slightly enlarged with distant and indistinct sounds. There was a small pedunculated growth on the right side of the abdomen.

The pupils failed to react to flashlight but they reacted to sunlight. They both were slightly irregular but were equal in size, and reacted in accommodation. There was apparently almost complete blindness and extreme deafness. Arm-jerks and knee-jerks were absent; there was an occasional slight response of the left ankle-jerk, but the right ankle-jerk was absent; the left abdominal reflex was very feeble; the right absent; the cremasteric reflexes were absent, but there were no other abnormalities in the systematic examination. Hand grips weak; gait awkward, with right leg held somewhat flaccidly.

It was significant that percussion over the left frontal and parietal regions was able to elicit great pain. Either through the patient's deafness or through sensory aphasia, spoken language was not understood. The serum W. R. was positive, the fluid W. R. negative.

Diagnosis: The clinical symptoms seem clearly to indicate syphilis. The local skull tenderness and impairment of vision might well suggest intracranial pressure. Uniting these suggestions, we might automatically arrive at a diagnosis of cerebral gumma. We have learned to be rather cautious of making a diagnosis of gumma of the brain through its mere rarity.

Decompression was suggested and executed. A deep growth resembling a GUMMA, in the view of the surgeon, was discovered. No attempt could be made to remove it. The patient died without recovering consciousness.

1. What is the significance of the negative fluid W. R. in this case of cerebral gumma? The W. R. producing substances not infrequently fail to appear in the spinal fluid from a gumma of the brain. The serum W. R. was positive in this case, but even the serum W. R. may be negative in cases of gumma, both of the brain and of the body at large. It must be remembered that the serum W. R. may be negative in paretic neurosyphilis (general paresis); the serum W. R. is even more apt to be negative in cases of gumma.

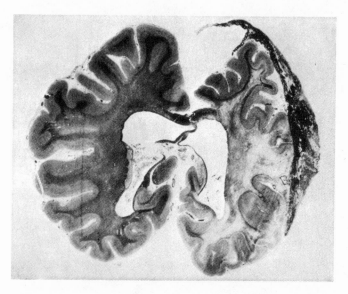

Gummatous meningitis. Compression of hemisphere. Tissue destruction of underlying cortex.

2. Is operative procedure to be advised in cerebral gumma? There are cases in which the acute and threatening symptoms of heightened intracranial pressure require operative treatment simply because the therapeutist cannot wait for the effect of antisyphilitic treatment. Moreover, antisyphilitic treatment of cerebral gumma is not always as successful as that of most syphilitic lesions.

3. Could the intracranial pressure be caused by other syphilitic lesions than gumma? A heavy meningitis may cause symptoms such as produced by an intracranial tumor. In such a case one will usually find evidences of inflammation in the spinal fluid. Cysts caused by syphilitic lesions may also produce identical symptoms.

4. What is the significance of cranial tenderness? Where sensitiveness to cranial percussion is not due to a scalp lesion it is very suggestive of a tumor underlying this point. A gummatous lesion of the cranium itself, may occur without causing pain or increased sensitiveness.

CRANIAL NEUROSYPHILIS (focal syphilitic extraocular palsy) without mental symptoms.

Case 28. A chef, Paolo Marini, 28 years of age, reported that on awaking one morning, everything appeared double to him and that his right eyelid had begun to drop. In the following month Marini had begun to feel weak and to have difficulty in swallowing, as well as at times difficulty in breathing. The diplopia was found to develop when Marini looked to the right. Mentally, the patient was in all respects normal, and no other physical signs were found except the diplopia and ptosis above mentioned. The W. serum test was positive, but the tests of the spinal fluid were negative.

Diagnosis: " CEREBRAL SYPHILIS."

1. What is the anatomical cause of this condition? It is thought to be due in a number of cases to a small diffuse gummatous lesion at the *basis cerebri*. In the case of Marini this lesion appears to have been a little more extensive and to have interfered with the tenth and twelfth nerves also.

2. Why is the spinal fluid negative in such a case as that of Marini? Head and Fearnsides believe that intracerebral lues is characterized by a negative spinal fluid, under which circumstance one has always to consider the possibility of brain tumor or migraine in addition to the suspicion of syphilis.

3. What other causes besides syphilis should one consider for the sudden diplopia? Brain tumor, multiple sclerosis, cerebral arteriorsclerosis, tuberculous meningitis, trauma and migrainous ophthalmoplegia, are not infrequently at the bottom of this condition. Cases also occur in which the etiology remains obscure, even at autopsy.

Under anti-syphilitic treatment, Marini slowly improved.

The SIX TESTS in TABETIC NEUROSYPHILIS (" tabes dorsalis ") may run milder than in paretic neurosyphilis (" general paresis ") and characteristically run somewhat like those of diffuse (meningovascular) neurosyphilis; in particular, the fluid Wassermann Reaction and the gold sol reaction are apt to run milder. The clinical course of tabes dorsalis is protracted and the prognosis as to life is good.

Case 29. Mario Sanzi, 55 years of age, had been having what he called rheumatism since his 43d year. This rheumatism affected only the hips and legs, had at times been very severe, and for two years past had been almost constant. Before that time, pains had come at intervals, lasted a variable period, and suddenly disappeared. They were of knife-thrust character, and could probably be called " lancinating." In a given attack, these pains would come at intervals of seconds or more. There was also a certain unsteadiness in locomotion and inability to control the vesical sphincter.

Physically, the patient was entirely normal so far as could be made out except **neurologically.** Argyll-Robertson pupils, absence of knee-jerks, and ankle-jerks, Romberg sign, and characteristic gait, left no cause for doubting the diagnosis of TABES DORSALIS. The blood and spinal fluid both proved positive to the W. R., though the W. R. in the fluid gave a negative reaction with 0.1 cm. and became positive with 0.3 cm. or more. The globulin was somewhat increased though less markedly so than in paresis. The gold sol reaction was " syphilitic " but weak. It is to be noted that the disease had run a 12-years' course before a doctor had been consulted. The primary infection occurred at 32 years, namely, 11 years before the symptoms began. At the time of his primary infection, Sanzi had received several years of treatment, chiefly in the form of mercury by mouth.

1. What is the value of mercurial treatment of syphilis in the prevention of tabetic or other forms of neurosyphilis? " Fournier strove for many years to convince the medical profession that a syphilitic patient should be treated for at least two years after his infection, whether the syphilis seemed latent or patent. The method of treating only the symptoms he characterized as the opportunist method; treatment in the absence of definite symptoms the preventive method, as preventing the later manifestations. That prolonged treatment does prevent is shown by Fournier's figures analyzing 2396 cases presenting tertiary signs. These he divides into three groups: Group 1, comprising 1878 cases, or 78 per cent of the whole number, having no treatment or inadequate treatment — that is mercury for less than one year; Group 2, comprising 455 cases, or 19 per cent, having moderate treatment — that is, mercury for one to three years; and Group 3, comprising the remaining 19 cases which represent only 3 per cent of the whole number, having treatment for more than three years." *

In the light of what we now know concerning latent neurosyphilis, it would seem well for patients to be followed from time to time with the W. R. on blood and spinal fluid after the supposed completion of the treatment of primary and secondary syphilis. The examination of the spinal fluid is not superfluous, as our experience with the so-called *paresis sine paresi* abundantly shows. At the present day it is not good practice to assure a patient that he is cured after two years of ordinary mercurial treatment without resort to frequent spinal fluid tests, even though the serum W. R. be negative.

---

* Solomon: " How Shall Latent Syphilis be Treated? The Prophylaxis of Syphilis of the Central Nervous System." Interstate Medical Journal, XXIII, 8.

TABETIC NEUROSYPHILIS ("tabes dorsalis")
is often quite ATYPICAL clinically and may even
show no single symptom warranting the old clinical
name "locomotor ataxia."

Case 30. Stephen Green is a case of TABES DORSALIS with
active knee-jerks and without locomotor or muscle-sense
disorder. When observed at the age of 45, it appeared that
there were but two complaints: lack of control of the vesical
sphincter and shooting pains in the legs. It appeared that
the urinary disorder dated back ten years, when there had
been difficulty in passing the urine. Sounds had been
passed at the time; occasionally there had been incontinence
during after years, ascribed by Mr. Green to the passing of
the sound. However, the physician at that time stated that
the incontinence was a symptom of tabes dorsalis. The
incontinence had recently become worse, especially marked
at night, though also occurring in the day; much worse during
excitement, and very much worse after taking alcoholic
drinks. Besides incontinence, there is also difficulty at
times in passing the urine, as well as dysuria.

As for the pains in the legs, they had been first noticed
some three or four years ago and considered to be mild
rheumatic effects. Now, however, they have grown progressively worse and have been the effective cause of giving
up business. The pains are sharp, darting, pinching, and
burning, and last, say, about a second with an interval of
about the same length. The attack will continue sometimes
for many hours.

There is a strabismus of the left eye, ascribed by the
patient to an accident with an umbrella (there had been
operation without relief). The pupils showed the Argyll-
Robertson effect and were markedly irregular. Despite the
divergent strabismus with diplopia, the eye movements were
well performed although not in parallel axes. Ankle-jerks
could not be obtained even on reinforcement, but the knee-

jerks were lively, and the other deep and skin reflexes proved
normal. The blood and spinal fluid tests were characteristic
of tabes dorsalis.

It appears that the syphilis was acquired by this patient
15 years before; that is, 5 years before neurological symptoms
began. Three courses of treatment had been taken at a
well-known watering-place, and mercury pills had been taken
for two years by mouth. The patient is married; has no
children; there have been no pregnancies.

1. What causes may be assigned for the absence of children
   in the family of a tabetic? There may be lesions of the
   genital apparatus (orchitis, or more specialized toxic
   lesions). But impotence such as characterized the
   present case must also be taken into account.
2. What is the therapy for tabetic pains? Pyramidon is
   nowadays much in favor; morphine may be used;
   some authors recommend that the patients be in-
   structed to chloroform or etherize themselves slightly
   for relief of the pain. Surgery of the nerve roots
   may be resorted to in extreme cases. Intraspinous
   therapy, suggested by various authors, seems to exert
   beneficial effect in many cases.
3. Is the lack of control of the vesical sphincter an unusual
   initial symptom? On the contrary, the more careful
   the clinical observation, according to some observers,
   the more likely is the examiner to find that vesical
   symptoms were the earliest or among the earliest complaints of the patient. Baldwin Lucke found sphincter
   disturbances to be initial in $8\frac{1}{4}\%$ of his long Blockley
   series. He found sphincter disturbance to occur in
   some stage of the disease in 67.6%, being exceeded in
   frequency only by staggering gait (87.2%) and lancinating pain (71.6%). According to Lucke, the most
   frequent *initial* symptom is lancinating pain in the
   lower extremity, which, it will be noticed, occurred
   also in our case of Stephen Green as an initial symptom
   along with vesical disturbance. Lucke's figures show
   that paresthesia of the lower extremities (17.6%) and
   weakness of the extremities (16.4%) are the next initial
   symptoms in frequency.
4. Could the early treatment in the case of Stephen Green
   be considered as adequate? No better answer can be
   given to this question than by quoting from Dr. Joseph

Collins,* who probably has done more than any other one man in this country in insisting on the need of proper treatment of syphilis. As to the adequate treatment of syphilis he says:

" It consists in the proper use of salvarsan and mercury begun at the earliest possible moment after infection and kept up till all biochemical evidence of the disease has ceased, while the metabolism of the individual is maintained as nearly normal as possible. But the physician does not do his whole duty when he has accomplished this. He must solicitously watch the individual to see that no evidence reappears for months and even years after the apparent cure. As an index of such reappearance the Wassermann test of the blood serum and of the cerebrospinal fluid is the safest guide.

Until there is a definite unanimity of belief among physicians as to when the treatment of syphilis shall be begun, and some concert of action as to what constitutes the adequate treatment of syphilis, we cannot hope to make any considerable progress in the prevention of syphilis of the nervous system, save by educating the individual toward infection."

---

* Joseph Collins: Syphilis of the Brain, *Journal American Medical Association*, July 10, 1915, Vol. LXV, pp. 139–144.

TABETIC NEUROSYPHILIS may produce symptoms chiefly if not entirely in the region supplied
by the CERVICAL plexus ("cervical tabes").

Case 31. Paul Halleck, 35, was a salesman who had begun
to find it hard to carry his sample case, since he was unable
to tell whether or not he had it in his hand. There was not
only an anesthesia of the hands, but they felt numb and
there was often a tingling sensation. Of late it had become
hard for Halleck to dress himself or to write, and these symptoms had been slowly growing worse. There was no other
complaint. There was, however, a history of a chancre about
7½ years before, which had been followed by a rash and a
sore throat. There had been treatment with mercury and
potassium iodid alternating for a period of two years.

Physically, there was no evidence of disease except **neurologically.** The pupils were unequal (the right larger than the
left) and reacted slowly to accommodation and not at all
to light. A marked ataxia of the hands was shown in coat-
buttoning. The finger-to-nose test showed a marked dysmetria. Arm-jerks as well as knee- and ankle-jerks were
absent. There was a slight swaying in the Romberg position but no true Romberg sign. There was no difficulty in
locomotion. Both blood and spinal fluid proved positive
to the W. R.; globulin and albumin were increased. The
gold sol reaction was syphilitic, and there were 85 cells per
cmm.

This case is probably not a pure example of CERVICAL
TABES, since the knee-jerks are also absent, and we may
suppose a degree of lumbar spinal cord changes in addition to
the cervical changes. It well illustrates, however, that the
tabetic involvement of the cord may be quite generalized and
that it may strike high as well as low.

ERB'S SYPHILITIC SPASTIC PARAPLEGIA.

Case 32. Margaret Neal, a maid-of-all-work, 36 years of age, was committed to a home for inebriates on account of her excessive alcoholism, but she was shortly transferred to the Psychopathic Hospital on account of difficulty with locomotion. We found a very marked spasticity in walking, with a characteristic scissors gait. The pupils were somewhat irregular, and although both reacted to light, the left reacted far more slowly than the right and the reaction failed to hold well. The arm reflexes were very active, and the knee-jerks and the ankle-jerks were particularly exaggerated. There was a double Babinski reaction, as well as Oppenheim and Gordon reflexes and a bilateral ankle-clonus. There seemed to be tenderness over the nerve trunks in the back of the leg, below the knee. There was no evidence of incoördination, no Rombergism, no disturbance of sensation, no disorder of the special senses, and not even a tremor of the tongue or hands.

Mentally, the patient was entirely negative.

Diagnosis: Symptomatically, it is entirely clear that the patient was suffering from SPASTIC PARAPLEGIA. One would have to consider besides spinal syphilis, also amyotrophic lateral sclerosis, syringomyelia, and spinal cord tumor. However, there appeared to be no definite wasting of muscles, and the fact that the sensations were intact seems to rule out also syringomyelia. There was none of the characteristic pain associated with a cord tumor. There was, in fact, a strong clinical premonition that the case was one of spinal syphilis, simply because syphilis is the most common cause of spastic paraplegia in the adult. The pupillary anomalies were also highly suggestive.

The serum W. R. proved to be weakly positive, as was also the gold sol reaction in the zones characteristic of syphilis. The spinal fluid examination yielded 14 cells per cmm. There was a positive globulin test and a moderate increase in albumin. The W. R. of the spinal fluid was negative.

1. Why was the spinal fluid W. R. negative in this case of spinal syphilis? The explanation of negative W. R.'s in spinal syphilis is not easy. Possibly, however, in the course of years the intensity of the process has been reduced and possibly the W. R. has been one of the first tests to disappear.
2. How shall we explain the nerve trunk tenderness? We might consider this to be due possibly to an inflammation about the posterior roots. On the whole, partly on account of the situation of the pains below the knee, it seems probable that the nerve trunk tenderness of this case is the residuum of an alcoholic neuritis.

Treatment: Under injections of mercury salicylate, there was a rapid improvement. In fact, in the course of several months, the patient regained an ability to walk long distances. There still remains a certain spasticity, but the abnormal spinal reflexes above mentioned are no longer present.

SYPHILITIC MUSCULAR ATROPHY, probably
due either to spinal parenchymal lesions, or to root
neuritis, or to both.

Case 33. Joseph Graham, now 50 years of age, seemed
no longer to be able to do good work as a teamster. His
arms had become weak and the muscles had become tremulous
and apparently wasted. There was also pain in the left leg
and hip. It appears that this latter symptom had been
thought to be rheumatism, having begun about 8 years before
with a sudden sharp shooting pain in the left hip, about the
region of the sciatic notch. Graham had rubbed the hip
with liniment, but without reducing the so-called rheumatism.
The trembling of the hands had begun some years later,
but no wasting had been noticed except during the past year.
The pain in the leg had suddenly become so severe that a
month before medical observation he had quit work. The
question immediately arose whether Graham was not
suffering from some familial form of muscular atrophy;
but according to his representations, there was nothing of
the sort in the family.

Physically, there was little to note. **Neurologically,** there
was more. The pupils were somewhat irregular in outline,
and the right was larger than the left. The left pupil failed
to react to light, and the right pupil reacted very slowly
and with but a slight excursion. There was no tremor of the
tongue and no evidence of facial palsy nor was there smooth-
ing of the nasolabial folds. It was somewhat remarkable,
that in the absence of these signs, there was a marked speech
defect. The atrophy of arms, forearms, and hands was
well marked, especially the atrophy of the thenar and hypo-
thenar eminences of the right hand. The extended hands,
especially the right, showed a marked coarse tremor. Fibrilla-
tion was found in the muscles of the hands, forearms, arms,
and pectoral muscles. There was no dysmetria, and the dia-
dochokinesia was normal. Strength was diminished (dyna-

mometer right hand, 32 kg., left 31 kg.). There was little or
no atrophy of the legs, although the left thigh was perhaps
slightly atrophic and the gluteal muscles of the left side
were somewhat flabby. The patellar and Achilles reflexes
were absent on both sides. There was a slight swaying in
Romberg position. Gait was normal. There was a marked
tenderness on the left side of the sciatic notch, as well as
over the entire distribution of both external and internal
popliteal nerves. This area of skin was also hyperesthetic.
There were no other neurological signs on systematic examination.

Diagnosis: The sensory disorder, the speech defect, and
the pupillary abnormalities seem to render the diagnosis
of progressive muscular atrophy doubtful. Nor was there
any dissociation of sensations to suggest a syringomyelia.
Under such circumstances, one must fall back upon the question of syphilis. Both blood and spinal fluid proved to be
positive to the W. R.; the globulin was increased and the
albumin markedly so; there were 61 cells per cmm., and the
gold sol reaction read 4 4 4 4 3 2 1 0 0 0.

1. Is there a relation of SYPHILITIC MUSCULAR ATROPHY to
   amyotrophic lateral sclerosis? Spiller, some years since,
   claimed such a relation, and it would seem with some
   justice.
2. How shall the present case be classified? There is
   evidence of root pains (left hip). We may naturally
   suppose that these root pains are reasonably good
   clinical evidence of a meningitic lesion, of which the
   spinal fluid clinically gave a confirmation. The fi-
   brillation in this case somewhat suggests, however, a
   central origin for the muscular atrophy. Accordingly,
   it would be difficult to definitely classify the present case
   as either one of meningovascular syphilis or one of
   central syphilis. It will be remembered that Head
   and Fearnsides classify muscular atrophy under both
   these headings.

> The period of SECONDARY SYPHILIS is frequently (over a third of all cases?) MARKED BY approved signs of NEUROSYPHILIS precisely like those of full-blown paretic or diffuse (meningovascular non-paretic) neurosyphilis. These signs occur sometimes in association with severe clinical symptoms, sometimes without clinical symptoms.

Case 34. John Bennett, 28, was brought to the Psychopathic Hospital much confused. His brother, who came with him, said that he had been a very heavy drinker but had given up drinking about four months before. He had recently had a cold but was otherwise in good health up to the night before admission. On this night, Bennett had become suddenly excited and went into his mother's room, at the common home, and began to curse her. However, he was put to bed safely, but on the next morning began to moan continuously. After some hours of moaning, he was brought to the hospital. Here he remained difficult to manage, being irritable, noisy, and resistive. Questions he either would not or could not answer, and there was even no evidence that he understood questions. However, within a few hours, it was clear that he was slowly coming out of the confused state. On the following day, it was possible even to rouse him and get his name. The confusion gradually cleared still further and, by the end of three days, he had become mentally absolutely well so far as could be determined.

He then informed us that he had had a chancre about five or six months before, followed by a secondary skin eruption; that he had received four injections of salvarsan (the last, a month before admission) and three injections of mercury. At about the time of the last injection of salvarsan, he had developed headache with pain and slight stiffness in the back of his neck; and a fortnight later, he began to have dizzy spells, followed during the last week by difficulty in hearing. There was amnesia for everything that happened after his spell of sudden excitement on the evening before admission, and this amnesia was never lifted for the four days that followed.

Physically, Bennett was very well built and muscular. Nor were there any evidences of disease outside the nervous system. There was some slight stiffness of the neck and slight pain on movement of the head, which probably ought to be attributed to meningitis. The **neurological examination** showed tendon reflexes all normal, and normal sensations. There were, in fact, no neurological signs except that both pupils were dilated; the left was larger than the right. Both pupils reacted to light but reacted very poorly. They reacted much better to accommodation.

The W. R. proved to be positive, as might well be expected in a man whose infection had taken place less than six months before. The globulin and albumin of the cerebrospinal fluid were in great excess, of a degree which we clinically express by ++++ . The W. R. of the fluid also was strongly positive down to 0.1 of a cmm. The gold sol reaction was the " paretic " type, and there were 228 cells per cmm.

1. How early may clinical evidence of neurosyphilis set in after infection? Craig found one case of " brain syphilis " occurring one month after infection. Frye claims a case of tabes dorsalis developing six weeks after infection. Craig states that he has had three cases of brain syphilis occurring within six months, and six within a year of infection.

2. What effect did the salvarsan injections have in causing or preventing the symptoms in this case? Nonne sums up the neurorecidive question as follows: Since the introduction of salvarsan therapy for neurosyphilis, paralyses of various cranial nerves are seen more frequently. This higher frequency is in part only apparent since more attention has been paid of late to auditory and labyrinthine disorders. On the whole, however, it must be considered that salvarsan does mobilize spirochete foci which without salvarsan therapy would perhaps have remained latent. Probably we are here dealing in some instances with fresh infections of neurosyphilis, in other cases with a Herxheimer reaction.

Ehrlich believed that these latent foci occur particularly in places with stagnant blood current; as, for instance, in the narrow bony canals. This hypothesis, sufficient in some instances, is less satisfactory for cases of peripheral neuritis, for example.

3. What treatment is indicated? Intensive antisyphilitic treatment is strongly indicated. Whatever may be the truth concerning the production of neuro-recurrences (" neurorecidives ") it is certain that the symptoms usually vanish with a continuance of salvarsan therapy. The important point is to give efficient treatment, and in a case like Bennett's improvement is fairly certain unless some serious insult occurs before the remedial efforts have been given time. It is still an open question whether intraspinous treatment is more efficient in such cases than intensive intravenous injections of salvarsan. In Bennett's case diarsenol was injected intravenously twice a week in 0.6 gm. doses, reënforced with intramuscular injections of mercury salicylate and potassium iodid by mouth. Under this treatment improvement began slowly and in a few months he was symptomatically well and after three months his tests were practically negative.

JUVENILE PARETIC NEUROSYPHILIS (" juvenile paresis ") with OPTIC ATROPHY.

Case 35. Mary Coughlin, a blind girl of 16 years, was brought to the hospital in a state of great excitement, laughing and crying alternately. The neurologist is entitled to think of blindness, and particularly of the optic atrophy which Mary showed, as probably due to syphilis. However, there was no history of syphilis in the father, who died in an accident at the age of 40, or the mother, who died at 45, of heart trouble. An elder sister was married and well; two younger sisters were living and well. The fifth sibling, a boy, had died in infancy. There had been no miscarriages. In fact, the only point in favor of syphilis was the somewhat far-fetched point that the younger brother of the patient had died in infancy.

The patient's history was rather suggestive of some other diagnosis. Her birth had been normal, she walked and talked at 13 months, was at school from six to twelve, reaching the seventh grade, and was considered bright. At three years of age, she had been run down by a car and dragged under the fender for a considerable distance. Her head was hurt but the patient did not lose consciousness in the accident. Fainting spells began at 11, in which spells the patient would lose consciousness for a minute or two. About this time, the patient's eyesight had begun to fail, and for some four years she had been entirely blind. Headaches had come on of late.

The Coughlin case, except for the above-mentioned suspicion of syphilitic optic atrophy, might be regarded as an unusual example of a post-traumatic disease.

We found her to be fairly well developed and nourished; there was a deformity of the lower half of the sternum and of the third and fourth ribs on the right side. There were no other physical phenomena found upon systematic examination. The left pupil still reacted to light; the right failed to react, but this lack of reaction could not be regarded as of

Argyll-Robertson nature on account of the finding of optic atrophy with the ophthalmoscope.

Mentally, it appeared that the patient's retention of school knowledge was poor, though her blindness for four years had doubtless given her little opportunity to keep such information fresh. Rather strangely, Mary gave utterance to many delusions: first, expecting to receive her sight by an operation on the head; second, to write a book of her doings; third, to buy a house for the children; fourth, would pay $3000 for the house, earning the money by working at a tailor's or as a trained nurse; fifth, to go on the stage to earn money by dancing; sixth, will have lots of money.

One of Mary's characteristic statements is as follows: " Won't it be lovely when I can see Dr. H.'s face in heaven or some other lovely place? Dr. H. was a grand doctor to me, and when we get together again we are going to Tremont Temple and keep us together. I am going to do some dancing and play the piano. I am going to graduate at the high school and go to Trinity College in Washington, and I hope I shall be a faithful keeper of mother's tomb."

The patient was at times euphoric and expansive.

At this stage, what with optic atrophy, euphoria, and expansive delusions, we should perhaps be entitled, had Mary been an adult, to offer the diagnosis GENERAL PARESIS. In fact, on the whole, any other than a syphilitic cause for the optic atrophy was exceedingly doubtful. Brain tumor of a nature to produce optic atrophy might very improbably last so long as five years. There was no evidence of any intoxication at the time when the blindness occurred.

The W. R. was positive in the blood and spinal fluid; there was a positive globulin test, and an excess albumin as well as 15 cells per cmm.

1. What is the significance of Mary's trauma at three years? So far as we are aware, none.
2. What light could be thrown by a W. R. study of the family? In some instances, much light is thrown; in the present case all three living sisters of the patient have been examined and their serum W. R.'s have been found negative.

3. What is the prognosis of juvenile general paresis? Death within a few years, as in general paresis in adults. The patients live rarely more than four or five years after the onset of symptoms. Mary Coughlin died a year and a half after the above examination, namely, in her eighteenth year, some seven years after the onset of symptoms.

4. What can be said of treatment? A few favorable results have been reported after intraspinous therapy (Swift-Ellis). Too little work has been done with systematic treatment of juvenile neurosyphilis, both paretic and non-paretic, to permit important conclusions at this time.

5. How can we explain the infection of this sibling whereas the others, both younger and older, escaped? It would seem that we would have to discard the hypothesis of a congenital infection and consider that it was acquired accidentally during the lifetime of the patient. Considering the prevalence of syphilis it is rather to be wondered that more such cases of " innocent " infection do not occur in children. We may recall how many instances of juvenile gonorrhea occur. In a case as this where the symptoms calling attention to syphilis necessarily occur so long after the original infection it is practically impossible to trace the origin of the infection.

> The diagnosis of JUVENILE PARESIS is often easy.

Case 36. Theresa Mullen, an under-sized girl of 12 years, presented a remarkable appearance due to congenital amputations of the fingers and toes. She lay in bed, drivelling and making unintelligible cries. It appeared that the patient weighed about 12 pounds at birth and was very fat; that she had been fed on condensed milk, had survived cholera infantum, whooping cough, and, as the parents said, " two kinds of measles."

Theresa had gone to school at 5 years, reaching the third grade at the age of 9; but at this time, she began to lose ground and was put in a class for backward children. Moreover, at about this time, the teachers noticed spells of causeless laughter and meaningless twisting back and forth. Theresa would also scream at night, looking about the room; once, rising and crying, " Take him away, that black thing," though no appropriate object was present. There had been little or no complaint of headache. Theresa had been deteriorating for some time, and for a year past had been having increased difficulty in walking. For two months the child had not spoken intelligible words; for the last week, she had been incontinent.

The **diagnosis** was almost obvious from the manual and pedal deformities taken in connection with the saddle-back deformity of the nose. It was interesting in connection with the contentions of W. W. Graves, that the scapulæ were scaphoid in type.

Accordingly, the history given by the parents seemed consistent enough. The parents were both 36 years of age, having married at 23. The first pregnancy was a miscarriage at two months, of unknown cause. Theresa came next; thirdly, came a miscarriage at three months; fourthly, a girl, who is not strong or well physically, has suffered much from headaches and sore throat, but is fairly bright. The fifth pregnancy resulted in a boy, who is bright but of under-size. Three more pregnancies resulted in miscarriage.

Taking into account the above-mentioned physical characteristics, the personal history, and the family history of Theresa, the diagnosis could hardly be in doubt even in the absence of a lack of pupillary reaction to light on the right side, infantilism of genitalia, positive W. R.'s of serum and spinal fluid, positive globulin, and excess albumin, 34 cells per cmm. and the paretic type of gold sol reaction which were found.

The **prognosis** of this case appears to be rapid deterioration, terminating in death within a few months. Now and again, however, some such cases spontaneously improve. Such a case as that of Theresa Mullen is always disheartening in itself but suggests the social value of Wassermann tests in the other members of the family. The other children of the Mullen family proved to be suffering also from syphilis, since their blood sera all showed a positive W. R.

1. What is the characteristic age of onset in JUVENILE PARESIS? An impression has prevailed in some quarters that the typical onset of juvenile paresis is in the adolescent years, and Clouston's first case (1877) developed in a boy of 16. Thierry's 58 cases, developing from the 8th to the 20th year, averaged 14 years of age at onset. Mott's 22 cases from the 8th to the 23d year, averaged 17 years at onset. According to Clouston, juvenile paresis develops most often at puberty (15 to 17 years). It is sometimes claimed that cases developing symptoms early live longer, and that juvenile cases developing symptoms after the 20th year run a short course. For a case developing in the 5th year, see John Friedreich, Case No. 77.

2. What may be concluded from the physical signs (congenital amputations) present in this case before the development of mental symptoms? Some cases of juvenile paresis appear to show no physical signs whatever in childhood. While these amputations might be the accidental result of a difficult delivery, it is more probable that they are due to a syphilitic process.

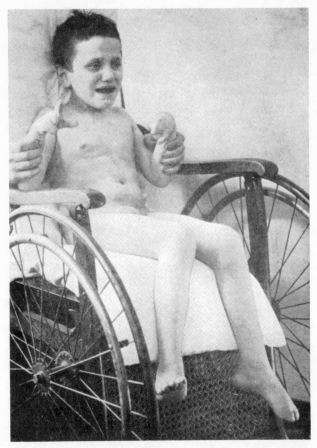

Juvenile paresis — congenital amputation of digits. This case reached fourth grade in school before deterioration.

CONGENITAL SYPHILIS is apparently capable
of producing simple FEEBLEMINDEDNESS (that
is, a form of disease non-paretic, non-tabetic, without special tendency to progression, and without
tendency to vascular insults).

Case 37. Isaac Goldstein was a small boy of six years and
seven months, with a father known to be suffering from general paresis. The child was very irritable and nervous and
very difficult to manage, but would hardly have been the
subject of medical attention except in a family study suggested by the paresis of the father.

The child had been born at term and had apparently
undergone a normal development. Physically, he showed no
definite signs of congenital syphilis. In fact, the physical
examination was to all intents and purposes negative. The
W. R. of the serum, however, proved to be positive. Mental
tests showed that his mental age was that of a child of a
little over five years. Taking all things into account, it is
probable that he should be regarded, therefore, as somewhat
retarded mentally.

1. Is syphilis answerable for the mental retardation in this
    case? Provided that the family is free from feeble-
    mindedness and mental disease, it would seem that
    the retardation of a congenital syphilitic should per-
    haps be regarded as syphilitic in origin. Of course, the
    institutions for the feebleminded have not shown ex-
    ceedingly high percentages of syphilitic children in
    various W. R. surveys; still, the percentage of positive
    reactions in institutions for the feebleminded is clearly
    higher than the incidence of congenital syphilis shown
    in the population at large. Hence, we may conclude
    that syphilis is one of the etiological factors in the
    production of feeblemindedness. Dr. W. E. Fernald,
    of the Waverley School for the Feebleminded, has re-
    cently pointed out that the syphilitic cases belong
    rather in the lower grades (idiots and imbeciles) of
    feeblemindedness than in the higher (morons).

2. Can we guess what the pathological anatomy and histology of the brain may be in such cases? The Waverley studies now in process seem to indicate that some cases have little or no gross alterations, but show a few slight traces of lymphocytic accumulations discovered upon extended search, and a certain tendency to the appearance of rod cells in various foci. But the whole matter is still *sub judice*. It is a question whether these traces of chronic inflammation are the residuals of a more active process or the beginnings of a process that is about to be more active.

3. How characteristic is a positive W. R. in the serum of a child without physical stigmata of congenital syphilis? If we limit the term *stigmata* to the major and more important signs, we must reply that it is not unusual to find positive W. R.'s in sera of physically normal looking children. Except in family studies, such cases will often escape notice, either because there are no stigmata whatever, or because such stigmata as exist are of a minor nature and regarded as unimportant anomalies. Some of these cases occur in the clinics later in life as so-called *syphilis hereditaria tarda*. If one wishes to discover these cases with late development of symptoms before their full bloom, the most obvious method is to examine carefully the children of known syphilitics.

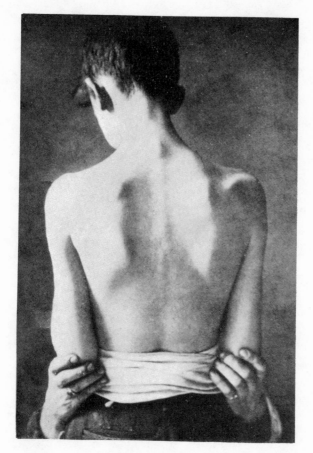

Scaphoid Scapulae.

JUVENILE TABETIC NEUROSYPHILIS ("juvenile tabes"); TREATMENT.

Case 38. The point in presenting Archibald Sherry, a JUVENILE TABETIC of 12 years on admission, is perhaps to exhibit pride in therapeutic results.

There was little or no doubt of the diagnosis; in an adult, the phenomenon would be called tabes dorsalis with a question of general paresis. The right pupil was larger than the left and reacted neither to light nor to distance. There was a slight tremor of the tongue and of the outstretched hands. The knee-jerks and ankle-jerks could not be obtained, nor could the periosteal reflexes in the legs. There was a slight unsteadiness in the gait and in various finer movements, and a slight ataxia of the legs. There was not a classical Romberg sign but there was slight swaying in Romberg position. The teeth were Hutchinsonian. For the rest, the physical examination was practically negative.

The family history was of interest. On the paternal side there was nervousness as well as alcoholism and degeneracy. The maternal grandmother had cancer. Archibald's father was immoral and alcoholic. There was a girl four years older than Archibald, who, though nervous and unstable, has shown no signs or symptoms of syphilis and does not yield a W. R. in blood or spinal fluid.

Archibald himself was born at term, a large child, who, however, lost weight rapidly, developing a marked skin eruption on head and back three weeks after birth. This skin disease lasted for a month and a half and then spontaneously disappeared. Archibald remained weak and sickly, not walking until three years of age. However, he did well in school up to the end of his 11th year, when he failed to keep up with the children. He had been an amiable child and had gotten on well with his playmates. Some time in his 10th year physical disability had begun; there was numbness in the legs with weakness; at times, actual inability to walk. The right pupil was noticed by the mother to have increased in size; the eyelashes had turned white. There was pain over the left eye and a feeling of weight on top of the head. Speech became difficult or even confused.

Consistently enough, the W. R. both in blood and spinal fluid was positive. Globulin and albumin were present in large amounts; there were 150 cells per cmm.

Granting that this be in some sense a case of juvenile tabes we may raise a doubt whether the case is one of congenital syphilis. The W. R.'s of the blood of both father and mother are negative. Syphilis is denied by them. The nervous and unstable older sister failed to show definite symptoms of syphilis or a positive W. R. There had been no miscarriages or stillbirths. The question arises whether the Hutchinsonian teeth do not indicate congenital syphilis. It appears, however, that it is possible to develop Hutchinsonian teeth if syphilis is acquired before the teeth are formed. We have no data as to how or why this particular baby should have acquired syphilis, if he did so acquire it, at the age of three weeks. On the whole, sceptics may doubt our suggestion that the case is one of acquired juvenile tabes. Possibly the question is academic so far as treatment is concerned.

Prognosis: The rarity of juvenile tabes is such that little can be said as to prognosis. Three and a half years have passed since a few injections of salvarsan were made. The pains above mentioned rapidly disappeared, the gait became steadier, the attacks of confusion ceased, and the speech improved. Unfortunately, on account of a lack of cooperation on the part of Archibald's mother, we have been unable to continue treatment. However, we have from time to time followed the patient in his home and he seems to have shown no falling back after the initial improvement. It would be of great value could we know the situation in the spinal fluid at the present time.

1. Is there any explanation why paresis should occur in some juveniles and tabes in others? There is no available explanation for this difference nor any for the characteristic early optic atrophy of juvenile tabetics.

Be frustrate, all ye stratagems of Hell,
And, devilish machinations, come to nought!

Paradise Regained, lines 180-181

III. PUZZLES AND ERRORS IN THE DIAGNOSIS OF NEUROSYPHILIS

This part of the case collection, dealing with puzzles and errors, is ushered in by six cases (39–44) drawn from a group of errors in diagnosis made some years since at the Danvers Hospital. These six are autopsied cases. Attention is called to the fact that modern methods of diagnosis might have prevented the errors.

DIFFUSE NEUROSYPHILIS (" cerebrospinal syphilis ") versus **PARETIC NEUROSYPHILIS** (" general paresis "). Autopsy.

Case 39. Caroline Davis, dead at 49 years, was a case of error in the diagnosis of general paresis. Like Cases 40 to 44, Case 39 was diagnosticated by the full Danvers staff as a case of general paresis; however, it must be added, before the days of the W. R. and the modern methods of systematic diagnosis. As will transpire in the sequel, there is a large question whether Case 39 is not after all really a case of neurosyphilis, possibly not of the paretic group. The details are as follows:

Caroline Davis was a normal school girl till 15, apt in studies, mill worker till marriage at 18; one child, dead (cause unknown). Habits good. Moderate deafness set in in the forties and in 1901 patient became completely deaf in three months' time. In 1905 she became unable to take care of her house and had a shock in which the right leg was affected.

On commitment patient showed good development and nutrition with slight enlargement of capillaries of cheeks, redness and roughening of skin of right ankle. Teeth absent. Slight radial and brachial arteriosclerosis. Urine negative. Sluggish pupil reactions to light both directly and consensually. Deafness absolute, bone conduction defective. Arm reflexes brisk, knee-jerks equal, brisk. Bilateral Babinski reaction more marked on the right side, tremor of tongue, Romberg's sign, gait defective. Speech stumbling, writing clear, without tremor.

Communicated by writing only. Consciousness normal, disorientation for day of month, for place (misnames hospital) and for persons (recognizing nurses, not patients).

Patient wrote many letters complaining of pain, headaches and especially of pain in the abdomen and side. The patient was thought to show a slight defect of memory, but her deafness rendered diagnosis difficult. The patient died suddenly on May 23, 1908, shortly after supper, falling backwards, and dying in five minutes with marked respiratory distress.

Post Mortem Findings. The **cause of death** was not clear. The heart's blood and cerebrospinal fluid were sterile. There was a small hemorrhage in the anterior part of the right ventricle derived from a small artery of the caudate nucleus. There was about 400 cc. of blood between the dura mater and the pia mater. There was a slight sclerosis of the basal and Sylvian arteries. The brain substance was uniformly softer than normal.

It is possible that the hemorrhage had taken place some time before the patient's fall and that the brain substance had swollen in consequence. Just before the fall she had a weeping spell.

The **anatomical diagnoses** were as follows:

Obesity, unequal pupils, fresh wound near left ear, edema of legs, slight focal adhesive pleuritis, hypostatic congestion of lungs, chronic endocarditis, chronic myocarditis, congestion of kidneys, congestion of pancreas, subacute splenitis, chronic adhesive pelvic peritonitis, hematoma and cystic condition of Fallopian tubes, **calvarium dense** and thick, subdural hemorrhage, slight **chronic leptomeningitis,** general **cerebral atrophy,** marked in tips of **frontal lobes,** old **cyst of softening** between left corpora albicantia and optic chiasm, small punctures of left ear drum, drums opaque, **chronic spinal leptomeningitis;** brain weight, 1190 grams.

There were marked firm interadhesions between dura and pia throughout. A lumbar puncture soon after admission in 1907 had shown:

	Per cent
Endothelial cells	10
Lymphocytes	30
Plasma cells	0
Phagocytes	0
Polymorphonuclear cells	51
Unclassified	9
Fibroblasts	0
Cells in 100 fields	125

It will be noted that the lumbar puncture yielded no plasma cells and yet showed 30% of lymphocytes. Alzheimer, in 1904, attempted to distinguish the histology of the cerebral syphilitic from that of the general paretic, maintaining that *lymphocytosis was the characteristic feature of the ordinary neurosyphilitic, whereas plasma cells were associated with the lymphocytes in the paretic.* This case showed **lymphocytic** deposits. To be sure, they were decidedly subordinate in the cerebral cortex, cerebellum, and basal ganglia, to the marked evidences of nerve cell destruction, although there were perivascular infiltrations about a few of the larger vessels in the white matter of the cerebral cortex.

The spinal cord, however, showed a most severe infiltration, especially in the gray matter, where the infiltration accompanied severe nerve cell changes and arterial changes. The pia mater of the spinal cord was also packed with mononuclear elements, among which, however, no plasma cells could be found.

But although the inflammatory changes in the shape of lymphocytosis were relatively more prominent in the spinal cord than in the cortex, yet the cortex yielded evidence of an exceedingly marked destructive process. Perhaps no layer of any of the areas of the cortex examined failed to show some atrophic alteration. The upper layers of the cortex were everywhere more severely diseased than the lower layers. Here we are dealing with an instance of an active meningomye-

litis and subcortical encephalitis. It is, of course, probable
that the W. R., had it been performed, would have been
positive in this case. On the basis of the histology, we are
inclined to regard the clinical picture in this case as belonging
among cases of NON-PARETIC DIFFUSE NEUROSYPHILIS.

This case, as also the next several, is especially instructive
in teaching the difficulty in differentiating paretic and non-
paretic neurosyphilis. Not only is this difficulty met in
clinical diagnosis, but in pathological diagnosis as well.

The histological diagnosis depends in large part on the
work of the Nissl-Alzheimer school, which has received great
recognition. At the present time, however, there is beginning to be considerable doubt as to the entire validity of this
teaching. At any rate there are many borderline cases in
which the differentiation is well nigh impossible. In this
case note chronic meningoencephalitis, with cortical degeneration, in the absence of plasmocytosis.

From the clinical standpoint the intensity of the W. R.,
the character of the gold sol reaction, and the result of
therapy have added new points in differentiation. Much
more work controlled by autopsies is still needed, however,
to put us on sure ground in borderline cases.

VASCULAR NEUROSYPHILIS(?)versus PARETIC
NEUROSYPHILIS ("general paresis"). Autopsy.

Case 40. Case 40 like Case 41 was an error in the diagnosis of general paresis which might be regarded as academic
rather than practical. Both were cases of arteriosclerotic
brain disease with severe cerebellar involvement. Case 40
had a spinal cord that was not quite normal. There was a
tabetiform lesion in the cervical spinal cord (not elsewhere),
together with a unilateral degeneration suggesting in some
respects a radicular origin. The most striking feature, however, of Case 40 as in Case 41, was a lesion of the cerebellum.
In Case 40 the dentate nuclei were in large part destroyed
by cysts of softening, although the cerebellar cortex was
fairly well preserved on both sides. The details of Case
40 are as follows:

H. F., male, gear maker, born 1850.

Heredity. Maternal grandmother insane. Mother insane
at 52, became demented and lost use of limbs, died at 71.
Aunt insane.

Personal History. Common school education. Capable
workman till within a few months. Early in life alcoholic.
Drunk almost every week until 1899 or 1900. Irritable,
nervous, selfish, loose in relations with women. Venereal
disease denied by wife. Married in 1883. Three frail
children. No miscarriages. Neuralgia in 1901 or 1902.

January, 1904, patient left carriage shop on account of
mistakes in work, became more pleasant, childish, fearful,
talkative, did funny things, later became vagrant, stole from
fruit stores, smoked cigarettes picked up in the street, and
became restless and irritable.

Committed to Danvers, June 24, 1904, with slightly
enlarged heart, somewhat heightened blood pressure, and a
slight sediment of epithelial cells in urine.

Romberg's sign was present, but there was little or no
demonstrable incoördination otherwise. Very slight tremor

of fingers. Left knee-jerk absent, right obtained on re-enforcement. Achilles jerk absent. Triceps, wrist and normal plantar reflexes present. Pupils react to accommodation, but very slightly, if at all, to light. Sensations normal except in legs. The legs show preservation of tactile and temperature senses, but abolition of pain sense except over dorsum of foot.

Speech showed slurring of syllables and " brigrade " for " brigade." Disorientation for time, place and in part for persons. Admitted that his work had been deficient but regarded himself as well. Emotionally variable, crying at times and suddenly becoming jocular. Eloped July 3 and somehow reached his wife's house in a neighboring city.

Euphoria persisted. The pupils continued Argyll-Robertson, and the knee-jerks remained absent. Became oriented for place and partially as to time (month and day of week correct).

During 1905 failure became rapid, with ataxia of legs, persistent euphoria, and loss of weight.

Convulsions, regarded as general paretic, developed in 1906. Death sudden, December 7, 1906.

Post Mortem Findings. The **cause of death** was streptococcus septicemia, probably derived from a gangrenous bronchopneumonia or related with a small thrombus of the right auricular appendix. There was also an acute purulent otitis media, mastoiditis and sphenoidal sinusitis, as well as extensive decubitus. From this decubitus or from the intestinal tract may have been derived the numerous colonies of *bacillus coli communis* which developed on plates from the cerebrospinal fluid.

Arteriosclerosis was little in evidence, being confined to the coronary, right vertebral and carotid arteries (slight in all). *Cysts of softening existed in the posterior part of each dentate nucleus* and may probably be interpreted as indicating vascular disease.

Chronic disease outside the nervous system was prominent and in part suggestive of senile findings; milky patches of pericardium, adhesions about liver and gall-bladder, adhesions about spleen, adhesions and fibrous thickening of parietal peritoneum, adhesions in both pleural cavities, chronic diffuse nephritis, hypertrophy of bladder wall, dense calvarium, dural adhesions.

The **nervous system** showed several unexpected features. The *absence of chronic leptomeningitis* was striking: the pia mater was everywhere delicate and transparent except that the walls of the cerebellar and chiasmal cisternæ were thickened and that there were slight opacities along the sulcal veins of the convexity. Brain weight 1090 grams. There was a generalized **sclerosis and pigmentation of the cerebral cortex.** The sclerosis varied in degree and was most marked in the prefrontal regions, the anterior halves of the superior frontal gyri, the middle third of the right precentral gyrus, the region of the splenium on the left side, and the sagittal rami. If the *bacillus coli communis* found in the cerebrospinal fluid had any effect upon the consistence of the brain, obviously hard to prove in a brain of leathery consistence at the outset, it was shown only in the right Rolandic area in the vicinity of the sclerotic part of the precentral gyrus. **Granular ependymitis** of all ventricles. Weight of cerebellum, pons and bulb, 135 grams.

Perhaps the most remarkable feature of all in the case was the occurrence of **cysts of softening** in the posterior part of each **dentate nucleus.** For discussion, see Case 41.

VASCULAR NEUROSYPHILIS (?) versus PARETIC NEUROSYPHILIS ("general paresis"). Autopsy.

Case 41, like Case 40, was one of arteriosclerotic brain disease with severe cerebellar involvement. Here is another case in which the Danvers staff made a diagnosis of general paresis without dissenting voice. There were some tabetic symptoms, and the spinal cord at autopsy did show a moderate lymphocytic infiltration of the meninges, entirely consistent with the picture in the spinal fluid. In this case, the dentate nuclei of the cerebellum were not destroyed as in Case 40, but were affected by cell atrophies of variable degree in different parts of the nuclei. There was also a severe gliosis of the cerebellar cortex. The left hemisphere of the cerebellum was more severely diseased than the right. The cortex showed far more marked and generalized cell atrophies throughout the layers than did Case 40. The details of this case, which was that of a colored coachman, Samuel North, are as follows:

He was born in 1871. Learned to read and write at school. Stableman and coachman. Alcoholic till 1902. Took much quinine, possibly impairing hearing thereby. Memory impaired and growing worse since 1902. Gait unsteady for a longer but unknown period. August 13, 1907, wandered about, instead of attending boot-black stand, muttered, talked incoherently. In the next few days talked about religion and apparently had hallucinations of hearing. Committed August 16, 1907.

On commitment stoop-shouldered, flat-chested. Gait staggering. Unsteadiness in Romberg's position. Incoördination of arms and fingers. Coarse tremor of tongue. Tremor of lower jaw. Exaggeration of left knee-jerk and diminution of right. Exaggerated Achilles jerks. Spurious left ankle clonus. Questionable Babinski reaction of left side. Abdominal and epigastric reflexes present but cremasteric absent. Left pupil smaller than right and fails to react to light. Reaction of right pupil sluggish. Moderate defect of hearing of both sides.

During the first week the patient developed hallucinations of sight and hearing, but of no other senses. Disorientation for time, place, and persons. Answers to arithmetical problems given with assurance but as a rule incorrectly (as 17 and 32 are 90; 18 divided by 3 is 88). Handwriting scarcely legible. Memory poor, especially for recent events (recalled a lumbar puncture as an exercise in baptism). Impressibility and attention poor. Euphoria.

Death after gradual failure July 29, 1908.

Lumbar puncture showed: Per Cent.

	Per Cent.
Endothelial cells	9
Lymphocytes	81
Plasma cells	6
Phagocytes	0
Polymorphonuclear cells	4
Unclassified	0
Fibroblasts	0
Cells in 100 fields	700

Post Mortem Findings. The cerebrospinal fluid showed a pure culture of *Bacillus coli communis*, and the heart's blood showed many colonies of an unidentified bacillus. Culture from mesenteric lymph nodes sterile.

The **cause of death** is somewhat in doubt. There was an early pneumonic process with fibrinous pleurisy, and there was an early acute hemorrhagic ileitis with a very slight overlying peritonitis and slight corresponding enlargement of mesenteric lymph nodes. There was an infection of the meninges with *Bacillus coli communis*.

Evidences of **chronic disease outside the nervous system** were: coronary and pulmonary arteriosclerosis, chronic fibrous endocarditis, mitral sclerosis, aortic sclerosis with calcification, chronic splenitis, chronic interstitial nephritis, hepatic atrophy (wt., 900 grams), thickening of cartilaginous portion of right auricle (old trauma), scars of apices of lungs.

The **calvarium** was dense and the **dura mater** everywhere adherent. The **arachnoidal villi** were but slightly developed, but there was one small focus of cortical herniation through the dura mater of the left middle cranial fossa. The pia mater was delicate except for slight opacities along sulci. There was some pial thickening over the region of the inter-parietal sulci on both sides. There was pial pigmentation anteriorly and superiorly.

There is no gross evidence of intracranial arteriosclerosis, except (1) that afforded by the lesions of the dentate nuclei of the cerebellum mentioned below and (2) the swerving to the right of the basilar artery, possibly due not to arterio-sclerotic lengthening of the artery but to an unusual shape of the pons (see below).

The **brain** weighed 1245 grams (cerebellum and pons 165 grams). **The anatomical diagnoses of central nervous system** were:

Slight general encephalomalacia (post mortem imbibition of fluid, 31 hours). Slight gliosis of right prefrontal and frontal gyri. Slight gliosis of right optic thalamus. General-ized granular ependymitis, especially near fornix and about foramina of Monro. Anomaly of pons (not gliotic, but possessing far more white matter on the left side than the right). Severe arteriosclerosis confined to the dentate nuclei of the cerebellum.

As we now look over the data in Cases 40 and 41 we are inclined to ask the question, whether modern systematic diagnosis would not have shown these cases to be NEUROSYPHI-LITIC? One is inclined to answer this question in the affirma-tive, on the basis that Case 40 showed somewhat questionable Argyll-Robertson pupils, and Case 41 showed unilateral Argyll-Robertson effect. Both cases showed Romberg sign, but the dentate nucleus and other cerebellar disease in each case may in some way have contributed to or imitated this phenomenon. Whether Case 40 was a tabetic must remain a question, but Case 41 must be regarded as a case with spinal and meningeal changes highly characteristic of syphilis.

VASCULAR NEUROSYPHILIS plus TABETIC NEUROSYPHILIS ("tabes dorsalis") simulating paretic neurosyphilis ("general paresis"). Autopsy.

Case 42. The case of Elizabeth Brown was at one time carefully studied by Dr. A. M. Barrett in his work on mental diseases associated with cerebral arteriosclerosis and, like Case 43, was one in which tabes dorsalis was a factor. Elizabeth Brown's maternal grandfather and mother were insane; there had also been insanity in a sister. Mrs. Brown was struck on the head at 44, and was unconscious for an hour, but there were no sequelæ to this accident. At 48, there was a shock, or apoplectiform attack, followed by unconsciousness for two hours and by left hemiplegia, right ptosis, and thick speech. Mrs. Brown began to walk again after two weeks, but was found to be forgetful and fabulatory. She seemed at times to be hearing music, and somewhat repeatedly became helpless and unable to walk. She could not remember from day to day, showed incontinence of urine and feces, and was brought to the Danvers Hospital. The physical and mental deterioration was progressive. There were some signs of organic brain disease. The musculature was especially flabby on the left side. The left angle of the mouth drooped, and the left nasolabial fold was smoothed out. The arm movements were ataxic, the tongue protruded to the left, the right pupil reacted but slightly to light (eye blind from cataract), the knee-jerks, Achilles, wrist, and elbow reflexes, were absent. The patient was unable to stand, and there was a marked tremor of the hand, tongue, and lips. There was a zone of anesthesia for pain and tactile stimulation extending round the body, from the 3d to the 6th rib, and there were symmetrical areas of anesthesia on the inner surface of the forearms and the legs.

The **autopsy** showed a **general arteriosclerosis** with **chronic and acute meningitis.** The brain weighed 1110 grams;

the **pia mater** was moderately thickened; the basal vessels were highly arteriosclerotic. The brain itself, however, normal externally, upon dissection, showed a number of small cysts irregularly scattered in the white substance. The basal ganglia were porous, and there were several small cysts in the pons. **Microscopically,** there was evidence of severe vascular disease, involving not only the arteries but also the veins. It was the superficial rather than the deep arteries that were more often attacked. There was a marked **perivascular gliosis.** Extensive search yielded *no evidence of lymphocyte infiltrations*, either in the brain or in the spinal cord.

The spinal cord showed degenerations in both the lateral and posterior columns, of which the explanation may possibly be like that in our paradigm, Case 1.

Is the case of Elizabeth Brown one of neurosyphilis? We cannot definitely say on account of the non-availability of the modern systematic tests, but it may well be that the case, although certainly not one of paretic neurosyphilis, was one of TABES WITH VASCULAR COMPLICATIONS.

TABETIC NEUROSYPHILIS (" tabes dorsalis ")
with symptoms of cerebral origin producing a picture resembling taboparetic neurosyphilis (" taboparesis "). Autopsy.

Case 43. Robert Allen was the fifth case of error in the
diagnosis of general paresis analyzed some years since from
the staff meeting records of the Danvers Hospital. The
Allen case resembles the case of Elizabeth Brown in that
there was a combination of tabetic phenomena with cerebral
lesions of a non-paretic character at autopsy. But although there seemed to be an utter absence of inflammatory
cells (lymphocytosis) in the case of Elizabeth Brown (42),
there were some slight perivascular cell accumulations in
the Allen case, with a few mononuclear cells suggestive of
lymphocytes. The cerebrum, however, failed to show plasmocytosis. It was seriously diseased, showing a marked
neuroglia proliferation about the atrophic nerve cells.

Robert Allen was a printer coming from a long-lived race.
The following are the main facts:

Married in 1875 (two children, healthy); again married in
1893 (one child, healthy). Compositor from 1890. In 1898
and 1899 girdle and lancinating pains. Thereafter for
several years gait was unsteady. During 1904 and 1905
freedom from pains and improvement in gait but gradually
increasing irritability and nervousness. Stopped work on
last of March, 1905, owing to sudden increase of irritability,
emotionality, boastfulness, expansive schemes, and ataxia.

Habits: no tobacco, very little alcohol at long intervals.
No drug habits, no sexual irregularity known.

Committed to Danvers April 3, 1905, with slight muscular
development, poor nutrition, acne, irregular, poorly preserved
teeth, gingivitis, flat-foot, slight radial arteriosclerosis, slight
arcus senilis, a few hyaline casts, leucocytes, epithelial cells,
and trace of albumin in the urine, scar in sulcus, and enlarged
inguinal lymph nodes.

Ataxic gait, Romberg's sign, fibrillary twitching of chest, abdominal and facial muscles when standing; right pupil slightly larger than left, pupillary margins irregular, light reactions (electric bulb test) both consensual and direct absent, slight pupillary reaction in accommodation; biceps, triceps and wrist reflexes lively and equal; abdominal, cremasteric and plantar reflexes normal, knee-jerks, Achilles and front taps negative even on reënforcement.

The patient himself stated that his ataxia began in 1904, that he had been under treatment for swelling of legs and feet and pain in limbs since 1903, and that there had been some trouble with limbs since 1895. He had been told that his disease was lead-poisoning. About three weeks before commitment patient said he had had an attack of unconsciousness.

The patient's speech showed considerable defect. Words were pronounced slowly with slurring and tripping especially of the labials. Orientation perfect. School knowledge well retained. The easier arithmetical problems were accurately performed. Memory imperfect for minor recent events. Estimations of space and time often very imperfect. Variability of mood, sometimes euphoric, sometimes tearful and irritable. Occasional expansive estimates of personal powers ("Can lift three five-hundred pound weights with one finger"). Indistinct expansive financial ideas.

The patient continued oriented, euphoric, expansive, untidy, till October, 1905, but on October 12 developed an infection at the site of a callus on the sole of the foot and died with pyemic symptoms, October 17.

Post Mortem Findings. The **cause of death** was streptococcus septicemia with acute ulcerative colitis, acute splenitis, bilateral purulent pleuritis, multiple infarctions of lungs.

There were no signs of **chronic disease outside the nervous system** except a moderate thickening of the mitral valves, and slight dural adhesions.

The brain weighed 1450 grams. The vessels at the base showed a slight degree of sclerosis. There was a slight opacity of the frontal, parietal, and temporal pia overlying slightly atrophied convolutions, whose surfaces showed in a few places slight cuppings. The ependyma over the thalami and the floor of the fourth ventricle was finely roughened. The spinal cord showed a typical TABES DORSALIS.

Although we probably cannot regard either Case 42 or Case 43 as a case of paretic neurosyphilis, and although it must remain doubtful whether they are cases of any form whatever of neurosyphilis (in the absence of the modern tests), yet it seems clear that both these cases may very well have been cases of neurosyphilis on account of the existence of a definite tabetic process in each. The symptoms of these cases, like those of Cases 38 to 41, suggest how difficult it must be *to make a clinical diagnosis of general paresis safely without employing available laboratory tests.* Yet how frequently in the past have neurologists brought data concerning various phenomena in long series of so-called paretics in which the error of diagnosis was certainly between 5 and 15% and frequently still greater. The entire question of the symptomatology of paretic and non-paretic neurosyphilis, therefore, needs re-opening and revision.

CEREBRAL GLIOSIS (probably non-syphilitic)
producing the clinical picture of paretic neurosyphilis (" general paresis "). Autopsy.

Case 44. John Hughes was a hostler, and later assistant
with a wholesale drug company, with which he remained
for 32 years. He had been moderately but constantly alcoholic all his adult life up to 50 years of age, and at 45 had
had an attack of so-called nervous prostration, in which his
head had troubled him and he had been seclusive. At 49,
he had a serious attack of otitis media, associated with
delirium, swelling of the feet, and what was called rheumatism. After this attack of otitis media, Hughes appears to
have been not altogether right.

At 53, after a quarrel with his employer, Hughes quit
work, began to trade a little in hens and pigs, became forgetful, especially of recent events, and did " a variety of
peculiar things." He was a married man but he had no
children. There had been miscarriages but of unknown
origin; venereal disease was denied. At 55, a week before
admission, Hughes had a spell of unconsciousness for several
hours, after which his speech was thick, and restlessness, insomnia, and a wandering tendency set in. Visual hallucinations, fabulation, tremors, " excited-looking " eyes, are
described. He would sweep things from the dining-room
table, pulled a hot stove into the middle of the floor, attempted to sweep paint off the floor, and cut up a carpet
with a knife.

The patient on commitment November 5, 1904, was well
developed and nourished. The mucous membranes were
rather pale. Bruises and excoriations of limbs. Harsh
breathing at the base of each lung. Enlargement of heart;
sounds irregular. Accentuation of aortic second sound;
tension fair, rate 80. Slight brachial arteriosclerosis. Abdomen slightly distended. The urine contained a faint trace
of albumin and many hyaline casts.

Moderate tremor of extended hands. Slight tongue tremor. Romberg's sign absent (slight swaying). Considerable ataxia of extremities (inability to stand with foot on opposite knee). Vision poor. Hearing could not be tested accurately. Prompt pupil reactions with direct light. Slight consensual reaction in left pupil, absent in right. Deep reflexes equal and lively.

Quiet and orderly at first. Later restless and noisy. Questions were answered at times relevantly, more often irrelevantly. Patient irritable, intractable. Required repeated urging to take nourishment. Consciousness clouded. Orientation imperfect. Attendants are possibly " officers." Date September, 1995. Slight errors in repeating alphabet. Mistakes in Lord's Prayer with rhyming tendency. Simple arithmetical tests answered automatically with many mistakes. More complex combinations incorrect. Handwriting tremulous (noted as " typical of general paresis "). Auditory hallucinations (answering invisible persons), " All right, I'm coming." Amnesia and confabulation. Q. " Have you had breakfast? " A. " No," (later) " Yes, I had a very light breakfast." Q. " What did you have? " A. " Anything that came along. A few green peas and beans that were left, bread and butter and pie. I had a good breakfast. Guess feed is very high." Q. " Give names of your sisters and brothers." A. " There are three or four I never see. I will have to think them up." (Later) — " Lillie, Abbie, Julia, George." On repetition of question, " Elizabeth, Julia, Annie and Lizzie."

Delusions somewhat doubtful. At no time euphoria.

The patient remained only nine days in the hospital, developing diarrhea a week after admission.

Post Mortem Findings. The **cause of death** was bilateral bronchopneumonia of hypostatic distribution, accompanied by bronchitis and acute splenitis. The intestinal tract was normal (despite the diarrhea). No cultures. The heart showed acute myocarditis.

The vessels in general showed no sclerosis, except that the aorta showed a few patches with calcification near bifurcation. There was a moderate degree of mitral sclerosis. The kidneys showed a moderate degree of chronic interstitial nephritis. The heart weighed 530 grams and there was moderate dilatation of all the valves.

There were some evidences of chronic disease outside the nervous system, namely, an obliterative pleuritis on the right side, chronic perisplenitis, and chronic external adhesive pachymeningitis.

The **nervous system** showed a pia mater thin and transparent, with a moderate congestion of larger and smaller vessels. No noteworthy change of the brain substance or of the ventricles was found, except that the cerebral substance was of unusual firmness (autopsy twelve hours after death).

It is clear that the brain was not wholly normal, exhibiting a general induration due in part to subpial gliosis and in part doubtless to perivascular gliosis. **Microscopically** the tissues showed features of great interest, especially multiple focal neuroglia cell proliferations of a perivascular distribution, considerable subpial fibrillar gliosis of an unusually focal type, and a rather general subpial cellular **gliosis.** Histologically, it seemed that this chronic progressive process had started, not so much in relation with dying nerve cells, as in relation with blood vessels. The **perivascular** deposits of neuroglia cells were confined almost exclusively to the infragranular cortex layers. It seems plain that the diagnosis of general paresis was not justified. It is probable that the diagnosis neurosyphilis is not justified. The explanation may be that now and then cases of cerebral sclerosis may clinically imitate the neurosyphilitic process. It must be borne in mind that the diagnosis in this case was made, like the other cases at head of Part III, without the advantage of modern systematic methods. Clinically speaking, of course, there was no definite Argyll-Robertson pupil, although the consensual reaction, slight on the left side, was absent in the right pupil. The general picture appeared to be one of the so-called demented form of paretic neurosyphilis.

Differential diagnosis between NEUROSYPHILIS
and NEURASTHENIA.

Case 45. Albert Robinson, a man of 28 years, was ship-wrecked on one of the Great Lakes. The ship was on the rocks for eight days, and Robinson was under a great strain. Ever after the wreck, Robinson had felt severe pain in the head, neck, and back, and a feeling of great weakness whenever he exerted himself physically or mentally, and seven months after the wreck, he had several attacks of fainting.

For a number of weeks he had worried a good deal about his inability to make money, especially as money was badly needed on account of his wife's approaching confinement. A few days before entrance, Robinson had become very forgetful, and was unable to recall, the night before entrance, where he had been during the day. On the whole, however, on mental examination no actual evidence of memory defect could be shown to exist.

Physically, Robinson was entirely negative, except for some hard glands in each groin. **Mentally,** there was little to show except depression, worry over his financial condition, and his inability to work. The serum W. R. proved negative.

Diagnosis: On the whole, the diagnosis of psychoneurosis (see case Harrison (9)) due to the shock at the time of the shipwreck seemed to be proper. To be sure, the patient gave a history of a chancre at 25, treated for two years, after which he was declared cured.

However, following up the clue of admitted syphilis, rigorous questioning elicited the fact that a few months before there had been diplopia, lasting part of a day.

Lumbar puncture seemed desirable. The fluid was clear but contained 125 cells per cmm. with appropriately increased amounts of albumin and globulin. The spinal fluid W. R. was positive. The diagnosis of CEREBROSPINAL SYPHILIS seemed established.

The lesson of this case appears to be that perhaps we should never exclude syphilis until we have made an examination of the cerebrospinal fluid. The W. R. of the blood in meningo-vascular (non-paretic syphilis) is negative in many cases (the figure is sometimes set as high as 40%).

Treatment: After a half dozen injections of salvarsan, all symptoms disappeared and Robinson went back to work, claiming to be in a better condition than for some time past.

1.   How shall we explain such a symptom as the transient diplopia? This diplopia is probably an example of a neurorecidive, but it will be observed that it occurred without salvarsan therapy. See discussion above under the case of Bennett (34), where the general result of the neurorecidive inquiry launched by Ehrlich early in the history of salvarsan therapy showed that precisely similar phenomena had always occurred in neurosyphilis, whether under treatment or not. The anatomical and histopathological explanation of such phenomena is, of course, doubtful, but a review of the findings in the case of Alice Morton (1) will show how many apparently serious symptoms in neurosyphilitics are actually irritative or at least due to lesions which are entirely recoverable. We may suppose, first, a local proliferation of spirochetes; second, a local over-formation of toxic substances, directly or indirectly the product of spirochetosis; thirdly, a local exudation; fourthly, a local proliferation; fifthly, a combination of these phenomena, any or all of which may be regarded as but transient. We have sometimes found at autopsy very little exudate except in small areas; sometimes not more than a few mm. or cm. in superficial extent. Note, for example, the small areas of lymphocytosis demonstrable in but two foci in the case of Alice Morton, the paradigm placed at the beginning of this book.

NEUROSYPHILIS(?) in the SECONDARY STAGE
of syphilis.   HYSTERICAL symptoms.   Diagnosis?

Case 46. Alice Caperson was a colored girl of 18 years.
She had acquired syphilis five months before admission to
the hospital, and the secondary symptoms of this syphilis
had just disappeared before admission.

Very shortly after acquiring syphilis, the young negress
began to act peculiarly. She describes herself as having
a sort of nightmare, both when asleep and also when awake.
For instance, she saw her dead grandmother. It appeared
at first like a seraph; then it came nearer to her and seemed
to fill out; and then was dressed precisely as her grandmother
had been. This seraph appeared as though trying to tell her
something, but she could not make out what the something
was. The vision had appeared on two or three occasions.

Our examination detected little beyond instability and
irritability of mood with some depression. The patient
readily fell to weeping. She soon made friends in the wards,
however, and got on well. **Physical examination** was entirely negative but the W. R. of the blood serum was positive.
The W. R. of the spinal fluid was negative, as was the gold
sol reaction; there was an excess of albumin and a positive
globulin test; there were seven cells per cmm.

The psychiatric diagnosis of a case like that of Alice Caperson would waver between hysteria and dementia præcox.
However, as for dementia præcox there are hardly any
typical symptoms. There is insight into the hallucinations,
which are hypnagogic. There are, however, no hysterical
stigmata.

The spinal fluid reaction is typical of the secondary stage
of syphilis. It is commonly said that in every case of syphilis the nervous system is involved at some period, if only
to the degree shown in the present case. However, such
involvement tends to disappear both with and without antisyphilitic treatment, just as do the secondary skin symptoms.

So far as syphilis is concerned, the prognosis under radical treatment is as good as usual. We are inclined to regard the case as one of the HYSTERICAL or PSYCHOPATHIC group and inasmuch as cases occurring in the developmental stage of a patient's life are of fairly good general prognosis, we are inclined to regard the prognosis in this particular case as good under proper therapy and hygiene.

1. What is the relation of neuroses to syphilis? Neurasthenia, chorea, hysteria, and epilepsy are often grouped (for example, by Nonne) as neuroses bearing at times important relations to neurosyphilis. (For the relations of neurasthenia, chorea, and epilepsy, see cases of Greeley Harrison (9), Margaret Green (72), and David Borofski (49), respectively.) As for the hysteria shown in Caperson, Charcot enumerated syphilis among *agents provocateurs* of hysteria along with alcohol, lead, arsenic, and the like. Fournier has also considered the problem. It is clearly necessary to show that before infection there were no hysterical symptoms, and that the hysteria developed during the operation of the syphilitic process, and it is probably necessary to show that the symptoms will clear up under antisyphilitic treatment, if we are to concede the existence of a syphilitic hysteria.

2. What are the evidences of neurosyphilis in the secondary and primary stages of syphilis? As above stated, the findings in Caperson are typical enough. Wile and Stokes at first stated that 60 to 70% of the secondary syphilitics show changes in the spinal fluid; in a further article they maintain that probably every case shows such changes and that clinical symptoms of neurosyphilis of the secondary period can probably be determined. They claim that it is probable also that the same holds for primary syphilis itself. The importance of these claims lodges partly in the relation of these early signs of neurosyphilis to the whole question of latency and to the question of *paresis sine paresi*. For a discussion of *paresis sine paresi* see cases Lawlor (25), Vogel (52).

Differential diagnosis between **NEUROSYPHILIS**
and **MANIC-DEPRESSIVE PSYCHOSIS.***

Case 47. As in other instances (compare Martha Bartlett
(21) and Annie Monks (85)) so also in the case of Ethel Hunter,
a woman 61 years of age, there was no initial suspicion of
neurosyphilis. Mrs. Hunter was brought to the hospital
stuporous as a result of an overdose of paraldehyd. The
paraldehyd had been administered by a physician to combat
insomnia and agitation. As soon as Mrs. H. had recovered
from the drug stupor, this agitation appeared once more, and
it was clear that she was suffering from marked depression.
There was tremendous worry over the sickness of a woman
with whom the patient lived. The patient was very self-
accusatory, blaming herself for many things that had happened in the household. Besides her agitation, depression,
self-accusations, and insomnia, the patient showed a good
deal of the symptom frequently termed " retardation " —
a kind of lagging of all mental processes found, according to
Kraepelin, in manic-depressive psychosis.

Accordingly, the diagnosis of manic-depressive psychosis
might well have been rendered. The fact that the psychosis
so far as known began in the involution period was not against
the diagnosis since the so-called involution-melancholia of
this period is at least in a certain fraction of cases nothing
more or less than a form of manic-depressive psychosis.
However, the **physical examination** made the diagnosis of
manic-depressive psychosis a little doubtful. There was a
superficial thickening of the arteries (blood pressure: systolic,
170; diastolic, 104), which thickening would not in itself be
against the diagnosis of manic-depressive psychosis. (In
point of fact, arteriosclerosis is rather common late in this

---

* A. M. Barrett has recently discussed this subject in a
paper in the *Journal of the American Medical Association*,
Vol. LXVII, Dec. 2, 1916.

disease and previous attacks could not be excluded on the basis of available history.) The contracted pupils were irregular and both reacted sluggishly to light, although better to accommodation; the right pupil was larger than the left. The arm reflexes were pretty active. The left knee-jerk could not be obtained, nor was the right knee-jerk more than very sluggish. The Achilles reflexes could not be obtained. Although there was not a positive Romberg sign, there was a considerable swaying in Romberg position. There was no speech defect. The other reflexes showed nothing abnormal. On the whole, we had to conclude that, although Mrs. Hunter might be an instance of manic-depressive psychosis, still there was much of neurological interest in the case.

This conclusion was emphasized when the W. R. of the blood serum was found to be positive. The spinal fluid W. R. was also positive, and the gold sol index was of the " paretic " type. There were 74 cells to the cmm. Globulin stood at +.+++, and albumin at ++++.

This case, therefore, again illustrates, as well the protean nature of GENERAL PARESIS (the diagnosis rendered), as the doubtful value of making a psychiatric diagnosis without due consideration of the physical examination and laboratory findings. How easy might it have been, at least some years ago, to consider that this patient of 61 years had suffered a slight shock at some previous time (left knee-jerk absent), but was as a matter of fact a case of manic-depressive psychosis with a vascular complication!

Note: We must again duly insist that the merely sluggish light reactions of the pupils in such a case as this do not especially point to general paresis. The literature seems to establish that sluggishness of light reaction precedes the classical Argyll-Robertson pupil. Yet it does not do to say that, if the Argyll-Robertson pupil pretty conclusively points to neurosyphilis (for exceptions see cases Falvey (55), Murphy (60)), then a sluggish pupillary reaction to light looks in the same direction. Sluggishness may precede stiffness in many, or perhaps all, cases, but sluggishness of pupils is a frequent phenomenon outside the syphilitic group of cases.

1. What part is played by emotional shock and psychic causes in the starting up of general paresis? The answer to this question cannot be definite. That a paretic process can be started up after trauma is admitted on all sides; but we here suppose actual physical or chemical brain disturbance permitting increased spirochetosis or inflammatory reaction. In the case of psychic shock, or what might be called *psychogenic general paresis*, our best resort will be to the indirect effects of hormone action, or of vasomotor and other autonomic disturbances produced directly or indirectly by emotion. We are clearly here dealing with material too speculative to be of practical service at this time.

2. Was the depressive drug therapy in the case of Hunter justifiable? The paraldehyd had been administered by a physician apparently on purely symptomatic grounds to combat the insomnia and agitation of this woman of 61 years. With all due acknowledgment of the difficulties of private practice, we must insist that when ordinary measures in the relief of insomnia and agitation are insufficient to curb these conditions, then a positive danger ensues with the larger doses. As a rule, with these larger doses and with the withdrawal of sensory stimulation, the patients relapse into a stupor of grave moment. We need only recall the situation in delirium tremens where adequately depressive drugs often tend to kill the patient.

Case for diagnosis. Errors in the diagnosis of
NEUROSYPHILIS are possible even when abundant clinical and laboratory data are available.

Case 48. The first error chosen for demonstration is that
in the case of the machinist, Milton Safsky.

Safsky, about 8 months before his entrance to the hospital
in the 42d year of his life, had begun to lose strength, to grow
thin and pale, and to suffer from an extreme and continuous
thirst. He was said to have drunk as much as 6½ gal. in a day,
and passed appropriately large quantities of urine. After a
time, his management at a general hospital became difficult,
as Safsky became confused, cried "hysterically," and was at
times very noisy. He sustained a marked memory loss,
seemed to show visual hallucinations, and complained of
headache, both frontal and occipital, and of pain about the
eyes. Sometimes the patient was very euphoric and expressed what seemed to be delusions of grandeur, saying he
was wealthy and owned many machine shops.

Some symptoms, e.g., polydipsia and polyuria amounting
to a diabetes insipidus, associated with headache and arrested
attention, suggested possibly a new growth in the pituitary
region. The mental symptoms might naturally be supposed
to be due to some infiltration or pressure effect of intracranial
growth. After admission to the Psychopathic Hospital, the
patient was found difficult to arouse, although he could
eventually be aroused. His orientation proved to be as poor
as his memory. From time to time, the patient became a
bit more intelligent and able to execute requests.

The **physical examination** was in general almost entirely
negative. **Neurologically,** the pupils were markedly contracted and reacted slowly to light, though they were otherwise normal. The deep reflexes were all somewhat lively,
though equal. The umbilical and cremasteric reflexes in
particular were present. Systematic examination revealed
no other reflex disorder, nor any disturbance of sensation.

There was a coarse tremor of the extended hands. There were no phenomena of importance in the visual fields.

As against the diagnosis of growth, pituitary or extra-pituitary (diabetes insipidus and headache), a hypothesis of neurosyphilis had to be considered. Not only were the con-tracted, slowly-reacting pupils and the active deep reflexes suggestive, but the euphoria with grandiose ideas looked entirely consistent. As for the polyuria, one had to think of the so-called syphilitic polyuria of the textbooks, which is regarded as a more or less characteristic result of syphilitic involvement of the *basis cerebri*. Moreover, the W. R. in the spinal fluid proved to be slightly positive; 146 cells per cmm. were found therein; there was a large quantity of globulin, and a very marked increase in albumin. These observations seemed to be exceedingly suggestive of a cerebral syphilis.

However, as the case progressed, the diagnostic situation changed. The W. R. upon a second puncture fluid proved negative. After some weeks, characteristic symptoms of in-tracranial pressure developed; the diagnosis of BRAIN TUMOR had to be taken as established, and there is no doubt of its correctness.

1. What is the explanation of the weakly positive W. R. in Safsky's spinal fluid? An explanation is not easy to find. Possibly we may regard the reaction as an ex-ample of error in technique. It is even possible that it may have been produced by exudative products in the spinal fluid.

2. What precautions may be taken against an error in diagnosis such as was first made through the positive spinal fluid Wassermann in the case of Safsky? First, repetition of the W. R.; secondly, it is very unusual to find a weakly positive W. R. in a case with such marked excess of albumin and such very marked in-crease of globulin as was shown by this case.

3. How can we explain the inflammatory products in the puncture fluid? Superficial brain tumors are fre-quently associated with a so-called *meningitis sym-pathica*. The products of such meningitis are ex-hibited: *viz.*, globulin, albumin, and pleocytosis, exactly as shown in Safsky.

Can PARETIC NEUROSYPHILIS ("general paresis") appear clinically EARLY (e.g., two years) after the initial syphilitic infection?

Case 49. David Borofski, a street car conductor, 27 years of age, suddenly had a convulsion while at work in his car. For four months Borofski continued to have rather numerous convulsions, was finally compelled to discontinue work, and resorted to the Psychopathic Hospital. It appears from his own story that, about two years before, he had had a chancre, for which he had been treated at a general hospital syphilis clinic, and of which he was told he was cured. With a progressive loss of memory and with convulsions, Borofski became much concerned about himself, and was finally persuaded by his fellow-workers to come to the Psychopathic Hospital.

The convulsions were described as follows: The patient gives a short cry, has convulsive movements for about ten minutes, remains unconscious for perhaps half an hour, and wakes with headache, dizziness, and a feverish appearance. Sometimes the attacks were more severe, with frothing at the mouth, biting of lips, and loss of sphincter control. There were also slight attacks, occurring almost every day, without loss of consciousness; these latter attacks consisted of dizziness, inability to speak for a few seconds, and some arm twitching.

Physically, Borofski was well developed and nourished, with a blood pressure of 160. The only abnormal phenomena **neurologically** were absent knee-jerks and ankle-jerks, sluggish pupillary reactions, and slight tremor of the hands.

Mentally, despite suggestive complaint of amnesia, the memory was found to be fairly good but knowledge of current events and school knowledge was poor. The simplest problems in arithmetic Borofski gave up.

The first diagnosis in such a case would naturally be epilepsy. However, when an epileptic or epileptiform attack occurs for the first time in adult life, the chances are probably against an idiopathic epilepsy. (This is not a universal rule but will serve.) Borofski himself, moreover, gave a history of syphilis. And the very nature of the attacks, with arm twitching and without loss of consciousness, would not readily fit into the frame of the idiopathic group. The absence of certain reflexes and the sluggish pupils are naturally also suggestive of syphilis, although not convincing.

The W. R. of the serum proved positive, as did that of the spinal fluid. The gold sol reaction was characteristically " paretic"; there was an excess of albumin and a positive globulin, and there were 15 cells per cmm. There could be little or no doubt of the diagnosis of some form of neuro-syphilis. The laboratory picture was consistent either with general paresis or with cerebrospinal syphilis. So far as we are aware in the present stage of knowledge, the two conditions can hardly be differentiated unless we choose to rely on therapeutics. However, it is exceedingly rare for general paresis to occur only two years after the original infection. If we can trust this statistical fact, we shall perhaps be wiser to term the case of Borofski one of DIFFUSE CEREBROSPINAL SYPHILIS, and not one of paresis.

Treatment: Borofski was put on antisyphilitic treatment consisting of 0.6 gram of salvarsan twice a week and potassium iodid, together with intramuscular injections of mercury salicylate. The convulsions then ceased. After four months Borofski returned to work, and he has remained at work for a year. He has never regained his former health.

Fifteen months after beginning of treatment the laboratory tests were again made (there had been more than 60 injections of salvarsan), and the cell count and gold sol reactions were found to be negative. Globulin and albumin were also in smaller amounts than in the original examination. However, the W. R. of the serum and the spinal fluid remained positive.

Head and Fearnsides state that cases of cerebrospinal syphilis should return negative spinal fluid tests after six months of treatment. Upon this criterion of Head and Fearnsides, Borofski would not be a case of cerebrospinal syphilis; but it is probably impossible to separate various forms of neurosyphilis into categories on any such grounds.

1. Shall case David Borofski be regarded as one of paretic neurosyphilis ("general paresis")? He has returned to work and has remained at work, though without regaining his former health. In any event, however, he does not offer the typical picture of inevitable decline and death presented by the typical case of Pietro Martiro (15) presented in our discussion of systematic diagnosis. However, we could not upon laboratory grounds, or even upon the ground of clinical observation, distinguish Borofski from Martiro; Borofski has greatly improved; Martiro is dead. Borofski developed his obvious neurosyphilis only two years after the original infection. The conservative syphilographer might, accordingly, reply that David Borofski is not a typical case of paretic neurosyphilis ("general paresis") either in the length of the incubation period for his neurosyphilitic symptoms, or in his outcome.

2. What is the cause of such convulsions as those developed by David Borofski? Evidence from clear cases of general paresis with convulsions leads to the hypothesis that such convulsions as those developed by Borofski are not necessarily based upon frank destructive lesions such as would be produced by the plugging of terminal arteries. They may well be produced through the activities of minor lesions, only demonstrable by microscopic methods, either through properly disposed cell losses or by the pressure of exudate, or even by endotoxins or other substances derived from the bodies of dead or living spirochetes.

3. Aside from the well-known syphilitic epilepsy due to meningitis, is there a non-meningitic epilepsy (such a disease as Fournier formerly described under the term parasyphilitic epilepsy)? We dismiss from discussion the so-called symptomatic epilepsies which are the result of a gross organic disease of the brain substance or its membranes, and which do not differ so far as we are aware from organic epilepsy produced by other gross lesions of an identical size and structure. These symptomatic epilepsies may be partial, or even may present the appearance of generalized epilepsy. We may also leave out of account those epileptic pictures which are produced in general paresis itself, and which

may be viewed as nothing but partial phenomena of general paresis. The kind of so-called "parasyphilitic" epilepsy that Fournier described is a kind of epilepsy that cannot be distinguished from genuine epilepsy, in which the sole disease-phenomenon throughout a long period of time consists of epileptic convulsions. It appears that these "parasyphilitic" imitations of genuine epilepsy occur in individuals with a very long post-infective "incubation period," but that there are some cases in which the epilepsy appears, on the contrary, in the very earliest stages of syphilis. The attacks are a little less common than those of idiopathic epilepsy; they have the same apparently causeless beginning; are associated with complete amnesia; and are followed by characteristic dazed states. The patient's intelligence, however, suffers little. Now and then a case reacts well to antisyphilitic treatment energetically pushed. (Spontaneous long remissions in non-syphilitic epilepsy must be remembered.) Petit mal attacks occur sometimes between the more severe attacks. In short, it would appear that there is a group of syphilitic epilepsies in which the brain shows no gross structural lesions, which accordingly do not exhibit any Jacksonian appearances, and which last a comparatively long time without changing their character, and often without being especially altered for the better by any form of antisyphilitic treatment. This condition is sometimes known as a post-syphilitic epileptic neurosis. Nonne had been able to collect up to 1902 some 12 cases from his own service.

4. Would it be proper to call Borofski a case of taboparesis? Absent knee-jerks in a victim of paretic neurosyphilis should not be used to suggest a diagnosis of taboparesis. This question of terminology has been discussed above, under Sullivan (16).

5. What is the mechanism by which the amnesia of a case like Borofski is produced? The answer runs in the same terms as the answer to the questions concerning the cause of convulsions. The amnesia in general paresis has surprising functionality. A study of autopsied cases of general paresis has shown that amnesia is practically as common in cases without marked destruction of brain tissue as in cases with atrophy of classical extent and depth. The clinical recovery in this case was practically complete in respect to memory. We must regard the amnesia as not due to the destruc-

tion of storage cells bearing the so-called neurograms (Morton Prince).

6. What is the explanation of the persistently positive W. R.'s of the serum and spinal fluid associated with diminished globulin and albumin tests, a negative gold sol reaction, and normal cell count? See discussion under Case Martha Bartlett (21).

7. How atypical is the early development of paretic symptoms in David Borofski? C. B. Craig has collected, in 100 cases of brain syphilis (a list including both paretic and non-paretic cases), some data on this point. The shortest period reported by Craig was in a case in which the neurosyphilitic symptoms appeared one month after infection. Craig found three cases where symptoms appeared in six months, and six cases within a year. The longest post-infective period of Craig's list was thirty years. Our case of Chatterton (73) developed symptoms 33 years after infection and Washington (66), forty years after infection. Nonne casts some doubt on statements to the effect that tabetic symptoms may occur three to four months after infection. It seems to be admitted that pupillary anomalies and reflex changes may occur in the early secondaries and may recover under antisyphilitic treatment. Nonne's case of longest post-infective interval, like that of Craig, was one of 30 years.

Myerson has reported a 20-year old patient who acquired chancre April 1, 1911 (spirochetes demonstrated); salvarsan was administered April 20th. There were no secondary symptoms, but in May, headache, visual disturbance, vertigo, and other symptoms developed (neurorecidive). Upon June 20th, that is, 11 weeks after development of the chancre, aphasia and astasia developed, with numbness of the left side. At this time, the pupils were slightly irregular and unequal but reacted normally. The signs in the fluid were positive. Upon this question see our cases of Bright (121) and Bennett (34).

HEMITREMOR following hemiplegia in PARETIC NEUROSYPHILIS (" general paresis "). Autopsy.

Case 50. Achilles Akropovlos, 39 years, had symptoms six months before commitment to Danvers Hospital. There were attacks of confusion, difficulty in walking, and speech defect, resulting in an entire incapacity to work and eventual commitment. Rather unusual and striking was a very marked tremor, apparently limited to the right side of the body. **Physically,** Akropovlos was normal, but **neurologically** he showed, in addition to the marked right-sided tremor, a marked speech defect, and a degree of ataxia. The tendon reflexes were very active, but there were no abnormal reflexes, and the pupils reacted normally. According to the history, the difficulty had followed a slight attack of apoplexy. **Mentally,** there was a marked confusion. The blood serum and the spinal fluid were both positive to the W. R.; globulin was present, and albumin was increased; there were 43 cells per cmm. There was hardly any diagnosis to make except general paresis.

Death followed 18 months later, or two years after onset of symptoms. Increasing weakness, emaciation, and dementia preceded death. Autopsy confirmed the diagnosis of PARETIC NEUROSYPHILIS.

1. What is the usual cause of death in general paresis? Intercurrent disease very frequently occurs in general paresis, and such intercurrent disease is then given as the cause of death. As a matter of fact, however, one feels that in many of these cases the intercurrent pneumonia or infection — frequently of the bladder, — bedsores, sepsis, and the like, are merely accidental incidents in a condition that is leading to death, and which has caused a lowered resistance to infection. In certain instances where nursing is exceptionally good and where no such infection occurs, the patient continues to grow weaker and weaker, paralyses of all the muscles follow and finally paralysis of deglutition or

respiration may lead to death. The emaciation and paralyses may be of such a grade that the patient is entirely devoid of fat and unable to move at all. Not infrequently vascular crises occur, and one of these may be responsible for death.

2. What was the cause of the hemitremor? The hemitremor suggested an irritative or destructive lesion in the motor path. Delving into the history it was learned that the patient had had a shock followed by a right hemiparesis. This had cleared up leaving the tremor as a residuum. The autopsy disclosed a reddish-brown pigmentation and fibrous thickening of the pia over the left motor area, confirming the idea of a previous hemorrhage. As a rule the shock phenomena occurring in paresis clear up more completely and no gross lesion is visible post-mortem. However, cerebral hemorrhage must be expected in any person suffering from syphilis, and is no rarity in paretic neurosyphilis.

PARETIC NEUROSYPHILIS (" general paresis ")
with NORMALLY REACTING PUPILS. History
of trauma. Autopsy.

Case 51. Daniel Wheelwright, a barber of English extraction, 57 years of age, had had a sunstroke at 15. At 42, there had been pneumonia, after which an attack of rheumatism was said to have kept the patient from work for a year. There was trauma of head (falling wrench) at 44. This blow on the head was the assigned cause of the mental disease, symptoms of which, however, did not develop until about the first of September, 1905, about three months before entrance, January 9, 1906, and about six months before death, March 20, 1906.

It seems that the patient had begun to change in manner; he had become despondent and apathetic, silent, and somnolent. Two weeks later, he stopped working, began to read the papers once more, and became somewhat more cheerful.

About Thanksgiving, Wheelwright got up at midnight, and remained up, lighting all the fires and talking continuously. During the next two weeks, he talked much to himself, laughing out at times. About two weeks before Christmas he went out and started to make a sidewalk of old boards, working in his shirtsleeves, without a hat. He would work until midnight making screens for windows. During the day, he would go out and give money to passing children; would offer to pay the grocer twice as much as articles were worth.

On the day before Christmas, he put out all the fires and lights in the house, sent all the family to bed, and opened all the doors. Christmas morning, he rose early and got the washtubs ready. He helped his compliant wife to do the washing, then put out all the fires and opened the windows. After Christmas, he began to tell how rich he was going to be through starting a garden and by making butter. He bought six or seven quarts of milk daily, and procured carrots and oranges, grinding them up to color the milk. January 9th he was committed to Danvers Hospital.

Physically, there were few symptoms. **Neurologically,** there was a tremor of tongue, fingers, and face. The knee-jerks were lively. The pupils reacted normally; the patient was restless, pacing up and down. There was a speech defect demonstrable with test phrases. Orientation was imperfect for time and for place. Hand-writing was poor, memory impairment was marked, but the patient was given to fabrication as to past events. A characteristic sample of statements:

" Do you know that this is an insane hospital?" " Yes; there are two or three men here out of their heads. I could cure them with my hands but they won't let me. I could get all the sick men on their feet just by rubbing them. I can do anything with my hands. I can build a house by just sitting down and thinking about it. I can whip all the men in this place. I have better sense now than I ever had in my life."

Again, " How long have you been here?" " Over three months; they have put me in heaven three times since I have been here. They killed me, crushed my heart, and turned my blood to water. I am all right now. I let the sun shine on my heart and it brought it together. I can whip every man in here as fast as they come up."

Again, " I will make a million dollars on my garden when I get it. I can make a million dollars on half an acre. I can do anything. I can move this house by just thinking of it."

During a special examination, the patient told how he had fastened wings on his hands and feet, and how he had gone to heaven; he told how he had soared high above the earth, and how differently the stars look when up near heaven than they do from the earth. He spoke of seeing angels and of the beauties of heaven.

The diagnosis of PARETIC NEUROSYPHILIS was confirmed at autopsy.

1. What is the significance of the normally reacting pupils? While it is usual to find pupillary anomalies in neurosyphilis, these changes are not an essential part and it is not rare to find normal pupils in all forms of neurosyphilis. It is less frequent to find a normal pupil in tabetic than in diffuse or paretic neurosyphilis. In paretic neurosyphilis it is the rule to find pupillary changes during some stage of the disease, but not necessarily early. At times the pupillary sign may be one of the earliest signs of neurosyphilis — again it may occur only as a late symptom, if at all. One of the most important of the pupillary signs is irregularity of contour. While this does not always mean neurosyphilis it is highly suggestive and certainly indicates careful examination even though the W. R. in the blood be negative.

2 What was the relation of trauma to the development of the neurosyphilitic symptoms? It is, of course, the rule in all forms of mental disease to have some factor offered by the patient or relatives as the cause of the psychosis. Often these assigned causes are minor events thought of only after the later appearance of symptoms. In this case it was not thought that the trauma had any causal effect. For a discussion of trauma and neurosyphilis see cases Joseph O'Hearn (90), Levi Sussman (91), and Joseph Larkin (92).

NEUROSYPHILIS, probably PARETIC, with
symptoms highly suggestive of MANIC-DEPRES-
SIVE PSYCHOSIS.

Case 52. Bessie Vogel* was admitted to the Psychopathic hospital New Year's day, 1915, in a very much excited condition. The family history is very meagre, and all
that is of significance is that mother has always been very
" nervous." The records in part:

Past History. Very healthy as a child, and except for occasional throat trouble and headache had no physical ailments
until eight years ago, when she had an operation for appendicitis, and two and one-half years ago was operated upon for
hernia and adhesions. Following this she began to show a
lack of energy, neglected her housework, was much depressed,
wept frequently, complained constantly of pain in various
places, and was ill-tempered. In about five months she
improved, and then after a couple of weeks at the shore
seemed entirely well.

Present Illness. In November, 1914, that is, about
seventeen months after the recovery from the previous depression, she again began to show practically the same
symptoms. She was depressed, could not sleep, and would
get up in the night and sew; was self-centered and hyper-
sensitive, then became restless and nervous; wanted to go
shopping and out for dinner; went to New York and then to
New Bedford. Symptoms became more marked; she became very ill-tempered, threatened her husband when angry
over trifles, threatened suicide, then began to get active and
spent money extravagantly. At the end of two months, that
is, Jan. 1, 1915, she was admitted to the hospital.

Physical Examination. A small, thin woman, appearing
to be about 45 years old (actual age 37). Aside from the

---

* Reprinted from an article by Southard & Solomon:
" Latent neurosyphilis and the Question of *Paresis sine
paresi.*" Boston Medical and Surgical Journal, XXIV, 1.

absence of teeth and the operation scars, the general examination is negative. **Neuromuscular system:** The pupils
are round, regular, equal, and react to light and accommodation, but do not hold very well. Extraocular movements well performed, no palsies of facial muscles, tongue
protruded medially without tremor. Uvula is raised symmetrically. Biceps and triceps and supinator reflexes are
present and brisk. Patellar and Achilles reflexes are equal
on the two sides and brisk. Abdominal skin reflexes not
obtained. Plantar reflex active and flexor in type. No
Babinski, Gordon, or Oppenheim. No tremors.

Wassermann reaction serum positive. Examination of
spinal fluid: clear, globulin $++++$, albumin $++++$;
cells, 130 per cmm.; small lymphocytes, 79.9%; large lymphocytes, 14.1%; polymorphonuclear leucocytes, 4.6%;
plasma cells, 0.7%; endothelial cell, 0.7%. W. R. positive.
Gold sol reaction, 55555522 $+ -$.

Mental Examination. On admission patient showed great
psychomotor activity, was very playful, marked flight of
ideas, was expansive, very emotional, very erotic. She
slept very little, appetite was poor, and she lost weight
rapidly. Orientation and memory intact. No hallucinations
elicited. In about three weeks improvement began, and at
the end of eight weeks she appeared practically recovered.
On April 9, 1915, — that is, 13 weeks after admission, —
she was allowed home on visit. On leaving, she appeared
normal in every way. There was no evidence of psychotic
symptoms, she had good insight, and physically there was
absolutely nothing of a neurological nature that was abnormal.

This case, with the history of a previous depression and its
clinical picture during the acute stage, and its recovery,
is certainly in every respect typical of manic-depressive insanity, and only the positive result of the six tests causes us
to put it in the group of GENERAL PARESIS. Only the further
course will shed any light as to the correct significance of
these findings, and even then we shall not be too sure that we
had not been dealing with a manic-depressive psychosis in a
latent neurosyphilitic. We would strongly emphasize the
point that at the present time this patient presents no mental

or physical signs of cerebrospinal syphilis or general paresis; but the six tests are still positive. This case differs from the ordinary general paresis remission in that there is not a single physical sign of paresis present.

There are many transitional cases between this case which shows no symptoms or signs of neurosyphilis except the laboratory tests, and the typical case of general paresis. Thus we have cases with slight character change and no physical signs except rare " seizures." On the other hand, in many cases the presence of abnormal neurological phenomena without definite mental signs is first noted. Certain remitted cases show only some slight pupillary or reflex abnormality. We believe we have here added the last link in the chain between the primary and quaternary symptoms.

This case is illustrative of several which we have published elsewhere under the name of *paresis sine paresi* or latent neurosyphilis to illustrate how all the laboratory signs of neurosyphilis may be present in a patient without any physical or mental symptoms that may be correlated with these findings.

We summarize our discussion of this as follows:

1. There is a group of cases showing the laboratory signs characteristic of central nervous system syphilis: (a) positive W. R. in the serum, (b) positive W. R. in the spinal fluid, (c) pleocytosis, (d) excess of albumin, and (e) of globulin in the spinal fluid, (f) gold sol reaction of central nervous system syphilis, and which show no sign or symptom of neurosyphilis.

2. We believe these cases represent a form of chronic cerebrospinal syphilis, probably paretic in type.

3. They have the greatest theoretical and practical significance in the consideration of the life history of neural syphilis, in the concept of *Allergie*, in regard to results of treatment, and finally as to the evaluation of the laboratory tests.

4. Here is perhaps offered the last link to form a complete chain between the symptoms of the primary stage of syphilis and its final termination of life as the result of the diseases cerebrospinal syphilis or general paresis.

**SYPHILIS (?); EXOPHTHALMIC GOITRE; neu-
rosyphilitic old lesion of optic thalamus; unilateral
induration and atrophy of left cerebral cortex.
Autopsy.**

Case 53. Carrie Pearson, a housewife 25 years of age, died
at Danvers Hospital less than a week after admission, and it
was at first stated that her symptoms had lasted but two
weeks before admission. In point of fact, a further investigation showed an important succession of symptoms, lasting
some four years.

Carrie had been considered a healthy child, going to school
at the usual age, and progressing well with her studies. She
however, left school in the ninth grammar grade, at the age
of 15, and went to work in a milltown. She married a worth-
less person at the age of 18, and lived with her husband
for three years. There was one child born a year after
marriage. Two years later, however, a tremendous goitre
had developed such that her neck was described as " out
square with the face," and at the same time the patient's
eyes had become prominent.

About two weeks before admission, she had gone to a
neighboring town to take care of a sick woman, but during
her endeavor to be a nurse, she had broken out into a mania,
tearing up furniture and bedding, and talking irrelevantly
for a period of four days. She also showed insomnia and
continually tore off her clothing from her body.

Upon **examination,** the marked enlargement of the thyroid
gland together with the prominent eyeballs, husky voice, and
pulse rate of 150 per minute, were entirely consistent with
the diagnosis of exophthalmic goitre. The patient described
herself as " Carrie Nation." Asked to write her name,
she took the pen and tried to spatter ink, wrote hurriedly and
carelessly her maiden name and several words without apparent meaning. Asked to write, " God save the Commonwealth of Massachusetts," she wrote: " God save the

common pal U S Spe Manor Gen, or til pat. Since Lord, or
no prime in Hear to the God Tel. Ho. n and or Mabel, or gal."
After this, she took paper and wrote meaningless scrawls,
saying that it was Japanese writing. There was much
motor restlessness with distractibility, pointing and grimacing, mimicking the actions of those about her.

Death occurred from exhaustion, and the case might not
have been regarded as unusual except for the autopsy, which
showed a peculiar brain lesion, described below. The point
of greatest interest in the case was the fact that syphilis is,
although not proved to exist by laboratory tests, beyond
question a factor in the case. Although the woman had
given birth to a normal child, who is still alive, yet in the
period of a few years her breasts had atrophied, her hair had
disappeared from the axilla and from the pubes; varicose
veins had developed in both legs. Whereas there was little
or no fat over the chest or back, the omentum and mesentery
were very plentifully supplied with fat. It is probable, then,
that we are dealing with a case of exophthalmic goitre somehow of syphilitic origin. The brain lesion is consistent with
this hypothesis.

Autopsy, March 3, 1907. Four hours post-mortem.
Body length, 165 cm. Body of a well developed and
well nourished young woman. Lividity in dependent
parts. Purplish discoloration of left thigh to knees.
Skin rough and scaly. Petechial eruption over chest.
Neck thick, protrudes anteriorly. Varicose veins over
upper parts of calves on both legs. Eyes protruding,
not covered entirely by lids. Pupils equal, dilated.
Subcutaneous fat very deep over lower part of body.
Very little fat over chest and back. Breasts are very
small, apparently atrophied. Normal amount of hair
on head, slight amount over pubes. Axillary hair absent. Fat on section of a light yellow color. Omentum
extends to pubes, plentifully supplied with fat. Large
amount of mesenteric fat. Appendix normal. Intestines smooth and glistening. Slightly injected. No
fluid in peritoneum. Uterus small, retroverted.

HEAD: HAIR in good quantity. SCALP normal.
CALVARIUM shows diploë. DURA MATER over left
cerebral hemisphere inseparably adherent to calvarium,

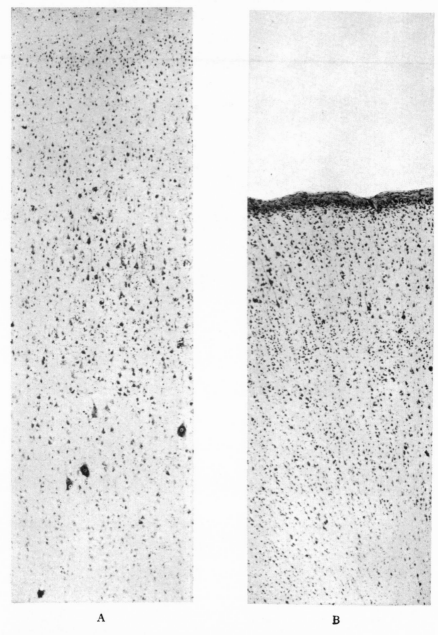

A   B

Cortical hemiatrophy — A, relatively normal right precentral ("motor") cortex; B, atrophic left precentral.

Note in B:

1. Absence of giant pyramids of Betz (corticospinal, upper motor neurones).

2. Superficial (subpial) condensation of tissues with sclerosis (gliosis). The tissues in all areas examined *on the left side* yielded this effect.

over right hemisphere normal. Arachnoidal VILLI
moderately developed. PIA MATER shows injected
veins, notably in the sulci of the right hemisphere.
Pia mater everywhere thin and clear. VESSELS at base
of normal appearance.

BRAIN weight 1180 grams. Spread on a board, the
right hemisphere tends to flatten so that it measures
1.5 cm. more from side to side than its fellow. Besides more marked venous injection, the right hemisphere shows also flatter and slightly more plastic
convolutions. The posterior poles of the hemispheres
are a little firmer than the parts anterior. The orbital
and hippocampal gyri on the right side are a little
firmer than the surrounding parts. On section the
gray and white matter shows no lesions, excepting the
slight plasticity of the tissues at large on the right side
and a well marked induration, with retraction under
the knife, of the occipital and hippocampal white
matter. The basal ganglia of the left side are
normal. On the right side a sagittal section demonstrates a rounded area of induration, with ill-defined
borders, measuring perhaps 1.5 cm. from above downwards by 2 × 2 cm., situated largely in the lenticular
nucleus and involving the greater portion of the globus
pallidus, a small segment of the putamen below and
behind and the regionary part of the anterior commissure with surrounding tissues. The most striking
feature of this lesion is the occurrence in the middle
of a cluster of vacuoles or cystic clefts, with smooth
pale interiors, ranging from pin-head to 0.25 cm. or even
0.5 cm. in greatest diameters. There are six to eight
clefts to a surface of section. The color of the lesion
differs little from that of the globus pallidus itself, but
the tissue is a trifle translucent. It is impossible to
demarcate the lesion with the eye. Induration is demonstrable several mm. beyond the visible part of the
lesion. The consistence of the lesion slightly surpasses
the usual consistence of the olivary bodies.

CERREBELLUM, PONS and BULB weight 165 grams.
Cerebellar tissue a trifle more plastic than usual.
The right olive is not so prominent as usual.

Note. THYROID: Weight 125 grams. Both lobes
and isthmus enlarged. One lobe more than the other;
lobe on one side measuring 6 × 4 cm.

Anatomical Diagnoses

Enlargement of thyroid gland.
Exophthalmos with dilated pupils.
Fatty degeneration of thoracic muscles.
Slight aortic sclerosis.
Dilatation of right heart.
Hypertrophy of left ventricle.
Slight tricuspid endocarditis.
Bicuspid aortic valve.
Hypostatic pneumonia.
Acute and chronic splenitis.
Fatty liver (central necroses?).
Acute nephritis.
Chronic gastritis.
Small breasts.
Axillary hair absent.
Petechial eruption of chest.
Varicose veins.
Chronic external adhesive pachymeningitis of left side.
Moderate swelling of right hemisphere with venous injection.
Slight occipital gliosis of both sides.
Slight gliosis of orbital and hippocampal gyri of right side.
Sclerosis with atrophy of occipital and hippocampal white matter of right side.
Gliotic lesion (1.5 × 2 × 2 cm. of right lenticular nucleus involving anterior commissure).

1. Was the exophthalmic goitre in Carrie Pearson due to syphilis? Unfortunately we have no clear proof that Carrie Pearson was syphilitic. She was stated to have been syphilitic by the physician who treated her before her commitment to Danvers Hospital. There is, however, no proof of syphilis, inasmuch as the patient died in the pre-Wassermann period.

2. Is the thalamic lesion probably syphilitic? No lymphocytosis or plasmocytosis characterizes the lesion, which is the only lesion of the sort in the Danvers collection. It would not do to call a lesion syphilitic just because it is *sui generis*. In any event, the clinical analysis of the case faced the claim of syphilis as an actual factor in the patient's life and as a possible factor in the goitre.

It is well known that the ARGYLL-ROBERTSON
PUPIL is characteristic of the so-called " PARA-
SYPHILITIC DISEASES " (" general paresis "
and " tabes "); does this sign occur in other neurosyphilitic conditions?

Case 54. Julius Kantor was a shoemaker of 35 years,
who came to the hospital for treatment because his family
physician had found a positive W. R. in Kantor's blood
serum. He had had a cough for a number of years, and
during the last year a little blood had been found in the
sputum; whereupon Kantor had been placed under active
anti-tuberculosis treatment. The enterprising family physician had found the positive W. R. in the first days of his
treatment for tuberculosis. There was, in fact, a history
of a chancre nine years before, which had not been followed
by any secondary or tertiary symptoms, and which had
been but scantily treated.

There were no mental symptoms.

Kantor was **physically** fairly well developed and nourished.
There were a few piping râles in the left upper chest, both
in front and back, and also a slight dulness with increased
vocal and tactile fremitus. No tubercle bacilli, however,
could be found on repeated sputum examination.

Neurologically, the pupils were myotic and both showed
the Argyll-Robertson reaction. There were no abnormal
reflexes whatever, and there was neither ataxia nor speech
defect. Not only the blood but also the spinal fluid W. R.
proved to be positive; there was a marked increase in the
albumin and globulin; there was a gold sol reaction of the
syphilitic type, and there were but three cells per cmm.

1. In view of the headache in case Kantor, what other
   causes of headache are to be considered? It is certain that irritations of the dura mater can produce
   headache, and the physiological observation of the
   sensitiveness of the membranes and the non-sensitive-

ness of the brain substance is an ancient and classical observation. Internal hemorrhagic pachymeningitis produces severe headache. The relations of this disease to trauma, to arteriosclerosis, and possibly to syphilis (alcohol perhaps should also be considered) in certain instances have not been entirely cleared up. Syphilitic headaches are, according to Lewandowski, dependent also upon a dural affection or upon a periosteal affection. The headaches of brain tumor are also commonly related to dural conditions, either directly due to the pressure of the tumor itself, or indirectly to the heightened intracranial pressure consequent upon the tumor. It is clear that the tension under which the dura mater lies is not always localized in the region of a brain tumor or a syphilitic lesion. Head has claimed that brain tumor produces headaches of two kinds, according to whether the disease affects the dura mater or is dependent upon an increase of pressure in the brain. It does not appear that the pia mater has any relation to headaches, but meningitis, in which the inflammation is confined to the pia mater, is nevertheless associated with headache; the headache is here supposed to be due to the increase in brain pressure, and thus actually to an effect wrought upon the dura mater. Vasomotor disorders and various types of cephalic hyperemia are thought to produce a kind of headache, but Lewandowski calls this kind of headache somewhat in question. Reflex headaches are stated to be produced indirectly by a process of radiation from interior lesions in the brain. There are certain headaches called nodal headaches (*Schwielen-Kopfschmerz*). Hypermetropia, caries of the teeth, adenoids, and diseases of the nose and axillary cavities, to say nothing of thoracic and abdominal diseases, are also counted among conditions that may produce headaches. In this connection, Head has claimed differential zones of headache corresponding to certain diseases.

The brain itself may produce headache through intoxications, through conditions produced by a variety of diseases; may follow neuroses. Alcohol may produce headaches in some persons even when it is taken in very small doses. Certain uremic cases yield headaches, as do also gouty and chlorotic conditions. According to Lewandowski, the headaches of arteriosclerotics are due possibly to vasomotor disturbances in the membranes, or one may think of nutritive cerebral disorders. A peculiar form of headache is that of fatigue after mental work, allied to which is the neurasthenic headache; constitutional headaches have been assumed to occur, to say nothing of hysterical headaches. There remains also the important question of migraine, for which a vasomotor explanation has been proposed.

2. Was Kantor suffering from tuberculosis of the lungs? The hypothesis of lung syphilis ought certainly to be very seriously considered. Upon repeated sputum examination, no tubercle bacilli have yet been found.

3. Is Kantor a case of general paresis? In the absence of mental symptoms, and in consideration of the mildness of the reactions, it is certainly not easy to make the diagnosis of general paresis. However, the diagnosis of tabes dorsalis is not justified either. Accordingly, we may answer our question: whether the Argyll-Robertson pupil occurs in other neurosyphilitic diseases, by pointing out that in the case of Julius Kantor, as in the case of Henri Lepère (105) and Frederick Stone (106), the Argyll-Robertson pupil has been found in syphilitic conditions that are neither typically paretic nor typically tabetic.

Does the Argyll-Robertson pupil necessarily indicate neurosyphilis?

Case 55. Daniel Falvey, 44 years of age, was an almshouse transfer to the Danvers State Hospital in the year 1904,
when the principle of state care was adopted in Massachusetts. As in most of the almshouse transfers of that day,
little could be discovered as to antecedents. He had been a
mill-worker from the time of his immigration in 1890, at 30
years of age. He had been somewhat alcoholic. There was
a shock some 17 months before his death, which occurred
about seven weeks from the date of transfer.

Not only was he unable to walk unsupported, but when
supported there was a slight dragging of the left leg and the
gait was noted to be somewhat propulsive. The tongue and
hands were tremulous, and the left grasp was somewhat
weaker than the right. Both knee-jerks were increased
although neither more than the other. There was no sensory
disorder.

Although but 44 years of age, Falvey presented the appearance of a much older man. His heart was somewhat enlarged
and there was a degree of peripheral arteriosclerosis. On the
whole, no special attention was attracted to this case clinically and he was regarded as an example of arteriosclerotic
dementia, like many another among the transfers. However,
we owe to Dr. H. M. Swift the important observation of the
Argyll-Robertson pupils. The case was studied long before
the Wassermann method was available, and is here reported
merely to call attention to the fact that the stiff pupils may
have other neural origin than neurosyphilis.

The autopsy material in the case was worked up by one of
the authors.* The autopsy had been performed by Dr. A. M.
Barrett, who found on section through the brain stem at the

---

* E. E. Southard. A case of glioma of the pineal region,
Am. Jour. of Ins., Vol. LXI, 1905.

anterior border of the pons a mass springing from and continuous with the pineal gland, lying in the third ventricle and the
aqueduct of Sylvius. Upon further study, this mass was
found to begin posteriorly in the pineal body itself, from
which the mass could hardly be told in the gross except by an
injected border.

This mass proved upon microscopic examination to be a
psammoma, which histologically resembled a glioma rather
than a sarcoma. Throughout the mass there was a variable
content of fibrillary intercellular substance having the histological reactions of neuroglia fibrillæ. The histological
details (mitosis, large giant cells with multiple nuclei, etc.) do
not here concern us. We deal with a neoplasm springing from
the pineal gland growing on the posterior half of the third
ventricle, the anterior orifice of the aqueduct of Sylvius, and
the space between the velum interpositum as far back as the
posterior corpora quadrigemina. There is no evidence in the
body of old syphilis; although it is possible that the stiff
pupils were neurosyphilitic, it seems probable that they were
related to the pineal tumor. At all events, there are in the
literature evidences that the pineal-quadrigeminal group of
tumors and other lesions may bring about pupillary disturbances. On this account, we here include the case. The
tumor hardly led to an error in diagnosis since neither neurosyphilis nor brain tumor was at all expected clinically.

1. Can alcoholism produce identical results? See Case
   Murphy, (60), one of alcoholic pseudoparesis.
2. What is the nature of stiff pupils? A pupil is called
   stiff in the sense of the Argyll-Robertson pupil if it
   fails to react to illumination either of itself or of the
   other eye and at the same time if it reacts properly in
   convergence and accommodation. Of course the stiffness of a blind eye must not be regarded as an Argyll-
   Robertson pupil. In a case of right-sided Argyll-
   Robertson pupil, therefore, the left pupil reacts properly
   both to direct illumination of itself and to illumination
   of the right eye, but the right eye fails to react to illumination of either eye. Such an Argyll-Robertson right
   pupil will remain of the same width both in darkness
   and in light. Clinicians agree that the Argyll-Robert-

son is diagnosticated rather too frequently than too seldom, and this by reason of the fact that a sluggishness of light reaction is interpreted as stiffness. The sign, as is well known, has come to be regarded as almost pathognomonic of tabetic or paretic neurosyphilis. Nonne, however, has found among 510 cases of alcoholism, nine instances of Argyll-Robertson pupil and 19 cases of sluggish light reactions. The pathological anatomy of this sign is still doubtful although a number of schematic accounts are available; among hypotheses, one may think of an elective effect of the tabetic or paretic degeneration upon reflex collaterals. The explanation would then resemble that for absent kneejerks and kindred reflex disorders. We should then hypothesize a loss of the finer processes of the terminal aborizations about the cells of the nucleus of sphincter nucleus iridis. However, the situation of the sphincter iridis has not yet been absolutely determined.

When a pupil is said to be entirely stiff it means that it reacts neither to light nor accommodation. This condition not infrequently follows the partial stiffness or Argyll-Robertson reaction.

3. Is the Argyll-Robertson pupil more tabetic than paretic? This has been claimed at times, but in point of fact, the Argyll-Robertson pupil is very frequent in paresis, and so also are posterior column changes. According to statistics of Bumke, 36% of tabetics fail to show the Argyll-Robertson pupil, and 38% of paretics. When, however, finer methods, such as those standardized by Weiler, with photographic records, are employed, the number of cases without at least a tendency to the Argyll-Robertson pupil becomes much smaller.

In connection with the important question as to the classical Argyll-Robertson pupil and pupillary sluggishness to light, it may be inquired what are the ocular signs in neurosyphilis? Joffroy has tabulated the signs in 300 general paretics as follows:

Sign.	No. of cases.	Per cent.
Alterations of light reflex..........	235	78
Inequality......................	205	68
Abolition of light reflex...........	156	52
(bilateral or unilateral)		
Abolition of light reflex...........	133	44
(bilateral)		
Irregularity of pupil..............	117	39

Sign.	No. of cases.	Per cent.
Irregularity of both pupils	109	36
Diminution of light reflex	108	36
ditto (bilateral)	79	26
Alteration in accommodation reflex	79	26
Diminution of accommodation reflex	52	17
Mydriasis	41	13
Myosis	40	13
Diminution of light reflex (unilateral)	35	11
Abolition of accommodation reflex	35	11
Diminution of accommodation reflex (bilateral)	29	9
Abolition of accommodation reflex (bilateral)	26	8
Diminution of accommodation reflex (unilateral)	23	7
Fundus changes	21	7
Vascular changes	16	5
Abolition of accommodation reflex (unilateral)	12	4
Paresis of the third nerves	10	3
Ptosis	9	3
Irregularity of one pupil	8	3
Nystagmus	7	2
Visual acuity lost	7	2
Atrophy of disc	6	2
Total blindness	5	2
Paralysis of the fourth nerves	1	1

Can neurosyphilis exist in the absence of positive findings in the spinal fluid?

Case 56. There was no great difficulty in setting up a diagnosis of general paresis in the case of James Burns, a mechanic of 31 years of age, who came voluntarily to the Psychopathic Hospital for treatment. The point in Burns' case was that the spinal fluid proved entirely negative in all respects despite the fact that the serum W. R. was positive, and despite the following facts of history and mental examination.

The patient claimed syphilitic infection seven years before, namely, at 24 years of age, and also claimed that he had infected his wife, who was in fact at the time undergoing anti-syphilitic treatment. He complained of insomnia, worry, depression, hypersensitivity to noises (such as those made by his own children), thoughts of suicide, and amnesia. The amnesia, however, might be regarded as subjective since our tests failed to show amnesia. Nor was there any diminution in arithmetical ability. Despite the patient's claim that he had been " way off in his way of thinking," there appeared to be no delusions. Beyond a certain flightiness in conversation, we could hardly get any evidence of psychosis unless of the neurasthenic order.

Physically, however, the left pupil failed to react to light though it was found to react to distance, and the right pupil exhibited a diminution of its reaction to light. There was no ataxia of gait, yet there was a complete Romberg reaction. There was a moderate tremor of the hands and of the tongue. Otherwise there were no reflex disorders upon systematic examination, nor was there any demonstrable disorder in the rest of the physical examination.

1. What is the diagnosis in the case of James Burns? On the whole we agree with Nonne, that negative spinal fluid findings (of course, in the absence of treatment) preclude the diagnosis of general paresis. The symp-

toms might possibly be explained, however, by means of a localized syphilitic involvement of the cerebrum, no cells or products of inflammation having penetrated to the spinal fluid. According to Head and Fearnsides, this condition may be found especially in the anterior or middle fossa. Accordingly, going upon these views of Nonne and of Head and Fearnsides, we should be entitled to make, perhaps, a diagnosis of cerebral syphilis.

2. What is the significance of the Argyll-Robertson pupil in James Burns? Nonne states that if one follows cases with Argyll-Robertson pupil over a sufficient period of years, they one and all eventuate in active symptoms of cerebrospinal syphilis (not necessarily of the cortical type), and this despite the fact that the pupillary change may have been present a number of years before any other symptom had developed.

Neurosyphilis ("DISSEMINATED ENCEPHA-
LITIS") within seven months of initial infection.
Autopsy.

Case 57. We borrow the main features of a remarkable
case examined at the Danvers State Hospital clinically by
Dr. H. W. Mitchell and reported elaborately by Dr. A. M.
Barrett. This case, whom we shall call John Summers,
acquired syphilis at about the end of the third week in May,
1902, and consulted a physician on June 12, at which time
a characteristic initial lesion of syphilis was plain. Summers
was excessively alcoholic at times and was not seen by a
physician again until July 2, just after an alcoholic debauch.
At this time there was ulceration of the primary lesion, and a
papillary eruption had developed over the arms, chest,
abdomen, and legs. Mercurial treatment and mixed treatment were given. Arthritis occurred but disappeared with
increased dosage.

About six months after infection, the patient developed
severe headaches, hardly controllable by treatment. Amnesia
and a certain stupidity, with neglect of personal habits, and
even of eating, developed, whereupon Summers was admitted
to the Danvers Hospital, December 11, 1902. He weighed
124 pounds, was extremely feeble, with dull and expression-
less face, coarse purposeless movements of arms; left pupil
larger than right; right external strabismus and ocular ptosis;
increased knee-jerks, crossed adductor reflex, coarse tremors
of arms and hands; and extreme clouding of consciousness.
It was doubtful whether the pupils were stiff to light or not.

The patient died on the ninth day, December 18, in a
state of coma. After admission, his stupor had become more
marked; there had been incontinence of urine and fæces,
and the patient could be aroused only by loud tones.
Difficulty in swallowing had developed; the right-sided
ptosis had become more marked, and muscular twitchings
had developed on the right side. When the left leg was

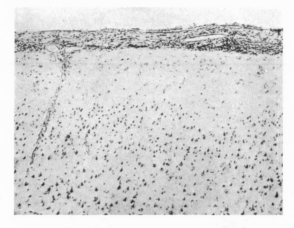

1. Exudate in pia mater — mononucleosis.

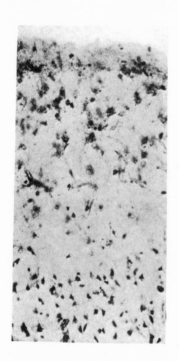

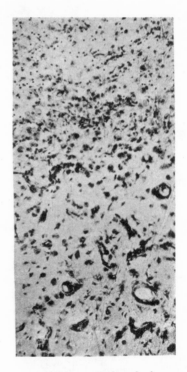

2. Superficial (subpial) cellular reaction of neuroglia tissue (expanded cell bodies).

3. Cellular gliosis of deeper layers of cortex. Apparent increase in capillary supply, possibly relative to loss of neural elements.

Case 57. Neurosyphilis ("disseminated syphilitic encephalitis" of A. M. Barrett), fatal seven months from initial infection. (Photographs by A. M. Barrett.)

pinched, there was twitching of the left leg and arm. There was slight spasticity of the right arm and leg. An examination upon the day of death definitely showed a lack of reaction of the pupils to light.

Dr. Barrett was able to find in the literature a case of Bechterew which histologically resembled his own case, but though in the instance reported by Bechterew the first symptoms developed within the year following infection, death did not occur until two years later.

In view of a total duration of symptoms clearly not over seven months, it is interesting to inquire how far microscopic brain changes could have proceeded. Neither calvarium nor dura mater showed changes. There was a slight haziness of the pia mater over the convexity, but the pia mater over the base (especially below the cisterna and from thence spreading out over the pons and into the fissure of Sylvius) was not only hazy but definitely thickened and hyperæmic. The thickening was most marked about the root of the right third nerve (corresponding with the eye findings in life). There was also a macroscopic thickening of the left Sylvian artery. Section of the brain showed nothing abnormal except a small area among the pyramidal fibres of the right side of the pons, where there was a single hemorrhagic area about 7 mm. in diameter around which there were small punctiform hemorrhages. (Compare twitchings of left leg and arm upon stimulation of left leg, and note also the muscular twitchings and slight spasticity of right leg and arm noted just before death.) This case was examined and reported upon in 1905. We learn from Dr. Barrett that a re-study of the case with modern methods has failed to demonstrate a spirochetosis.

The meninges show infiltration and destructive and proliferative changes of the blood vessels. Condensed extracts from Dr. Barrett's full report follow:

> There were local variations in the severity of the meningitis. The sulci showed the most marked infiltration. The slighter degrees of exudation were made up largely of lymphocytes with a few plasma cells, occasionally large mononuclear cells, and rarely

a polymorphonuclear leukocyte. Where the exudation was more extensive, the large mononuclear cells became more common and the polymorphonuclear leukocytes increased in number. The large mononuclear cells were often phagocytic, containing from one to six leukocytes. The exudate was always most abundant about the blood vessels. The plasma cells were always most numerous in the adventitia of the veins, here greatly outnumbering the leukocytes. The polymorphonuclear leukocytes were relatively infrequent except where there were necrotic areas, which areas were usually continuous with an infiltration of a vessel wall.

As to vascular changes, the media was not often involved, nor was the adventitia so often affected as the intima. Such lesions as appeared in the intima and adventitia were infiltrative rather than proliferative. The elastica of the blood vessels proved to show but slight changes.

A characteristic change was the endarteritis, — of a focal nature with a few large mononuclear and lymphocytic cells pushing the intima inward at the edge of a lesion. In the more marked portion of the focal process, the thickness of the intima was greatly increased by proliferation. Great numbers of large mononuclear cells could be seen between the intima and the elastica. About these cells and interlacing among the other elements of the proliferating tissue was an excess of connective tissue fibres.

The meningeal veins were more often diseased than the arteries; there was adventitial infiltration with lymphoid and plasma cells; sometimes the vein walls had become necrotic and infiltrated with polymorphonuclear leukocytes.

It will be remembered that the left Sylvian artery was grossly thickened, and microscopic section of this vessel showed a partial thrombosis.

The brain showed diffuse and focal changes. The *diffuse* process was one of nerve cell degeneration and proliferative changes in the neuroglia and blood vessels, and no section of the many examined proved to be free from such changes, although in the majority of instances, these diffuse changes were slight. The cortical layers showed more of these diffuse changes than did the white substance. Barrett considered that the glial cell changes were more delicate indicators of the cortical changes than the nerve cell changes. He found rod

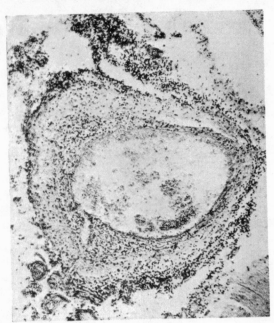

4. Arteritis of pia mater.

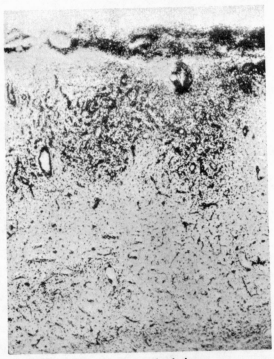

5. Focal vascular lesions.

Case 57. Seven months from infection. "Disseminated syphilitic encephalitis," Barrett. (Photographs by Barrett.)

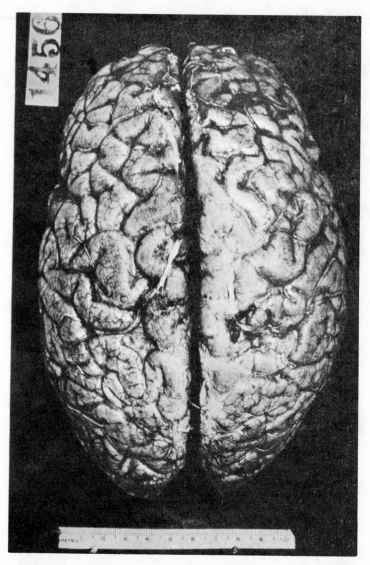

Paretic neurosyphilis ("general paresis") — cerebral atrophy, *without* meningitis.   Therapeutics cannot hope to restore lost tissue.

Duration.   3 years from beginning of well marked symptoms; 6 years from beginning of obvious symptoms; 12 years from a so-called " nervous prostration."

cells, satellitosis, superficial gliosis, and a large gamut of changes in the neuroglia. There were two rather characteristic nerve-cell changes: a shrinkage change going on to almost complete destruction, and a type of cell swelling, also apparently proceeding to complete destruction.

Among *focal* changes, there were four main types: Areas of encephalitis, having the general appearance of granulation tissue, areas of simple necrosis or softening, apparently directly related to vascular changes near by, hemorrhages, and certain foci regarded as gummatous.

Save for pial infiltration and a few vascular changes, there was very little change in the medulla and spinal cord. There was a hypertrophic gliosis of the margin of the medulla and cord throughout, and a focal lesion of well-marked gliosis at one point in the bulb. There were no fibre degenerations in the medulla or cord, nor were there any coarse fibre degenerations in the cortex itself except in one locus, the left gyrus rectus. This case is of peculiar value in showing to what extent lesions may proceed in a period of six to eight months after primary infection.

Of course the case is in one sense entirely atypical. The lesions were not confined to the nervous system. Aside from the maculo-papular eruption and ecchymosis of the skin, there was a diffuse hemorrhage of the inner half of the conjunctiva of the left eyeball, a small hemorrhagic focus in the mitral valve, a caseous nodule, one cm. in diameter, in the apex of the left lung whose tuberculous or syphilitic nature is left in doubt; a broad milk-colored patch of thickening of the capsule of the liver. It is to be noted that there were no gross lesions of the aorta.

On the classical assumption that PARETIC NEU-
ROSYPHILIS ("general paresis") is a fatal
disease, is there a disease PSEUDOPARETIC
NEUROSYPHILIS ("pseudoparesis") which may
recover or pursue a long course like that of a case
of diffuse neurosyphilis ("cerebrospinal syphilis")?

Case 58. Peter Burkhardt had been an efficient highway
inspector, but in his forty-fifth year he had begun to be unable
to do his work satisfactorily. His wife had become somewhat
afraid of him. He had had somnolent spells in his chair and
had squandered money. The mental symptoms had lasted
for some six months, but had become more marked during
the month preceding admission. Burkhardt would at times
fail to recognize his friends.

The general **physical condition** of Burkhardt was very good.
The pupils were irregular and reacted sluggishly both to light
and to accommodation. The knee-jerks and ankle-jerks were
absent. There were no other neurological disorders upon
systematic examination. There was a speech defect. **Mentally,** little could be determined except a certain sluggishness.

History and physical examination at once suggested general paresis. The serum W. R. was doubtful, but the spinal
fluid reaction was positive, as was the gold sol reaction (which
was "paretic"); the globulin and albumin were greatly
increased; there were 48 cells per cmm. Antisyphilitic
treatment, consisting of salvarsan twice a week and potassium
iodid by mouth, was followed by a rapid mental improvement. After two months, Burkhardt was discharged apparently normal, with all the blood and spinal fluid tests negative. He has been taken back into the highway service.

1.   What is the proper definition of pseudoparesis? Fournier
termed pseudoparesis certain cases that looked like
paresis but were not syphilitic in origin. Of these
cases the most characteristic group is that of alcoholic
pseudoparesis. It is clear that there will be no diffi-

culty in the definition of a disease pseudoparesis whose entity is presented in the adjective that precedes the term (*e.g.*, alcoholic pseudoparesis). According to this usage, a case of pseudoparesis would be one in which the symptoms and possibly some of the signs somewhat resemble the symptoms of paresis itself but for which another etiology could be fairly established.

2. Are there any cases of syphilitic pseudoparesis? We are of the opinion that the term should be dropped. It is true that there are cases which clinically look like general paresis and exhibit the appropriate laboratory signs of general paresis but seem to differ from paresis in their course even when they receive no treatment whatever. In the present phase of doubt as to the classification of paretic and non-paretic forms of neurosyphilis, it seems to us of doubtful utility to characterize a case as pseudo simply because it differs in its course, particularly as the literature has always duly recognized that a number of cases of general paresis have had long courses and sometimes very long remissions.

There is also another group of cases that have been termed cases of pseudoparesis, namely: certain cases of neurosyphilis which clinically look like general paresis and seem to be following its classical course but are interrupted by treatment. Here again it seems to us doubtful whether the designation pseudo should be attached to this group of cases, particularly while the whole therapeutic question in the paretic group of neuro-syphilis cases remains *sub judice*. Accordingly we are tempted to include in the group of paretic neurosyphilis cases that either get well of themselves, or get well under treatment, or pursue a very long course, or are subject to very long remissions. But we make this decision in terminology without prejudice to the therapeutic question and it is open to any critic to throw these cases into an atypical non-paretic group of neurosyphilis cases.

3. How shall we explain the absence of ataxia of case Burk-hardt when knee-jerks are absent and when, therefore, we are entitled to conclude a certain degree of spinal disease? As stated in connection with case Sullivan (16), the absence of knee-jerks is not a warrant for terming a case — paresis of the tabetic form. The fact is that the lesion in paresis tends to be intraspinal, just as the higher brain lesions tend to occur within the brain substance. The meninges are relatively spared both within the cranium and within the spinal canal.

The characteristic degeneration of posterior nerve roots which we find in tabes dorsalis is not necessarily found in general paresis even when there are somewhat extensive spinal lesions. Accordingly the absence of sensory returns by way of the posterior nerve roots which characterizes tabes dorsalis is not necessarily a phenomenon of general paresis. The mechanism by which the knee-jerks are lost depends upon histological detail. They may be lost when under tabetic conditions the posterior roots are severely diseased and when under paretic conditions only intraspinal collaterals or a small portion of fibres are affected. The whole question hinges upon where and to what degree the various reflex arcs are cut in the disease. The tabetic phenomena are, as so commonly stated, intradural; that is, the sensory or gangliospinal neurones at certain levels are affected all the way in from the points at which they pierce the dura mater. The affection of these and other neurones in general paresis is an intraspinal and parenchymatous affection.

Neurosyphilis; auditory hallucinations; ideas of persecution; attacks of excitement. SYPHILITIC PARANOIA (Kraepelin)?

Case 59. Bridget Curley was a case that was discharged from the Psychopathic Hospital, recovered, after 26 days in hospital. The symptoms so resembled those of alcoholic hallucinosis that the diagnosis was made despite the fact that the patient consistently denied the use of intoxicants. There was, in fact, no proof that she drank alcohol. The case was, however, not clearly one of alcoholic hallucinosis or of any other well-defined form of mental disease. A provisional diagnosis of manic-depressive psychosis, manic phase, had, in fact, also been made.

The illness had begun with depression and inactivity, Bridget's friends accounted for these conditions on the ground that a lover had departed for Ireland. A few days after the depression began, Bridget became dizzy and refused to give a boarder his breakfast, stating that she had lost her memory and had begun to hear bells ringing and people talking. She then became greatly excited and was brought to hospital, where the prolonged baths quieted her.

It seems that Bridget had had stomach trouble and head-aches at the top of her head or sometimes in her temples. **Physical examination** showed the left pupil to be larger than the right, a slight tremor of the lips, a slight systolic murmur at the apex, slightly irregular pulse, and moderate edema of ankles. The blood serum was negative to the W. R., but lumbar puncture was executed and the fluid showed a positive W. R.

The patient was tested by the Binet and other methods, and although 35 years of age, seemed to be by the mental tests hardly over 11 years old. She was inclined to be feverish, somewhat restive, and pugnacious; rather slow of speech, sometimes refusing to answer and grimacing. Her pugnacity was, however, easily controllable, and the excitement was largely at night. This excitement subsided rapidly in the course of a few days.

1. What is the diagnosis in this case? The following diagnoses and suggestions for diagnosis were made at the staff meetings:

>Unclassified mania.
>Manic-depressive psychosis, manic phase.
>Toxic delirium.
>Dementia praecox.
>Bacterial infection of the brain.
>Unclassified delirium.
>Acute delirium.
>Infectious psychosis.
>Acute confusional psychosis.
>Psychopathic personality by use of alcohol.
>Mental deficiency with atypical mental state.
>Syphilitic paranoia.

2. Is this a case of syphilitic paranoia? The so-called syphilitic paranoia of Kraepelin is a rare and uncertain type of syphilitic mental disease. Delusions and hallucinations are prominent. As a rule, the onset is stated to be slow and insidious, or at any rate there are a variety of indefinite prodromata. Jealousy is a prominent feature, sometimes attended with marked sexual excitement. Auditory hallucinations and ideas of persecution are particularly in evidence. The most striking feature in Kraepelin's group was a sudden occurrence and equally sudden disappearance of violent excitement, with or without external cause. Thus, an excitement would be produced by a few words spoken, and immediately after, the phase of excitement would pass and the patient would become entirely friendly and accessible once more, as if nothing had happened. About half of Kraepelin's cases showed a positive serum W. R. He does not report lumbar puncture findings, and grounds the existence of disease upon certain autopsied cases. The speech and writing disorder of paresis as well as the characteristic disorientation for time and muscular weakness of general paresis were absent in the group. It appears that most cases of the group have hitherto been placed in dementia praecox.

The clinical symptoms of CHRONIC ALCOHOL-
ISM are sometimes largely identical with those of
PARETIC NEUROSYPHILIS ("general paresis"):
differentiation by means of the laboratory findings.

To demonstrate this proposition, the cases of Francis
Murphy (60) and David Collins (61) are in point, being
sharp foils to one another.

Case 60.   A laboring man about 44 years of age was brought
to the Psychopathic Hospital one summer day, in a stupor.
This patient, Francis Murphy, had been at his regular work
as axeman in the Park Service, when he suddenly fell in a
heavy convulsion. He was carried to a general hospital,
still in convulsions, and ether was administered to quiet
the movements. The convulsions shortly ceased, but the
patient's consciousness failed to clear; hence his transfer to
the Psychopathic Hospital.

Here he remained much disturbed and was placed in a room
with a mattress on the floor. On this mattress he would
crouch on all fours for a considerable time, looking fixedly
downward as if at an object on the floor, unresponsive to
questions but compliant with efforts to place him on his back.
He gave the impression of daze and either disorientation or
confusion.

Within twenty-four hours the patient became more tranquil and consciousness became clearer, but the patient was at
a loss to bring to memory either recent or remote events.
However, he replied to questions, giving some different story
each time he was approached. Curiously enough, the patient
seemed very contented and good natured and would even
laugh foolishly at times, saying that he felt fine and all
ready to go out to work.

The general impression conveyed by Francis Murphy at
once suggested the possibility of neurosyphilis. Convulsions, perhaps initial in middle age, with a post-convulsive

stupor, followed by a partial clearing up, with persistent amnesia and a suggestion of fabrications with euphoria, bore out the suggestion.

The **physical examination** strengthened the impression of neurosyphilis. Well developed and nourished, florid, with a manual tremor and sweating of the palms, the patient was in general without physical symptoms. **Neurologically,** however, whereas the left pupil was larger than the right and reacted properly to light, the right pupil was a bit contracted, somewhat irregular, and either reacted not at all to light or very slightly so (reacting perfectly to accommodation). The knee-jerks could be obtained only with reinforcement, and several other reflexes could not be elicited (triceps, radial, ulnar, periosteal, Achilles, umbilical). Moreover, the heel-to-knee test was poorly performed; some of the common tests phrases were very poorly repeated; there was marked tremor in writing; and the paragraphia seemed to be not merely peripheral, for syllables were left out in words and ordinary words spelled incorrectly (psychographic disturbance).

We do not care here to insist that the right pupil was really an example of the Argyll-Robertson phenomenon since the slightest tinge of doubt is important if a positive diagnosis is practically equivalent to asserting syphilis. Practically, however, the right pupil was regarded as an Argyll-Robertson pupil under hospital conditions (flash-light reaction). Argyll-Robertson pupil, areflexia, speech disorder, writing disorder, memory disorder, conduct disorder, and euphoria, all with a history of convulsions, certainly warranted the tentative diagnosis of neurosyphilis.

As usual, resort was made to the W. R. in the serum and in the spinal fluid. One of the first results to come through from the laboratory was the absence of globulin, normal albumin, negative gold sol reaction, and a cell count of two cells per cmm. in the spinal fluid. Later the *W. R.'s* were returned *negative* for blood and spinal fluid.

In the meantime, an illuminating change had occurred in the patient, for two days later, — three days after the first convulsion in the park, — the patient had apparently quite recovered; his consciousness became nearly clear; he could remember every event up to the time of the convulsion, and his memory came back in appropriate degree for both remote and recent events.

The patient, it appeared, had for some time been drinking more and more heavily. In recent days, he had been taking five or six whiskeys and a half dozen beers daily on the average, and often much more. About ten years before, the patient narrated, there had been a convulsion at a ballgame, and this convulsion the patient himself called a " rum fit."

Here, then, is a case of ALCOHOLIC PSEUDOPARESIS. Without the W. serum test and without the spinal fluid examination, it is probable that the diagnosis of general paresis might have clung to the patient for some time on account of the apparent Argyll-Robertson pupil, which had to be accepted as such on the flash-light data. In point of fact, in this case the pupil later reacted more normally to light, and the speech and writing disorders measurably cleared up.

1. Can alcohol produce the Argyll-Robertson pupil? The majority of neurologists would today answer, Yes.

2. If in the case of Francis Murphy, the W. R. in the blood had happened to be positive on account of a non-neural syphilitic infection (spinal fluid negative), would the diagnosis *general paresis* be warranted? Probably the diagnosis *general paresis* would have been made. If the patient had been lost to observation, he might well have been regarded as an atypical paretic with prodromal convulsions.

3. Would positive globulin and excess albumin in the spinal fluid alone or in association with a positive serum W. R. warrant the diagnosis *general paresis* or *neurosyphilis?* The chances are that most neurologists would advocate proceeding to treatment in any case of positive serum reaction, whether or not there was globulin or excess albumin; but the positive globulin and excess albumin would probably not warrant the diagnosis *general paresis* or *neurosyphilis* in the absence of excess cells and the characteristic gold sol reaction and W. R. in the fluid.

4. Is the case of Francis Murphy one of alcoholic epilepsy (as suggested by Murphy's own phrase, " rum fits ")? It must be remembered that epileptics become alcoholic and that epileptic convulsions increase or become

more severe with alcoholism. On the other hand, the literature indicates that alcoholism can produce convulsions, as can many other factors. The literature also indicates that there is a condition of epilepsy in which the convulsive tendency sets in as a result of alcoholism in a patient not previously disposed to epilepsy; it appears also that sometimes, though very rarely, the epilepsy continues after withdrawal of alcohol, and even after giving up the habit. Francis Murphy appears to have had but two spells of convulsions, both of them following heavy bouts with alcohol. There is so far, then, no warrant for calling Francis Murphy's case one of alcoholic epilepsy.

5. Does the use of alcohol by a subject destroy the value of the W.R.? It has been held by some that alcoholism interferes with the accuracy of the W. R. This has not been our experience and for the present we are of opinion that the results have the same value in alcoholics as in non-alcoholics. The next case (Collins, 61) is one in which a positive W. R. occurred in an alcoholic. When dealing with paretic neurosyphilis it is especially true that the W. R. is disturbed very rarely, if at all, by toxins or drugs, except antisyphilitic drugs.

ALCOHOLISM may cloud the diagnosis of NEURO-
SYPHILIS. Differentiation by laboratory tests.

Case 61. David Collins was a steamfitter of about 43
years of age, picked up at 6.45 a.m. in the midst of convulsions
and talking incoherently, in a state apparently of fairly clear
consciousness. On arrival at the hospital, the patient was
able to tell how he had always been a hard drinker, and how
during the past week of unemployment he had taken large
quantities of poor whiskey, — perhaps an average of a pint a
day. Collins also told how he had had delirium tremens several times, but he said the present spell was quite unlike delirium tremens. There was no disorientation or impairment of
memory, and the patient did not in any wise suggest a mental
case a few hours after admission.

It appears, according to Collins, that he had obtained some
work the night before, and had quit work about 6.30, whereupon he stepped into a barroom, took one drink of whiskey,
left the barroom, walked down the street, and suddenly lost
track of the world, coming to consciousness in a carriage with
two policemen, but remaining, as he said, " dopy," inattentive, and confused. After a meal, however, the patient began
to feel better and soon felt quite all right.

The **physical examination** was quite negative except that
neurologically there was lingual and manual tremor, a speech
defect, apparent only with test phrases, unsteadiness of handwriting, left knee-jerk greater than right, a left-sided Babinski
reflex, and a difficulty in executing rapid successive movements (dysdiadochokinesis). This degree of neurological disorder in our experience warrants lumbar puncture as well as a
serum test. The lumbar puncture shortly disclosed a positive
globulin and excess albumin, and the returns from the W. R.'s
were positive for both spinal fluid and blood serum. The
data of the gold sol reaction were not available on account of
technical difficulties. However, it appears that the diagnosis
of neurosyphilis could hardly be avoided in this case.

David Collins differs from Francis Murphy, then, in showing a positive blood and spinal fluid reaction for syphilis as
well as a positive globulin and excess albumin. As above
remarked, it is probable that the positive globulin and excess
albumin would not warrant more than a suspicion of neurosyphilis taken by themselves.

Unfortunately, we were unable to persuade the patient to
submit to treatment, and from the patient's point of view
possibly his decision, not to submit to treatment, was a good
one since he has had no symptoms of any sort for a period of 18
months since his episode. However, as abundantly elsewhere demonstrated, we feel that the patient is wrong, and
that the physicians are right in urging treatment.

1. Is not the convulsive episode an alcoholic phenomenon
    in David Collins entirely separate from the patient's
    general and neurosyphilis? Possibly; however, an
    outbreak of neurological symptoms with spontaneous
    recovery is not only consistent with the diagnosis of
    syphilis, but somewhat characteristic of neurosyphilis.
    We suspect that another attack will occur in David
    Collins.* We shall from time to time make use of the
    social service to suggest his going under treatment, and
    shall employ his record of contact with a public institu-
    tion to drive in our suggestion. Still it is clear that
    there are numerous cases in the community that are
    not accessible to social service initiated from a public
    institution. Accordingly, educational propaganda is
    necessary for salvage of the middle- and upper-class
    victims of syphilis. It is a little unfortunate that the
    ethics of the private practitioner make such salvage of
    middle- and upper-class persons not very likely. Might
    it not be that an extension of state medicine to this
    field would incidentally increase the amount of success-
    ful private practice?
2. What may be the cause of such a convulsive episode as
    that of David Collins? It would appear that the con-
    vulsions of general paresis and of neurosyphilis in gen-
    eral often occur without gross structural lesions of the
    brain. It may be suggested that vascular irritation or

---

* Since this was written Collins has had further difficulties
related to his neurosyphilis, improving under treatment.

parenchymal irritation by spirochetes, acting in appropriate parts of the central nervous system, can produce such convulsions.

3. What is the significance of the unilateral phenomenon in David Collins (left knee-jerk greater than right; left-sided Babinski)? The current explanation of hyper-reflexia is that somehow inhibitory impulses from upper portions of the nervous system have ceased to influence the local arcs that mechanize reactions like the knee-jerk and the normal plantar reflex. The phenomena are commonly found in cases with pyramidal tract disorder, and in the case of David Collins one may suspect, therefore, that there was a central disorder affecting the right pyramidal tract above its decussation. One might suspect that the convulsions were initiated by a lesion (whether gross or microscopic in range) in the right side of the cerebrum; but whether in the white matter or in the gray matter must be left doubtful. The clearing up of all symptoms suggests either that the lesion was microscopic in range or that the phenomena were transient and functional.

4. Can the dysdiadochokinesis be used to indicate cerebellar lesion in David Collins? Possibly; but it does not appear that the difficulty in executing successive movements was unilateral. It seems impossible to bring into close topographical relation the basis for the Babinski and left-sided hyperreflexia, and the basis for the dysdiadochokinesis. Alcohol is sometimes asserted to exert an especial effect upon the cerebellum.

5. Must we suppose structural lesions, either (a) of the nature of cell losses demonstrable microscopically, or (b) of the nature of secondary degenerations demonstrable by Weigert myelin sheath methods, in the case of David Collins? It appears that we do not need to assert the existence of such lesions.

6. Could the hyperreflexia and the Babinski reaction be due to local spinal cord disease? Possibly; but the existence of other neurological symptoms (lingual and manual tremor, speech defect to test phrases, ataxic handwriting, and dysdiadochokinesis) makes it probable that there were lesions, or at any rate disordered functions, within the cranium; and there appears to be no basis for asserting local spinal cord disease.

**Differential diagnosis between NEUROSYPHILIS
and ACUTE ALCOHOLIC PSYCHOSIS.**

Case 62. Joseph Buck was a chef of 60 years who came in,
seeking advice because his memory was getting poor; he
was unable to remember names and what he was about to do.
He was tremulous and had much pain in his limbs. He had
been drinking heavily for weeks, — probably ten weeks;
in fact, he described himself as having had " the shakes "
and as having lately seen animals and people that were unreal.
He had had the shakes before and the condition had lasted
for two to three days after alcohol was discontinued.

Physically, Buck was tall, well developed, although poorly
nourished, with a skin suggesting alcoholism. There was
a slight acne over the back and chest; there was a slight
enlargement of the heart, with blood pressure, systolic, 180,
diastolic, 120. There was a corneal opacity of the left eye,
which the patient said was the result of syphilis following a
chancre, which he had acquired at the age of 27. There
was also a ptosis of the upper lid of the left eye. The right
pupil was irregular and reacted to light sluggishly, and with
a very small excursion. The patient was slightly deaf in
both ears. The deep reflexes were all lively and equal. The
tremor was most marked in finely coördinated movements.
There was a slight swaying in the Romberg position but the
sign could not be said to be present. The gait was unsteady.
There was a marked tenderness over the nerve trunks.

So far as **mental examination** went, it seemed that the
patient's claim of amnesia was subjective. There was certainly no more amnesia than a slight difficulty in recalling
details. The diagnosis of alcoholism with convalescence
from delirium tremens would certainly seem to have been
sufficient for the phenomena, and the suggestion of alcoholic
neuritis only confirmed the picture. To be sure, one might
expect a diminution or absence of deep reflexes; still, these reflexes may be over-active in an irritative stage of the disease.

Naturally, however, the history of syphilis and the pupillary phenomena and ptosis, made the consideration of neurosyphilis necessary. Both serum and fluid W. R.'s proved positive; there was an excessive amount of albumin and globulin, the gold sol reaction was typically "paretic," and there were 377 cells per cmm.

The patient improved upon a rest treatment and was given injections of mercury for his syphilis. After a few months he felt well enough to return to work, and continued at work throughout a season, receiving mercurial treatment throughout this time. A spinal fluid examination fifteen months later showed a weaker gold sol reaction, reduction in the amount of globulin and albumin, and but 26 cells to the cmm. The W. R.'s had remained positive.

1. What are the forms of syphilitic neuritis? According to Nonne, syphilitic neuritis and polyneuritis have at last acquired standing in neuropathology. The older claims depended upon findings on palpation and recovery after antisyphilitic treatment. Since the introduction of salvarsan, cases of ophthalmoplegia, facial, acoustic, and optic nerve disease, as well as neuritis of the extremities, have been reported in large numbers. These phenomena are to be regarded as neurorecidives in the modern sense of that term. The neurorecidive is not a salvarsan effect, but is an effect of the syphilitic process itself, settling in the peripheral nerves. Paresthesias are especially prominent in peripheral mono- or polyneuritis, and this point is of some value in differentiating the syphilitic peripheral neuritis from root neuritis. Root neuritis is more often characterized by neuralgic attacks. Objective hyperesthesia of neuromuscular origin is also found in these cases, demonstrated by pressure on the nerves. The motor phenomena consist in a flaccid paresis or paralysis, especially affecting the radial, ulnar, and peroneal nerves. Nonne states that it is rare for syphilis to affect a single nerve region, and he regards cases in which a single region alone is affected as usually due to a local gummatous process.

2. What is the significance of 377 cells per cmm.? See discussion of Washington (Case 66).

Differential diagnosis between NEUROSYPHILIS and CHRONIC ALCOHOLISM.

Case 63. Albert Fielding, 46, was an insurance broker, who was brought to the hospital for excessive alcoholism. Indeed, he showed all the signs, both of chronic and acute intoxication, except that there was no nerve trunk tenderness. Fielding was very loquacious though his speech was rather thick. He showed tremor of hands and an alcoholic skin. Physical and neurological examination proved entirely negative.

Fielding claimed that he had had a nervous breakdown at about 36 years of age, after disappointment in love. He had the drinking habit and began to drink more and more. He had now become nervous and tremulous and had to drink in order to brace himself. After a few days, the patient began to be much better, having recovered from acute alcoholism. **Mental examination** now showed good memory with orientation intact. There was a certain tendency to reminiscence and to somewhat childish actions. He had attempted to stop drinking but had been unable to quit. As a matter of fact, his mother and father had been excessive drinkers and he had inherited the tendency, etc.

The **diagnosis** seemed to be plain. The routine W. R. upon the blood serum was negative. However, the patient had remarked during the history taking, that he had had a chancre and secondary symptoms of syphilis. Accordingly, lumbar puncture was resorted to. The fluid showed a slightly positive W. R.; the gold sol reaction was of the syphilitic type; there was a considerable increase in albumin and globulin, and there were 20 cells per cmm. The diagnosis of neurosyphilis seemed clear.

Course: The patient received six months' treatment in a sanatorium but the symptoms remained almost as before, and the patient showed the same childishness and inability to take care of himself. Since the symptoms continued six months after the withdrawal of alcohol, it might well be suspected that the condition was more than a merely alcoholic one. However, in a number of purely alcoholic cases, such long-standing effects are found: even as long as six months or longer after the withdrawal of the alcohol, and one might conclude therefore that Fielding was actually a victim of alcoholic dementia. The spinal fluid after these six months (during which period antisyphilitic treatment was given) showed no change, and the prognosis was offered that the case would probably develop into one of paresis.

A year later, after six months sanatorial care and six months life in the community, the patient returned to the Psychopathic Hospital in an alcoholic condition. The lumbar puncture showed all signs negative except the W. R. which was slightly positive. The W. R. of the blood was negative.

In connection with this case, see the case of *paresis sine paresi* (25).

1. What is the relation of the syphilitic and alcoholic process in Robert Fielding? One does not like to break the so-called rule of parsimony in diagnosis, but it would seem that the effects in Fielding are the combined effects of syphilis and alcoholism.

Differential diagnosis between NEUROSYPHILIS,
DIABETIC   PSEUDOPARESIS   and   BRAIN
TUMOR.

Case 64. A large and imposing person, Calvin Hall, 55,
had been employed as a doorkeeper and guard, in which
position he was on duty for 12 to 14 hours daily. Eventually,
however, he had begun to have a good deal of pain in the legs
and a few months before observation, one day, his legs gave
way and he fell to the floor. There was, however, no loss of
consciousness, and he was carried to a general hospital. The
result of an examination there was that his family was informed that he had some nervous trouble.

Hall now began to be melancholy and wept a good deal.
His appetite and sleep remained intact. He felt too weak to
walk. At the end of about a year, he began to improve and
again became able to do a little light work. About a month
before coming to the Psychopathic Hospital, about two years
after the onset of symptoms, Hall suddenly began to talk
excessively, in a rambling and rather senseless way. A fortnight later, he began to suffer from insomnia and restlessness.

Some medical facts were available: It seems that at 25
years this patient had become infected with syphilis though
there had never been any secondary signs. He was married
four years later but there had not been any children. Moreover, for four years past, the patient had been treated for
glycosuria.

Upon admission, the patient's sensorium was clear, but
his orientation was only partial. He could give a fair account
of his life, but it appeared that his memory was somewhat
impaired. There were auditory hallucinations (voices of
relatives). He often mistook the identity of persons about
him. He talked in a grandiose fashion of his great strength
and especially of a God-given power to read minds. His
flow of thought was rapid, rambling, circumstantial, and with
traces of irrelevance. He was rather continuously busy and

at times restive. There was a good deal of emotional agitation and apprehensiveness, and again the patient would become suspicious and tearful.

Physically, there was a discharging sinus connected with the right humerus, close to the elbow. The pupils, though equal and regular, were sluggish in reaction to light. The knee-jerks and ankle-jerks were absent. There was no Romberg sign but there was some swaying in the Romberg position. There was a moderate ataxia in walking. Glycosuria to a moderate degree was determined. There were no casts or albumin in the urine. The W. R. of the blood and of the spinal fluid was negative. The albumin of the fluid, however, was considerably increased. X-ray examination of the skull yielded a suggestion of absorption of the posterior clinoid processes of the sella turcica. The X-ray examination of the arm in the region of the sinus showed a chronic osteomyelitis, possibly syphilitic (or diabetic?).

The diagnostic problems in the case of Calvin Hall are extremely intricate. There are clinical suggestions of general paresis, not confirmed by the laboratory findings.

1. Are we dealing with a case of diabetic pseudoparesis? Is the pain in the legs of like origin, and has a neuritic process led to the absence of the knee-jerks? The Allen treatment appears to have had no beneficial result in this case.
2. Is there a tumor of the sella region, which could account for the mental symptoms and the glycosuria? The spinal fluid albumin might be regarded as consistent with a variety of psychoses, including that of brain tumor. We have to remember the definite history of infection, the sterile marriage. and the possibly syphilitic osteomyelitis.

DIABETES AND NEUROSYPHILIS, relations?

Case 65. Donald Barrie, a man of 61, diabetic for several years, had begun to worry about the diabetes, feeling that he was about to die, and had gone so far as to make several threats of suicide. Hence he was brought to the Psychopathic Hospital for observation.

Barrie was rather well developed and nourished, although he looked far older than he was. There was a marked arcus senilis; the skin was dry and rough; the radial and other accessible vessels were markedly sclerosed; abdomen obese; right testicle very low with thickened and hard epididymis.

Neurologically there was little abnormal to discover. The pupils were irregular; both reacted fairly well to light. There was a slight tremor of the extended hands, and still less of the tongue. The voice was slightly thick and the patient stumbled somewhat on test phrases. Urine: specific gravity, 1029; sugar; no acetone; no diacetic acid. Sugar 2 to 11 grams for 24 hours on ordinary diet. It proved impossible to get the patient sugar-free, either by cutting down the carbohydrates or by using the Allen method.

Mentally, the depression with reiteration of wrong-doing and self-accusation because of the contraction of syphilis, were the striking features. There was, to be sure, a slight imperfection of memory for remote events; memory for recent events and knowledge of current events was very poor. Barrie claimed that his condition was entirely hopeless, that his memory was exceedingly bad, and that he was no longer capable of supporting his family.

1. What shall be said as to diagnosis in a man of 61 with glycosuria, depression, amnesia, sluggish pupil, slight tremor, slight speech defect, and a history of syphilis?
   The W. R. of the serum proved positive, and also the W. R. of the spinal fluid. The gold sol reaction of the fluid was of the syphilitic type. There were 112 cells

per cmm., there was an excess of albumin, and a large amount of globulin. Accordingly, the diagnosis of PARETIC NEUROSYPHILIS ("general paresis"), especially in view of the laboratory findings, seems necessary.

2. What is the cause of the glycosuria? First: possibly it has no relation with the syphilis; secondly: it may possibly be due to a syphilitic involvement of the pancreas; thirdly: it is barely possible that it is due to syphilitic disease of the fourth ventricle or of the base of the brain, involving the pituitary region. Perhaps our case is too complex for analysis. At all events, the case brings up the possibility of a syphilitic glycosuria.

3. Can the diabetes in the case of Barrie be explained as syphilitic? Warthin of Ann Arbor has recently described somewhat remarkable spirochete findings in his autopsy material. The order of organic infection according to frequency is: aorta, heart, testis, adrenal, pancreas, nervous system, liver, and spleen. Warthin has called attention to the relation of pancreatitis and spirochetosis to diabetes in a recent review * of findings in 41 autopsied cases from the University Hospital in Michigan. Warthin found active luetic lesions in the pancreas in 6 cases.

---

* Warthin: " Persistence of active lesions and spirochetes in the tissues of clinically inactive or ' cured ' syphilitics," *American Journal of Medical Sciences*, CLII, 1916.

Hemianopsia in a case of neurosyphilis.

Case 66. Lawrence Washington, a colored cabman, 58 years of age, began to forget addresses given him by his fares. Moreover, he could no longer see as well as before, especially on looking toward the right side. He himself states that the visual trouble dated back as long ago as his 39th year, at which time he had a terrific pain in both temples, leading back from the eyes. Washington thought that his vision had been getting slowly but steadily worse ever since.

We got the impression that the amnesia claimed by Washington was more or less subjective and he was found to be well informed. This association of amnesia and impairment of vision naturally suggests syphilis. The patient himself stated that he had had a chancre at the age of 18.

We found the W. R. of the serum to be appropriately positive. The W. R. of the spinal fluid was also positive though weakly so. There was an excess of albumin; globulin appeared in large amount; the gold sol reaction was of the syphilitic type; there were 186 cells in the spinal fluid.

Is this case one of paresis or of some other form of cerebrospinal syphilis? Let us consider the data of the **physical examination.** On the whole, the patient was well preserved. There was a slight radial arteriosclerosis, but on the whole the cardiovascular system was almost negative. The blood pressure was 100 systolic, 65 diastolic. **Neurologically** the visual field of the left eye was somewhat limited, and there was a temporal hemianopsia of the right eye. The ophthalmoscopic examination showed a disseminated choroiditis on both sides. The right pupil failed to react to light. The left pupil reacted slowly. Both pupils reacted properly to accommodation.

The knee-jerks could be obtained only on reinforcement, and when obtained, the right was apparently more active than the left. The left Achilles was absent; the right present. There were no other abnormal reflexes.

The motility of the facial muscles was somewhat impaired. Finger-to-finger and finger-to-nose tests were rather poorly done. The muscle sense was good; there was no swaying in Romberg position; and there was no speech defect.

We are unable to decide whether the case is one of the **parenchymatous** type (paretic) or of the **meningovascular** type of **neurosyphilis**. It is certainly rather unusual to find hemianopsia in a paretic.

We have been unable to get definite results from the treatment of this case, since the patient would not return for months after getting an injection or two of salvarsan, on the ground that he was improved enough and did not require further treatment.

1. What conclusion can be drawn from the 186 cells per cmm. in the spinal fluid? Ordinarily this finding would indicate an active process. Some writers have claimed that a cell count running above 100 per cmm. was an indicator of diffuse non-paretic neurosyphilis. It does not appear that this claim has been substantiated. It is remarkable that this case shows an interval of 40 years between infection and the occurrence of definite clinical symptoms. With respect to the cell count, both in untreated and in treated cases, the following conclusions from a recent article (Solomon and Koefod)* are in point:

    1. The number of cells found in the fluid of untreated cases offers no definite information of prognostic value.

    2. One is not justified in drawing any conclusions as to whether the case is cerebrospinal syphilis or general paresis, nor the time the process has been active, nor the severity of it, from the cell count.

    3. The cell count may vary greatly from month to month, or when the interval is but several days, while at other times it may remain very nearly the same after an interval of months.

    4. Cases showing natural remissions may show no reduction in the cell count, or other spinal fluid findings.

---

* " The Significance of Changes in Cellular Content of Cerebrospinal Fluid in Neurosyphilis," *Boston Medical and Surgical Journal*, CLXXIII, 27.

5. Cases treated with salvarsan, either intraspinously or intravenously, tend to show a more or less rapid fall in the cell count. This count will, as a rule, remain low during treatment, but is likely to rise when treatment has been discontinued, but may rise during treatment after having first fallen.

6. Cases may show remissions during treatment and still have a pleocytosis.

7. Treated cases having the cell count fall to normal may at the same time become very much worse and develop more marked paralytic symptoms.

8. In general paresis the cell count in no way parallels the other spinal fluid findings.

9. In cases in which the other tests show an improvement, for instance cerebrospinal syphilis, the cell count also readily and early drops to normal. At times it may drop to normal before other spinal fluid tests become negative; again it may be last to reach normal.

10. The change in cell count seen in syphilitic disease untreated is also found in non-syphilitic diseases, as brain tumor.

11. The cell count offers nothing of prognostic importance in syphilis of the nervous system unless accompanied by improvement of the other laboratory signs.

12. The cell count is not an index to the predominance of irritative or degenerative changes.

Case of CEREBRAL MALARIA and SYPHILIS: simulation of PARETIC NEUROSYPHILIS (" general paresis ").

Case 67. Joseph Temple, 45, who had been a sea-going steamboat steward, was brought to the hospital in a semi-stupor. He was entirely uncooperative, often resistive, attempting to bite the physician's fingers, and for the most part lying curled up. He was incontinent and tube-fed. This phase, it seems, had begun the night before entrance to the hospital. Twenty-four hours later, an extraordinary change was noted. Temple became alert and attended to his wants, began to eat well, and began to behave as normally as probably he ever behaved.

He was now able to give a coherent history. It was now January. In the previous September, he had left for Mexico; he was returning when he suddenly fell to the deck, unconscious. After this fall, he had not been well, having had chills and fever. At the Marine Hospital, he had been diagnosed as suffering from malaria, and was given quinin. He had been delirious a short time in the hospital, not being able to recognize his wife, who called. He shortly improved so that his wife was able to take him home. Nevertheless, headache, gastric distress, and intermittent vomiting continued. A spell of confusion took place, two days before admission. The patient tossed about, moaned, and failed to recognize anyone. Malaria of the æstivo-autumnal type was demonstrated in the hospital. The temperature always remained at normal. He was somewhat emaciated and pale. The pupils were small, somewhat unequal, and reacted though poorly to light and distance. The tendon reflexes were lively.

The W. R. of the serum was positive, and information from the patient's physician runs to the effect that there was a syphilitic infection some seven or eight years ago, followed by secondary symptoms, but the patient had refused to take any protracted treatment. The spinal fluid examination was practically negative.

Mentally, the patient was euphoric, expansive, boastful, and showed a marked emotional instability and considerable memory defect.

1. Can the diagnosis of general paresis be made in Joseph Temple? Certainly the acute confusion and the syncope are consistent enough with the diagnosis, yet the severe malaria makes it seem likely that the phenomena were due to a cerebral attack of malaria, and such occurrences are found in the æstivo-autumnal form of malaria. Yet malaria would hardly explain the euphoria, memory defect, and the pupillary findings, to say nothing of the irritability and the active tendon reflexes. Even if we regard the active tendon reflexes and the irritability as malarial, the other phenomena remain outstanding as exceedingly suspicious of paresis.

On the other hand, if we try to support forcibly the diagnosis of general paresis, we are hardly able to explain the negative findings in the spinal fluid.

In point of fact, a study of the patient's past life revealed a story that the mental traits of euphoria, irritability, and memory defect had been characteristic of the patient for many years. In fact, there is some question whether the patient is not really to be regarded as a moron of high grade.

Upon this basis, if we regard the confusional phenomena as malarial and the persistent mental phenomena as characteristic of a moron and somewhat exaggerated by the disease, we have merely to explain the suggestive pupils. As to these, it must be remembered that though they reacted poorly to light, still they reacted somewhat, so it is not a question of explaining an Argyll-Robertson pupil, but only an impaired pupillary reaction. Of course, some workers are of the opinion that pupillary changes, perhaps even the Argyll-Robertson pupils, may occur in syphilitic cases that are not neurosyphilitic, or at all events are not victims of central neurosyphilis. Finally, we must remember that there are cases of neurosyphilis of a vascular type which yield negative spinal fluids. The case leaves many questions unanswered.

> Can paretic and non-paretic neurosyphilis be dif-
> ferentiated by means of the gold sol reaction?
> The gold sol reaction in this case was an extremely
> mild one and would not at all have warranted the
> diagnosis GENERAL PARESIS, yet the discovery
> of a heavy meningeal exudate including an un-
> usually heavy deposit of plasma cells even in the
> spinal pia mater will perhaps warrant us in making
> a final retrospective diagnosis of paretic neuro-
> syphilis. Autopsy.

Case 68. We would like to give the full effect of our surprise at the outcome of the case of Margaret O'Brien, a
school-teacher, 26 years of age. To be sure, Miss O'Brien
developed symptoms at 22 or 23 which we can now explain
consistently with the outcome of the case; for at that time,
she began to complain of severe pain in the head, especially
in the forehead and temples, and also became nervous, unable
to remain quiet, and given to insomnia. She was markedly
depressed at the time and would refuse to talk at times.
However, only the headache in this prodromal period could
be regarded as particularly suggestive of syphilis, and headache in an over-worked school-teacher is not uncommon.

In fact, the picture presented by the patient was one of
catatonic dementia praecox. The patient was admitted to
the hospital after a sudden onset of excitement. At first she
was very restless, continually looking about and getting up
and walking away from the examiner, giving the impression of
understanding all questions but preserving an air of indif-
ference. A few days later, the patient was gotten to answer
more coöperatively. She remarked that the hospital was
heaven although in Boston; that it was summer time (correct)
and that her memory was greatly impaired. The physician
was a messenger of God (delusion later corrected). The
patient had not done God's will; her breath was leaving her;
God's voice was heard from time to time, and Miss O'Brien

had heard it for a long time. God tells her to do His will. However, as Miss O'Brien remarked, " I must think all this nonsense, turning against God."

The patient frequently attitudinized and would remain in an apparently catatonic condition for many minutes. For the most part, she was resistive and mute and non-coöperative as to examination. From time to time, she made impulsive suicidal attempts. So far as a somewhat inadequate **physical examination** was concerned, nothing abnormal could be made out; in particular, the pupils reacted normally to light and were otherwise normal. The routine W. R. of the blood serum, however, returned positive, and in accordance with the policy of the Psychopathic Hospital, the patient was subjected to a lumbar puncture. The lumbar puncture yielded a positive W. R., 109 cells per cmm., a positive globulin and a considerable excess of albumin, and an exceedingly mild gold reaction — syphilitic type.

Ten days after admission, the patient had a convulsion. She never regained consciousness, continued to have convulsions for a few hours, and died, apparently from paralysis of respiration. The heart continued to beat for a short period after respiration ceased. The **autopsy** was consistent with the diagnosis which had been rendered after the surprising results of the W. R. in the blood and the laboratory findings in the spinal fluid had been learned. There was a generalized encephalitis with congestion of all the smaller cerebral vessels and petechial areas in the meninges and upon the cortical surfaces. We regard the case as one of syphilitic encephalitis.

The brain weighed 1265 grams, indicating a loss of 79 grams by Tigges' formula (8 times the body length in centimetres). The pia mater was, in the gross, quite normal within the cranium; nor were any cells found in a smear from this pia mater; but the pia mater over the spinal cord was visibly edematous, and a smear from the spinal pia mater showed great numbers of lymphocytes and especially of plasma cells — a finding which was confirmed in stained section, by which a remarkable display of plasma cells was found plastered somewhat generally over the entire pia mater of certain segments. The brain substance was softer than normal, but displayed no differences of consistence. The stripping of the pia mater of the temporal lobes on both sides yielded the so-called " decortication " (that is, the adhesion of small bits of brain substance to the pia mater). The optic nerves were somewhat thinner than normal. No other gross lesions of the brain were found.

The dura mater, although dense and injected, was not otherwise abnormal. There was an early visible sclerosis of the middle meningeal arteries, more marked on the left side.

The cause of death, so far as the autopsy revealed it, was bronchial pneumonia. There was a diffuse nephritis.

1. Are the hallucinations in the case of O'Brien characteristic? Hallucinations are regarded as playing a minor rôle in general paresis. In fact, earlier workers sometimes denied that hallucinations occurred at all, and this denial has been made once more of late by Plaut,* but Kraepelin quotes Obersteiner as observing hallucinations in 10%, and regards that figure as approximately corresponding with his own experience. Junius and Arndt are cited as finding 17% of their cases hallucinated. Auditory hallucinations are somewhat more frequent than those of vision (alcoholic psychosis must be considered). The visual hallucinations of paresis are thought by Kraepelin to be related with atrophy of the optic nerves, and he states that they occur by preference in patients having such atrophy. Hallucinations though not common are more frequent in non-paretic neurosyphilis than in paretic neurosyphilis.

2. What was the cause of death in Margaret O'Brien? The autopsy, as above stated, indicated pneumonia. In point of fact, this patient developed convulsions and ceased respiration, the heart continuing to beat for some time after respiration had ceased. It may be that the death should be counted as one of neurosyphilitic seizure.

---

* Plaut: Ueber Halluzinosen der Syphilitiker, Berlin, 1913.

Tonsillar abscess associated with neurosyphilis
(Lues Maligna?).

Case 69. Frank Mason, 49 years, a rectifier of spirits, was admitted to the Psychopathic Hospital in a tremulous, mentally confused, depressed, and unhappy state. He was particularly concerned because he could not give an accurate account of his past life and because he found that he was continually contradicting himself.

Superficial examination shortly discovered the pupils to be much contracted, irregular, and non-reactive either to light or distance. Although these pupils showed more than the Argyll-Robertson phenomenon, yet the suspicion of syphilis was important.

Throat examination showed a large area of ulceration involving the whole of the right tonsil and extending even to the left side of the median line so that the whole of the faucial pillar was involved. In the midst of this ulcerative area was a mass of purulent necrotic tissue, about which the edges of the ulcer stood out sharply. There was, however, very little acute reaction about the margin of the area.

The association of pupillary changes (especially stiffness to light), what looked like tonsillar gumma, and mental disorder (including memory disturbance) heightened the impression of syphilis.

However, the remainder of the examination was not especially confirmatory of the diagnosis. The man was well developed and obese, with a slightly enlarged heart, with sounds of poor quality and the aortic second sound accentuated. The systolic blood pressure was 130; the diastolic, 90. There was no disorder of reflexes except that the arm reflexes were very lively.

After a time, a few facts concerning the patient's life became available. Although a rectifier of spirits, Mason could not be found to have over-indulged in alcohol. It appears that some five months before his admission to the hospital, a wisdom-tooth had been extracted. About four months before admission, the ulceration of the faucial pillar had begun, and this ulceration was immediately laid to infection from the wisdom-tooth cavity. Mason then had to discontinue work and a depression followed. But the account of this depression led us to think that he was a victim more of natural sadness than psychopathic depression. There was much worry and insomnia. To meet the insomnia, large amounts of hypnotics were administered. The sequence of these hypnotics was a tremendous disturbance and continual crying out by the patient. In fact, Mason became so excited that he was removed to the Psychopathic Hospital for temporary care in the condition above mentioned.

We naturally awaited the outcome of the serum W. R. The return was negative. However, the typical position of the ulcerative lesion and the non-reacting pupils, — to say nothing of the mental symptoms and the associated tremors, with incoördination (this incoördination was non-characteristic and apparently due largely to the tremor), — led to lumbar puncture.

The spinal fluid yielded a weakly positive W. R. There was a slight positive albumin, the globulin test was slightly positive, there were 14 cells per cmm., and the gold sol reaction was of the syphilitic type. We were, then, probably entitled to conclude that syphilis was active not only in the body at large but also in the nervous system. Looking back upon the case, we considered that large doses of morphine and hyoscyamus might well have produced the marked mental confusion and possibly the tremors that characterized Mason on his arrival at the hospital.

Improvement followed after a few days of rest; the confusion disappeared and the tremors diminished; the pupils returned to their normal size and reaction; depression persisted, and the patient was very properly much concerned about the tonsillar lesion. However, further improvement did not take place under antisyphilitic treatment and patient died after several weeks from what was believed to be an embolus from the tonsil.

1. What was the true interpretation of Frank Mason's pupillary changes? They were probably due to the opiates, despite the fact that, taken in association with the gummatous lesion of the faucial pillar, we had regarded them as possibly syphilitic.

2. How shall the negative serum W. R. be explained? Such a reaction is consistent with the diagnosis *gumma*. It is, however, a little surprising that with active neuro-syphilis and a relatively active non-nervous syphilitic lesion like that in this case, the serum W. R. should have been negative. Possibly a repetition of the test at various times would have shown a positive serum W. R. In any event, the fluid reaction was positive.

3. Could the tonsillar ulceration be due to dental infection? The chances are against this on account of the interval (2 months) between extraction of the wisdom tooth and the ulceration, which itself seems to be of a tertiary syphilitic nature. In point of fact, the patient admitted a syphilitic infection 27 years previously namely, at 28 years of age. At that time he took large quantities of mercury and potassium iodid by mouth.

4. Relation of the case of Frank Mason to the so-called *lues maligna?* The case closely resembled the cases reported by Bly. Frank Mason showed great destruction of tissue, toxemia, failure to react to antisyphilitic treatment. In both of Bly's cases, the tonsil was the starting point of the illness; and in both cases there was a trauma of the tonsil or peri-tonsillar structures (tonsillectomy and application of caustic). In our case there not only had been extraction of a wisdom tooth, but the tonsil had been cauterized.

Neurosyphilis versus multiple sclerosis.

Case 70. Annie Kelly is a young Irish woman, 21 years of age, who was perfectly well until three months before her admission to the Psychopathic Hospital, when suddenly one evening she became very dizzy. This was followed by a chill and vomiting. The next day she had a sore throat but was able to be about and do her work. The dizziness, however, continued and she began to feel rather queer. Gradually it became difficult for her to walk on account of staggering.

A little later she noticed a weakness of the left side, involving face, arm, and leg; then she began to find it difficult to talk. Finally the right leg became weak, making walking practically impossible. All these symptoms grew worse and the dizziness increased. At times her vision would be blurred; there were somewhat frequent attacks of diplopia. Finally she had to take to her bed, and at last she lost control of her sphincters.

At no time did she suffer any pain. She was taken to a hospital, and after a time improved somewhat; but she was told she had a brain tumor and had better be in a large city, where she could have surgical aid if this became necessary; consequently, she was brought from Montana to Boston.

On admission to the hospital, the examination disclosed no important symptoms outside of the nervous and locomotor systems. She was unable to walk unless assisted. The pupils were large but reacted well to both light and accommodation, were equal in size, and regular. Slight nystagmus was present; there was no ptosis or strabismus; vision in the left eye was poor. The other cranial nerves showed no involvement. The tendon reflexes were all present and very lively; Babinski, Gordon, and Oppenheim signs were present on either side. The ataxia was marked, especially of the lower arms, and she had some difficulty in the alignment of the fingers. The sense of position of the limbs was very poor. There was some tremor, which was not of the intention type. The writing showed some incoördination. The speech showed nothing abnormal. **Mental examination** disclosed nothing of note objectively, but patient stated she could not think so clearly as she could formerly.

The **diagnosis** would seem to lie between brain tumor, — which had been suggested to the patient by her physician, — multiple sclerosis, and neurosyphilis. The numerous neurological symptoms without any definite evidence of intracranial pressure were sufficient to rule out for the moment the consideration of brain tumor. The syndrome of multiple sclerosis is not complete, but the race, age, and onset, with the increasing and decreasing intensity of symptoms are very suggestive of this diagnosis. The symptoms, of course, are all consistent with neurosyphilis also, and while the patient denied any knowledge of syphilitic involvement, the examination of the blood and spinal fluid was made. The W. R. was negative in both the blood serum and spinal fluid. Further examination of the spinal fluid showed presence of globulin and an increase in the albumin content, 43 cells per cmm. and a " paretic " type of gold sol reaction. With the negative W. R. of both blood serum and spinal fluid, and with so much in favor of MULTIPLE SCLEROSIS, this diagnosis was made.

1.   What is the relation of multiple sclerosis to syphilis? There is no definite relationship between multiple sclerosis and syphilis, — that is, multiple sclerosis is not a syphilitic disease; but the complete syndrome of multiple sclerosis is often given by a syphilitic involvement of the central nervous system (see case Lauder, 71).

2.   Is the spinal fluid finding in this case consistent with multiple sclerosis? According to Nonne, about 19% of the cases of multiple sclerosis show globulin and pleocytosis in the spinal fluid. As a rule, the number of cells ranges between 10 and 20 per cmm. and the globulin is not present in large amounts. In this case, the amount of globulin, which was given as 2+, is only a moderate amount, — less than is usually found in cases of general paresis. There are not very many

cases of multiple sclerosis in the literature in which a gold sol reaction has been performed, but in the majority of those tested, the reaction is reported as mild. However, cases of multiple sclerosis giving a typical paretic curve have been described by a number of observers, among whom may be mentioned Kaplan and Solomon.

3. How frequently is it necessary to make a differential diagnosis between multiple sclerosis and neurosyphilis? Before the days of the W. R. this differentiation was much more difficult than at present. But we, however, still have to face a not very rare difficulty in separating the two conditions. Syphilis is prone to cause small localized lesions in the nervous system. The changes in the patient's condition, with improvements and regressions are equally characteristic of both diseases. How closely the symptomatology of neurosyphilis may simulate that of typical multiple sclerosis is shown in the next case (Lauder, 71). When the sclerotic area of multiple sclerosis occurs in appropriate parts of the cerebrum, symptoms of mental disturbances will occur. In its histological picture multiple sclerosis is at times highly suggestive of syphilis, even showing mononucleosis and meningitis.

> Optic atrophy; nystagmus; spasticity; intention tremor. Diagnosis: ?

Case 71. James Lauder began to lose his eyesight at 32 years, and was shortly determined to be suffering from primary optic atrophy. In the course of a year, he had become completely blind. No mental symptoms had developed.

Physically, Lauder was in very good condition. **Neurologically,** there was a complete optic atrophy with paralysis of the internal rectus muscle, marked nystagmus, and absent pupillary reactions. All the tendon reflexes were exceedingly lively, though the right arm reflexes were more lively than the left, and the left leg reflexes more lively than the right. There was an ankle clonus on both sides. The abdominal and cremasteric reflexes were lively. There was a slight intention tremor. There was, however, no ataxia and no speech defect.

Diagnosis: The nystagmus, optic atrophy, and the reflex disorder suggested multiple sclerosis, although the liveliness of the superficial reflexes, especially the abdominal reflexes, was a point somewhat against any advanced degree of multiple sclerosis. It would appear that the absence of pupillary reaction to accommodation is also rather unusual in multiple sclerosis.

The serum and spinal fluid W. R.'s proved positive. There were 25 cells per cmm., albumin was in excess, and there was a positive globulin reaction.

1. What is the significance of optic atrophy and other optic changes with respect to neurosyphilis? Canavan, from our laboratory, has reported that she found that 40 of 58 unselected cases of mental disease exhibited obvious and undeniably important changes in the optic nerve. She found that optic nerve changes were even more frequent than chronic spinal cord changes as detectable by the same method (Weigert myelin

sheath method); there were only 34 of the 58 cases which showed chronic spinal cord changes. Eighteen cases very probably syphilitic (although the clinical evidence was not in all cases supported by the W. R.) failed to show optic nerve changes in but three instances. The 15 syphilitic cases that did show optic nerve changes showed them in but one eye in three cases, in both eyes in 12 cases. Canavan incidentally demonstrated a spirochetosis in the pial sheath of the optic nerve in a case of neurosyphilis, possibly paretic.

2. What is the frequency of eye changes in neurosyphilis? Posey and Spiller ("The Eye and the Nervous System," 1906) quote Kéraval as finding 42 instances of fundus change in 51 cases of paresis. Clifford Allbutt found 41 cases of atrophy in 53 of paresis; other authors have found far fewer. Optic atrophy sufficiently marked to cause blindness is relatively rare in paresis. Compare table of eye changes from Joffroy under Case Falvey (55).

As for optic atrophy in tabes, Posey and Spiller record statistics as so various as to be on the whole unsatisfactory. The highest percentages found appear to be those of Mott, 80%, and Gross, 88%. It is evident that the standards for measuring optic atrophy must differ very much.

Atypical case of neurosyphilis. Picture of Huntington's chorea.

Case 72. Margaret Green, 28, was received at Danvers
State Hospital in an excited and frightened state. She was
very talkative and said that she was being bitten by snakes
and serpents. She thought every one approaching her was
the devil, and sprinkled what she called " holy water " about
her for protection. It was clear that she was hallucinated.
She heard her child crying, and she saw a woman carrying it
away.

After a few weeks, Mrs. Green grew quiet and more rational
except for a few spells of violence and noise; she gave the
impression of a rather pleasant and agreeable, though somewhat demented, patient. Physically, beyond a tremor of
fingers and tongue and lively knee-jerks and some evidence
of enlargement of the heart, there was nothing to be found.

Margaret Green is still in the Danvers Hospital, being now
48 years of age. During the twenty years, she has presented,
— besides the mental picture of impairment of memory —
occasional spells of confusion, a variety of delusions based,
at least in part, upon auditory and vivid visual hallucinations,
a certain irritability and psychomotor excitement, and a
picture of Huntington's chorea. The diagnosis of Huntington's chorea has always been in doubt by reason of the lack
of any evidences of hereditary taint; it has, however, not
been possible to secure a properly intensive account of her
relatives.

It appears that the choreic movements were first observed — in the hospital at least — about 16 years ago. The
patient has always been decidedly mixed upon dates. From
internal evidence derived from her obviously in part erroneous
statements, it may be that the chorea began at the age of
23. It appears that she had been often termed a victim of
of St. Vitus' dance, and had had to leave her work in the mill
on account of the disease. From one source of information,

it would appear that the patient began to have what was called St. Vitus' dance when she was 14 or 15 years of age; so far as this informant knew, no other member of the family had had the affliction.

The first movements observed in the hospital were irregular, jerking movements, more marked in the left arm but also occurring in the other extremities, as well as in the face, wherein were produced peculiar grimaces. The twitching movements would become decidedly worse during spells of irritability. Observation in the patient's early thirties left the question in doubt whether the left pupil reacted to light or not. In 1904, when the patient was 36, both pupils failed to react to light either directly or consensually. At this time, the jerky movements continued, especially in the left hand and forearm, the tongue was tremulous, test phrases were poorly pronounced, the knee-jerks were exaggerated (especially the left), and both wrist-jerks were exaggerated. The systematic examination, however, revealed no other neurological disorder. Within a year, slight spurious ankle clonus developed on both sides; the eyes, especially the left, gave the appearance of developing cataracts. A slight consensual light reaction was demonstrable on the right side, but all light reactions were absent in the left eye.

At the age of 42, the patient was still disoriented for time, place, and persons and subject to a deep amnesia; was tidy, tranquil, and of a pleasant demeanor, but many of her muscles were in continual motion. There were chewing movements and both hands and feet were rarely still. There were no longer any spells of irritability or violence; and once when found crying on the piazza, Mrs. Green, on being asked the reason, replied that a gray cat had come and looked at her so hard it made her cry. There were other crying spells at times for equally good reasons, or for no reason.

More recently, the patient has become fairly well oriented for time and place, and has acquired a fairly good insight into her condition and a good memory for past events. She has had occasionally auditory hallucinations, as of water running. In 1914, it was reported that the pupils reacted to light, and the rest of the systematic neurological examination was negative except that the knee-jerks were exaggerated; and a re-examination in 1916 showed the pupils still reacted to light. At present, the patient is disoriented for time, stating that her age is about 25; she is no longer subject to auditory hallucinations; she has a marked difficulty in enunciation, emphasized by the lack of teeth and in part due to continual movements of the tongue; the movements appear to be part of a generalized chorea.

In a systematic review of the Wassermann findings in the hospital population, the blood of Margaret Green was examined and found to be positive. Lumbar puncture forthwith performed showed a positive W. R. in the fluid; there was a positive globulin and an excess of albumin; the gold sol was characteristic of paresis; there were, however, but three cells per cmm.

1. Are the choreiform movements related to the demonstrable syphilis of the nervous system? Neither the fluid W. R. nor the gold sol reaction should be regarded as necessarily an indicator of tissue loss. The fluid W. R. is commonly thought to signify merely that the fluid contains substances which are somehow due to the presence of spirochetes in some region pretty closely related with the fluid. The gold sol reaction, although well established to be characteristic of neurosyphilis, is perhaps not so strong an evidence of the existence of spirochetes in the region from which fluid constituents are derived. There is no pleocytosis. However, the positive globulin test and the excess of albumin do indicate a certain amount of destructive process somewhere in the neural tissues. Are we to suppose that these substances have been continually found during the course of this disease? This question cannot be answered with the data in hand, and we can only suspect that these positive tests for albumin and globulin are an effect of tissue destruction caused by neurosyphilis. It must be admitted that the argument here is a little tenuous. The lesson is plain: that in the present stage of our knowledge the W. R. should not be omitted even in cases which present a fairly convincing picture of some well-known entity. Thus, a disease, which looks like Huntington's chorea,

as well as a disease suggestive of multiple sclerosis, requires investigation by the methods of the syphilographer.

2. How shall we explain the changes in pupillary reaction in this case? They cannot yet be explained. A few observers have reported changes in pupillary reflexes in the direction of normality. In our experience such changes have not been noted. It cannot be too strongly emphasized that it is very easy to make errors in judging pupillary reaction if care is not used. For instance, if the patient is accommodating for near vision, light will probably not cause contraction. A frequent cause of error in testing the light reflex arises from using a weak electric light. An electric flashlight is much less efficient than daylight. Probably the most satisfactory method is to take the patient to a window, ask him to look at a distant object, shade the eye with the hand, remove hand, and observe.

3. What is the chief triad of symptoms in Huntington's chorea? (1) Choreiform movements associated with (2) progressive mental enfeeblement, (3) occurring in a patient whose family history shows a similar condition in a preceding generation.

Differential diagnosis between NEUROSYPHILIS
and SENILE ARTERIOSCLEROTIC PSYCHOSIS.

Case 73. Marcus Chatterton was a retired sea captain, 75 years of age. At the age of 71, he had had a seizure with a slight right hemiplegia and inability to talk. He had been slightly confused for a short time but had rapidly recovered. During the intervening four years, there had been three similar attacks, and the last one had caused him to come to the hospital. He was, in fact, confused upon admission but had become perfectly clear by the next day. There was a considerable memory defect, which the patient himself did not entirely appreciate. Possibly his judgment had been deteriorating slightly. He had been irritable of late and sometimes sleepless.

Physical examination showed a rather well-preserved man with but slight senile changes. The pupils were equal and reacted readily to light and accommodation. There was no sensory disorder and no disturbance of coördination. There were no tremors. The systolic blood pressure was 205, the diastolic 135. The arteries were sclerotic upon palpation. A sufficient diagnosis would have seemed to be arteriosclerosis, and the hypothesis of syphilis would hardly have been raised off-hand by most practitioners. The W. R. of the serum was negative. What led to lumbar puncture in this case was the fact that the sea captain's wife had died 15 years before of general paresis. The lumbar puncture was rewarding since the W. R. was positive. There was an increase of albumin and globulin, a " paretic " type of gold sol reaction, and 56 cells per cmm.

Accordingly, we must regard the condition as one of neurosyphilis. Perhaps the arteriosclerosis was of syphilitic origin. If this is a case of general paresis as we suppose, it is one of very long-standing syphilis.

1. Do delusions of grandeur in the senile period suggest syphilis? Not necessarily; it appears that there is a small group of senile cases which might be called cases of senile pseudoparesis in which extravagant delusions of grandeur are entertained, and in which frontal atrophy is found although entirely without evidence of chronic inflammation. It has not been proved that these cases are of syphilitic origin. It is suggestive that the site of the most extensive lesion is precisely the site of the most extensive lesion classically found in paretic neurosyphilis, viz., in the frontal regions.

2. Is neurosyphilis frequently found in both mates? It can hardly be said that this is a usual finding. However, it is far from rare, and it occurs frequently enough to be used in support of the theory that there is a special strain of spirochete that has a predilection for nervous tissue. It must be remembered, however, that the wives of syphilitics are frequently infected without being aware of it. In such cases they receive no treatment and consequently have a larger chance of developing neurosyphilis. It is a good rule to consider the mate of every syphilitic a candidate for neurosyphilis.

An atypical case of recurrent dazed states resembling HYSTERICAL FUGUES. Probably an instance of NEUROSYPHILIS.

Case 74. Abel Bachmann, a man of 40 years, remains doubtful and perhaps belongs to the still unresolved group of mental cases due to syphilis that cannot be placed in any of the well-known categories. Bachmann had been found by the police, working in front of a cowbarn without the consent or even the knowledge of the owner. Bachmann had, in fact, spent the night in the cowbarn and was working with the idea of paying for his night's lodgings. The situation struck the police as so peculiar, and Bachmann was so confused and irresponsive, that he was brought to the Psychopathic Hospital. The afternoon of his admission, however, he entirely cleared up and was able to give a good account of himself.

His story was that he had been worrying a good deal about a divorce suit, and the morning of his episode he had awakened with peculiar feelings. He walked from Boston to Cambridge, feeling that he was in a strange city. He recognized the places he passed, yet they all seemed to be changed. Upon reaching Harvard Square, he determined to return to Boston and walked and walked, failing to reach Boston. All day he had eaten nothing; when night fell he stole into a field and dug out radishes. A postman stopped and said, " Hello, Bill," which awakened him as by an electric shock. A barn presented itself, in which he spent the night. In the morning, the barn looked different. In fact, his entire surroundings appeared mysterious. As he felt like working, he went to work in front of the barn.

It seems that in his life there had been two other episodes of a similar nature; in fact, Bachmann had been in a state hospital for six weeks after the first episode. The first episode had lasted a few days only, and followed worry when he learned that the girl with whom he was in love was married.

The second attack followed the death of his mother, whereupon he was taken to a state hospital although the total
duration of symptoms was only three days. Bachmann
had had a chancre or some other form of genital disease at
26, and had at that time been treated with mercury.

Except for irregular and absolutely rigid pupils, reacting
neither to light nor to accommodation, Bachmann showed
no physical and especially no neurological disease whatever.
Moreover, the W. R. in the blood serum was negative.

As to diagnosis, one might consider hysteria, of which,
however, there are no visible stigmata. It would not appear
that brain tumor would be likely to have lasted so long as
eight or nine years, even if we should attempt to make the
hypothesis of tumor cover both the non-reacting pupils and
the episodes. Bachmann was non-alcoholic, and there was
no sign of any other form of intoxication. The spinal fluid
showed a negative gold sol reaction, there were no cells in the
fluid, there was no globulin; albumin was normal. However, the W. R. was strongly positive.

The situation, then, in this case is that we have somewhat
peculiar psychopathic episodes, pupils rigid to light and
accommodation, a positve W. R. in the spinal fluid, and extremely little else to permit a diagnosis. We are ignorant
as to the course and pathology of such cases. However, we
cannot resist the temptation of the diagnosis of neurosyphilis,
although further classification is not ventured.

I. What is the significance of stiff pupil as an isolated
symptom? Nonne finds that in the end, after years of
observation, the Argyll-Robertson pupil turns out to
be an advance courier of other more functionally
serious signs and symptoms of neurosyphilis. We can
confirm this experience and regard it as an established
clinical proposition that the Argyll-Robertson pupil
cannot be neglected. In this connection, refer to the
case of alcoholic pseudoparesis (Murphy, 60), and also
to the case of pineal tumor (Donald Falvey, 35). En-
thusiastic reports have occasionally been made upon
apparent restoration of the true syphilitic Argyll-
Robertson pupil to normal light reaction. The difficulties in rendering the symptomatic diagnosis of

Argyll-Robertson pupil in a given case are so great, and the chances of complication so numerous, that we are inclined to attach little significance at present to these claims.

It may not be amiss to mention a somewhat humorous incident familiar to some local neurologists. A case was reported by the interne for a number of months as a victim of a pupil stiff to light and accommodation, and the entirely adequate cause of this phenomenon was actually only discovered at autopsy by the triumphant medical examiner, who demonstrated that the patient in question was possessed of a **glass eye.**

TABETIC NEUROSYPHILIS ("tabes dorsalis")
versus PERNICIOUS ANEMIA with spinal
symptoms.

Case 75. Mrs. Brown was a woman of 56, who for the
past eight or ten years had been complaining of trouble in
her legs. As she described it, at times her legs were so weak
she could hardly stand; at other times there was considerable pain and numbness. She has always been considered
"high strung"; that is, she had a very bad temper and
lost control of herself almost entirely when she became
excited. Her legs had been growing progressively worse,
and for about a month prior to admission she had been unable to stand or walk. She had also lost control of her
bladder. On account of her temper, it had been almost
impossible to nurse her; no nurse would stay with her because of her scolding and fault-finding. Recently, she had
been having fits of the blues.

Her husband, who was seen before Mrs. Brown, was an
old gentleman, over 70, who was chiefly remarkable from the
fact that he had unequal, irregular pupils, which reacted
neither to light nor accommodation; there was also a speech
defect.

The patient herself proved to be extremely irritable, as
had been stated, — so much so that at times it seemed
almost impossible to do anything for her. She was very
querulous, constantly complaining, and not satisfied with
anything that was done. Aside from this, her **mental examination** proved to be entirely negative; that is, there were
no psychotic symptoms.

The systematic **physical examination** gave the following
significant findings: blood pressure, 160 systolic, 90 diastolic;
no evidences, however, of peripheral arteriosclerosis. Patient
was unable to walk or stand, and had no control over her
bladder. The knee-jerks and ankle-jerks absent on both
sides; ataxia in the leg movements; loss of sense of localiza-

tion, with no tenderness over the nerve trunks; no atrophy, paralyses, or muscular asymmetry of the parts. The vibratory sense was maintained. Subjectively, the patient thought that the vibratory sense differed in the legs from that in the arms. Localization, touch, pain, heat, and cold responded to correctly. The arms showed nothing abnormal; there was no incoördination, dysmetria, or dysdiadochokinesis. Her pupils were equal, regular, and both reacted normally to light and accommodation.

Diagnosis: The first consideration in the case is naturally tabes dorsalis, especially when one considers that the husband had signs which suggested syphilis of the nervous system. The rapid onset of the acute symptoms in this case, and the absence of the characteristic signs of pain were at least atypical for this diagnosis, as was the absence of any pupillary signs. Further, the W. R. was negative in the blood and spinal fluid; there were no definite signs of inflammatory reaction as shown by the other spinal fluid tests. These findings made a diagnosis of tabes entirely improbable. After tabes, the most frequent cause of the symptoms above enumerated is perhaps to be found in pernicious anemia. Examination of the blood showed that the patient had 2,500,000 erythrocytes per cmm. The hemoglobin by Tallquist scale was 80%. The smear was practically negative; no blasts could be seen. Although this picture is not a typical one for pernicious anemia, at least it is significant in the low number of red cells to be found, and as no causes for anemia were to be found, it seemed probable that we were dealing with a primary anemia. The diagnosis in the case, therefore, is spinal sclerosis of primary anemia. The mental picture was not uncharacteristic of PERNICIOUS ANEMIA.

1. Could the diagnosis be rendered in this case without a lumbar puncture? In the first place, the emaciation is not entirely characteristic. The pupils react normally to light. Probably such a case might well have been regarded as one of tabes dorsalis in former days, or even at the present time, if a lumbar puncture had not been resorted to.

2. Could this case possibly have been one of tabes dorsalis with negative spinal findings? Such cases have been reported frequently, but, unlike the present case, are apt to be of long standing and non-progressive, in which the active inflammation is no longer present. The negative findings would not be consistent with tabes, in which the symptoms are of short duration and of sudden onset.

3. If the serum W. R. had been positive would the diagnosis have been neurosyphilis? We are loath to make the diagnosis of spinal syphilis when the spinal fluid is normal. Syphilis may produce a marked anemia, however, and thus produce symptoms such as shown by Mrs. Brown. It is even possible that such is the explanation of this case, taking into consideration the suggestive findings in the husband. However, there is insufficient evidence to make such an hypothesis rock firm, and we do not more than suggest it.

Atypical case of CONGENITAL NEUROSYPH-
ILIS — peculiar mental state.

Case 76. James Seabrook, 20 years of age, obviously showed a number of signs of congenital syphilis. The **physical examination** disclosed an old scar and indentation in the right mastoid region, another on the right side of the neck, another on the posterior surface of the right forearm, and two on the outer surface of the right upper arm. The lesions were about the size of half a dollar. There was a saddle-shaped nose and a perforation of the palate and uvula; there were palpable cervical and axillary glands, small but numerous. There was a dulness in the region of the right scapula, and slight dulness on both sides behind. There were loud whispering and piping râles and bronchial breathing throughout the chest, more marked on the left; there was much coughing, and the sputum was at times blood-stained. The pupils were irregular but reacted perfectly. The left knee-jerk was slightly more active than the right. The W. R. in blood and fluid was negative; the gold sol, globulin and albumin tests were negative. There were, however, 56 cells per cmm. in the fluid.

We learned that the patient had had several spells of great excitement, with pounding on the door and a desire to fight bystanders. There were spells of headache and vertigo. **Mentally** the tests showed him to be subnormal.

The **diagnosis** of CONGENITAL SYPHILIS seems established; possibly the pulmonary condition is syphilitic. The mental subnormality as well as the abnormal traits and episodes are probably to be accounted for on the basis of syphilitic involvement of the brain.

1. Are the headache and vertigo connected with syphilis? This is perhaps suggested by the pleocytosis in the spinal fluid.
2. How shall we explain the negative W. R.? This patient had received, shortly before his entrance to the hospital,

salvarsan and mercury. Possibly the drug treatment has little or nothing to do with the negative W. R.'s since they not infrequently grow weaker as congenital syphilitics grow older.

3. What is the explanation of the spells of excitement? Compare the spells of excitement in a form of neurosyphilis described by Kraepelin, namely: syphilitic paranoia, discussed in the case of Bridget Collins (59).

4. Is treatment indicated considering the W. R.'s to be negative in blood and fluid? Despite the negative ,W. R.'s in this case treatment is strongly indicated on account of the pleocytosis. This would seem to indicate that there is an active inflammatory process in the cerebrospinal axis, and it is more than probable that this process is syphilitic. How much real improvement of the symptoms would result from antisyphilitic treatment it is impossible to prophesy. Every case is a special problem, and this case is very unusual in showing a pleocytosis in the absence of other indications of syphilitic nervous disease, *viz.*, globulin, albumin and W. R.'s.

CONGENITAL NEUROSYPHILIS resembling
an undifferentiated case of FEEBLEMINDED-
NESS — actually PARETIC.

Case 77. John Friedreich, a 7-year old boy, was brought
to the Psychopathic Hospital by agents of a charitable society,
who found him a neglected child and quite evidently a subnormal one.

The dominance of syphilis in the situation was clear. The
boy's father had died but a few months before of syphilitic
heart disease, from which he is said to have suffered for five
years. The boy's mother (the parents were first cousins)
had also been treated for syphilis and was excessively alcoholic. The first child of this union — a girl — had died
at 6 years, of a disease diagnosticated spinal meningitis.
The history indicates that syphilis was acquired after the
birth of this first child; but in any event it is possible that
the meningitic condition of which the first child had died was
syphilitic. The second pregnancy terminated in a still-
birth; the third issued in a girl, who died two weeks after
birth of what was termed "inward convulsions." The
fourth pregnancy resulted in a miscarriage; the fifth in our
patient, John Friedreich. The sixth pregnancy resulted in
a girl, now 5 years of age, who is apparently normal. (Her
W. R. was negative and she shows no stigmata of syphilis.)

The patient, John Friedreich, at some very early age had
a rash on his body diagnosticated as syphilis. He also had
many seizures called fainting spells. Ever since birth he had
been taking mercury pills. He had not learned to talk
until his third year, and was able then to say only a few dis-
connected words. In fact, John has never been able to talk
in complete sentences, mumbling much that is quite unintelligible. However, he walked at 15 months in a normal
fashion and nothing peculiar in his gait was noted until he
was 5 years old, when he began walking on his toes, particularly those of his left foot. Shortly thereafter, the seem-

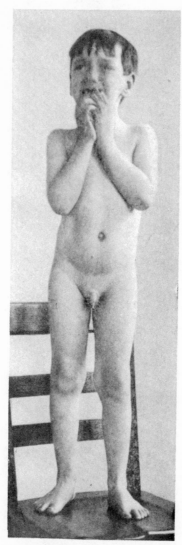

Juvenile paresis.   7 years.

ingly inevitable trauma appeared; John fell out of a window and severely injured his left leg, whereupon the peculiarity of toe-walking became more pronounced and associated with a limp.

The patient strikes one **physically** as having the development of a child of about five years (actual age, 7). There are a few lymph nodes palpable in the anterior triangles of the neck. The dilated and slightly unequal pupils react neither to light nor accommodation. There is practically complete deafness; loud sounds are not at all noticed.

Withal, the child in a general way presents a somewhat attractive appearance, being very playful and mischievous, lying about on the floor and playing with whatever comes to hand, talking to himself or making a few indistinct remarks to the bystanders. He walks awkwardly, on the toes of the left foot. He pays little or no attention to his toilet and needs to be dressed and cared for in all ways. He is quick-tempered and at times very difficult to manage.

There was, of course, little doubt of the **diagnosis** of CONGENITAL SYPHILIS and of FEEBLEMINDEDNESS. The W. R. was positive both in the blood and in the spinal fluid. The gold sol reaction of the fluid was of the " paretic " type; there were 44 cells per cmm. and there was a large excess of albumin and much globulin.

As to prognosis, there is doubt.

1. Is, or is not, this a case of juvenile paresis?
2. Is it, perhaps, a relatively permanent case of feeblemindedness due to congenital syphilis? On the whole, on account of the spinal fluid symptoms, we should be inclined to give the case a relatively poor prognosis, namely, of death in a few years. However, we may perchance be later surprised to learn that the patient has lived on, at least into early adult age.

    Note: Mercury tablets in some cases of congenital syphilis do not seem effective. John Friedreich was treated most intensively by syphilographers from birth.

    Dr. W. E. Fernald in a personal communication stated that syphilitic cases of feeblemindedness are rather those of the imbecile and idiot groups than of the higher levels. This statement emphasizes again that the true hereditary cases of feeblemindedness are rather those of the higher group, whereas the cases in which special causes have operated in the uterus or in early life eventuate in idiocy and imbecility. However, such a case as that of Friedreich shows that now and then a case of feeblemindedness without evidence of neurological disorder and looking in almost all respects like an hereditary case may be at times produced by syphilis.

3. How often is the central nervous system involved in hereditary syphilis? An interesting table bearing on this point is presented by Veeder.* The table concerns the lesions in various parts and systems of the body in 100 cases of late syphilis. It appears that in 47, or approximately one-half of Veeder's series of 100 late cases, the infection developed some form of lesion of the nervous system. As Veeder remarks, this result runs counter to the common statements of pediatricians, notably of Holt.

Bones:

Periostitis tibia...... 4
Periostitis skull...... 1
Osteomyelitis........ 1

Joints:

Acute arthritis knee.. 8
Acute arthritis ankle. 1

Skin:

Macular eruption.... 1
Condyloma anus..... 3
Gummata.......... 3
Alopecia........... 3

Eye:

Interstitial keratitis.. 24
Choroiditis.......... 1

Ulcerations:

Nasal.............. 2
Laryngeal.......... 1
Pharyngeal......... 1

Central Nervous System:

Mental deficiency........ 23
Cerebrospinal syphilis..... 14
Hemiplegia............. 6
Epilepsy............... 5
Spastic paraplegia........ 4
Chorea................ 2
Hydrocephalus.......... 2

Miscellaneous Conditions:

Ozena................. 1
Enlarged spleen (only symp- 1
  tom)................ 1
Torticollis............. 1
Aortitis............... 1
Obscure abdominal pain... 1
Obscure pain in legs...... 2
Endarteritis obliterans.... 1
Paroxysmal hemoglobinuria 1
Raynaud's disease........ 1
Hutchinson's teeth....... 4

---

* Borden S. Veeder: Hereditary Syphilis in the Light of Recent Clinical Studies; Am. Jour. of Med. Sc., CLII, 1916.

Juvenile paretic neurosyphilis. Quadriplegia.

Case 78. Gridley Ringer, 15 years of age, had the facies of a congenital syphilitic, including Hutchinsonian teeth, rhagades of the face, and the so-called Olympic brow. No secondary sexual characteristics had developed. There was a marked speech defect. **Mentally,** Ringer was a low-grade imbecile. He had been born at full term, and delivery had been normal. There had never been other pregnancies. He had never developed normally.

The father admitted syphilis 23 years before, namely, 8 years before the birth of his son, but the father had been treated for several years and had been declared cured.

1. What would be expected in the spinal fluid of this case? Without the history, it would perhaps be impossible to say whether the case was one of a quiescent imbecility or one of juvenile paresis. The spinal fluid of the juvenile paretic gives a picture identical with that in the adult. The spinal fluid in this case showed a positive W. R. (as did also the serum), a marked increase of albumin and globulin, 115 cells per cmm., and a " paretic " gold sol reaction. Accordingly, the diagnosis of GENERAL PARESIS was made.

2. What is the prognosis? The prognosis of juvenile paresis is currently regarded as entirely grave. There is probably less hope for improvement in juvenile paresis than in the acquired paresis of adult life, since it seems to be a general principle that congenital syphilis is always more difficult to cure than acquired syphilis.

   This case had seizures a few months after initial observation, and the seizures were followed by a transient right hemiplegia. This right hemiplegia was shortly followed by a left hemiplegia, which remained permanently. Moreover, a few weeks later, a right hemiplegia again developed, leaving the patient with complete paralysis and aphasia. Death followed in six weeks.

3. What effects were shown in the parents? Following up the parents was rewarded by the discovery that the

mother was suffering from nerve deafness, probably of syphilitic origin, and that the father had recently begun to suffer from what he considered rheumatism, but which on examination was shown to be tabetic neurosyphilis (" tabes dorsalis "). This family again supports the hypothesis that there is a strain of spirochetes especially prone to attack the nervous system. Here it would seem that the syphilis acquired by the father had infected the mother and been transmitted to the son. In all three infected by the same strain or strains of organisms the nervous system was involved. It is difficult, nevertheless, to explain on this hypothesis why in one case the disease took the form of tabes dorsalis, in the second, eighth nerve involvement and in the third, paresis. This question of strains is really more than academic because it enters deeply into the question of treatment, as well as that of the suggested increased viability of the neural strain.

Is there a relation between epilepsy and juvenile neurosyphilis?

Case 79. John Doran fell off the rear of an ice-wagon, at six years of age, and shortly afterward developed fits. It appears that John was not unconscious at the time of his fall, but that he complained of headache. Although the convulsions were fairly frequent at first, it appears that they later became rare and occurred only when the patient got into a temper. At the stage of exhaustion after violent excitement, John would fall.

Physically, at 9 years a fair development and nutrition were evident. There was a great exaggeration of the frontal bosses; the nose could not be said to be typically saddle-backed, yet there was a suggestion of a sinking of the bridge. The teeth slightly suggested the Hutchinsonian type, but only slightly. There was a slight roughening of the tibia, and there was a slight scar over either knee. The patient graded according to the Binet scale at 9 years, and he was regarded as definitely feebleminded.

The family physician states that, according to his information, the father contracted syphilis when the child was between three and four months of age, and that the mother also was infected at this time. However, the child had not been suckled except immediately after birth, and there had been no evidences, according to the family physician, that John had acquired syphilis.

Ordinarily, one might content himself regarding the case of John Doran as one of idiopathic epilepsy with mental defect or deterioration. However, the frontal bosses, suggestive teeth, the flattened bridge of the nose, the roughened tibiae, and the old scars, though singly not of great significance, collectively make one suspicious. Despite the family physician's belief that John could not have acquired syphilis from the parents, the infection seems entirely possible despite the fact that no symptoms developed early thereafter.

The W. R. in this case proved positive in both blood serum and spinal fluid.

1. What is the relation of trauma to this case of JUVENILE NEUROSYPHILIS? Probably none.
2. What would be the effect of treatment? For a number of years John Doran was lost sight of. He was, however, treated, according to our information, with intraspinous injections of salvarsanized serum, whereupon his convulsions shortly ceased. He has been recently examined mentally once more, and still grades as feeble-minded. He still has violent outbreaks of temper.
3. Is such a case as Doran typical? Shanahan has investigated conditions at Craig Colony. There were 22 out of 886 epileptics (at Craig Colony) or $2\frac{1}{2}\%$, who showed a positive W. R. Nine of these cases were regarded by Shanahan as cases of epilepsy actually caused by syphilis. Viet had found 7%, and Bratz and Lüth 5% of constitutional epileptics to be syphilitic, but the data of these German authors were obtained before the era of Wassermann tests.

Adrenal tuberculosis complicating juvenile paretic
neurosyphilis ("juvenile paresis"). Autopsy.

Case 80. When James Arnold appeared at the Danvers
Hospital in his 22d year, he looked as if he were but 12 or 14
years of age. He was excessively fat but of fair muscular
development. The left eye diverged outward, and the left
pupil was smaller than the right. An odd feature was a high
degree of pigmentation of the skin of the genitalia and the
groins (the axilla, the mammillary areas, and the oral mucosæ
were free from pigmentation). **Physically** speaking, the
patient was practically normal. **Neurologically,** however,
there was much of interest, in the light of which the clinical
history was of value.

It seems that after an apparently normal early childhood,
the boy had begun, at the age of 11, to experience difficulty
in carrying out every-day school tasks; and after this his
mental capacity had slowly but progressively deteriorated.
The deterioration was not merely intellectual, but the boy
became dishonest and untrustworthy and developed a number
of untidy and uncleanly habits, behaving at the age of 16, as
the parents stated, like a child of six.

In his seventeenth year, the boy had been taken with a severe
attack of what was regarded as an "attack of indigestion."
This attack ushered in a gradually developing muscular
weakness, especially involving the limbs. By the age of 21
he had become irritable and the paresis was so extreme that
the patient was unable to get in or out of a carriage.

This generalized muscular weakness was plain upon admission to the hospital though there seemed to be no actual
paralysis. The patient was unable to walk in a straight line
and Romberg's position could not be maintained. Marked
tremor was present in the hands and lips. There was bilateral impairment of vision and nystagmus. Reflexes and
sensations normal. Speech was markedly affected, all syllables being very much slurred. School knowledge and memory

for both recent and remote events very poor. The patient's habits were very untidy. He was very emotional, easily made to laugh or cry; and in behavior, extremely childish.

Two months after his admission to the hospital, the weakness suddenly became extreme. He was constantly nauseated, refusing food. The face and hands were cyanosed and the heart's action rapid, weak, and irregular. This attack lasted for a week and was followed by a period of improvement, during which, however, he still remained very weak and apathetic.

One month later he again became so feeble that he was unable to raise himself in bed. He complained persistently of feeling very "sick." His temperature was elevated and there occurred the same train of circulatory symptoms observed previously, viz., rapid and tumultuous action of the heart, with cyanosis of face and extremities. He soon became unconscious, remaining so until his death, which occurred on the seventh day of the acute attack.

This case was under observation before the days of the W. R., yet clinically the case had been diagnosticated JUVENILE PARESIS. There was no history of the acquisition of syphilis or any likelihood of its acquisition. Considered clinically, many of the classical features described by Addison were present, viz., marked asthenia and apathy; severe and frequent gastro-intestinal symptoms (the disease probably commencing with the attack of so-called "acute indigestion" six years prior to patient's death); attacks of extreme cardiac weakness with the characteristic small, low-pressure pulse. On the other hand, pigmentation of the skin (usually the most striking clinical feature) was limited to the external genitalia, these being colored a deep brown.

The most striking feature found at autopsy was a bilateral adrenal tuberculosis (caseation, giant cells, lymphocytosis, tubercle bacilli). The thymus gland was persistent ($7 \times 5 \times .5$ cm.), whereas the thyroid gland was smaller than usual. The brain showed macroscopic and microscopic features entirely consistent with the diagnosis of general paresis, including lymphocytosis, plasmocytosis, irregular degrees of nerve-cell destruction, and gliosis, with an especially characteristic microscopic picture in the frontal regions.

It may be of note to consider the degree of change undergone by a brain in 11 years or more of deterioration, and the following description of the head findings is therefore included:

Head: Hair abundant, dark. Scalp normal. Calvarium, weight 435 gm., transparent in bregmatic region only, elsewhere thick and dense. The average thickness of the vertical plate of the frontal bone is 7 mm. The frontal bone shows a moderate thickening and hardening of the inner table with obliteration of diploë. Dura mater moderately adherent to the bregmatic region of calvarium. Arachnoidal villi moderately developed. Sinuses not remarkable. Pia mater shows a moderate focal thickening with opacity, especially along sulci. Vessels well injected. **Brain:** Weight, 1200 gm. The brain shows marked focal variations in sulcation and consistence. Spread on a board, the right hemisphere is obviously somewhat bigger than the left. There is a difference of only 0.5 to 0.75 cm. on measurement of the greatest circumference of the cerebrum, taken from the median line superiorly to the median line inferiorly, but the right hemisphere is throughout slightly more convex than the left. Both postcentral gyri are much narrowed in their superior portions, and the sulci posterior thereto are deeper than the other sulci of the hemispheres. The sulci of the orbital surfaces are asymmetrical and, on the left side, show a tendency to microgyria. The cerebral hemispheres as a whole show a remarkable tendency to slight protrusion of the border gyri; especially those of the two poles, of the free edges along the great fissure, and most strikingly the gyri at the boundary line between the inferior and lateral surfaces. This *marginal prominence* is slight but obvious and is emphasized by a slightly paler color in some regions. The cerebrum shows a general induration which is greatest in the frontal tips and along the inferior borders of the lateral surfaces of the hemispheres, especially right. The orbital surfaces are firm, especially anteriorly and externally (prefrontal); the tips of the temporal lobes are firm, and the superior temporal gyri are firmer than adjacent gyri. The postcentral gyri are indurated more than

the other gyri of the superior surface. The hippocampal gyri are likewise firmer than adjacent gyri.

Cerebellum and pons: Weight, 145 gm. The inequality of the two hemispheres is more marked than in
the case of the cerebrum.

Greatest lateral diameter; left, 4.5 cm., right, 5.5 cm.

Anteroposterior diameter adjacent to notch: Left,
5.8 cm., right, 5.5 cm.

There is no appreciable difference in depth. The
diminution in volume appears to be chiefly at the expense
of the right clivus. The inferior surface is firmer than
the superior. The laminæ adjacent to the horizontal
fissure are firmer than the remainder of the cerebellum.
The pons is small.

There was also a lateral curvature of the spinal column,
as well as characteristic adhesions between spinal dura and
pia mater which are always suggestive of syphilis. For the
rest, there were few findings of note: some adhesions of the
left pleura, hypostatic congestion of the lungs, tracheitis, and
chronic gastritis. There were four lobes of the right lung
but it is doubtful whether this should be regarded as a stigma.

1. Can we separate the symptoms of Addison's disease from
    those of paresis in this case? The extreme cardiac
    weakness with a characteristic, small low-pressure
    pulse is in point. The asthenia and apathy are consis-
    tent enough with Addison's disease as well as with paresis
    itself. It would also be possible to ascribe the gastro-
    intestinal symptoms to either disease.

2. Of what significance is the persistent thymus? Persistent
    thymus has been observed in a few cases of Addison's
    disease, but that it plays any part in the symptoma-
    tology thereof is a matter of doubt.

3. How can the obesity be explained? It is of course of
    note that the thyroid gland was small, but micro-
    scopically there were no peculiar features in this gland.

4. Was the adrenal tuberculosis actually primary? Minute
    search failed to reveal evidences of tuberculosis else-
    where unless we regard the few adhesions binding the
    lower half of the lung to the chest wall as indicative
    of an old tuberculosis. In particular, the mesenteric
    lymph nodes were normal.

Neurosyphilis? Secondary stage of syphilis.

Case 81. Florence Fitzgerald, a woman 25 years of age, applied at the police station to be taken care of. She said she had been a prostitute for the last few months, was now ill, and wanted to reform. She appeared physically ill and was sent to the Psychopathic Hospital, where she remained at first almost mute, making answers chiefly by nodding the head. She gave the impression of daze or stupor, and in fact her condition was at first regarded as catatonic. This reaction, after a few days, changed and Florence became quite normal, giving a full account of her condition.

It seems that four months before going to the police station, she developed a chancre, which was locally treated. A careful physical examination showed a fine red macular eruption which was without much question a syphilitic roseola. The spinal fluid yielded a positive W. R. although other tests of the fluid were negative. Curiously enough, no physical sign of involvement of the nervous system could be discovered. We were inclined to regard the mental symptoms as partly due to the syphilitic intoxication, and partly due to a psychic reaction of the nature of defense. As for the positive W. R. in the spinal fluid, in early secondaries various observers differ as to the frequency both of the W. R. and of other changes, percentages being given that range from 25 to 90%. See case Caperson (45). It is of note that clinically there were symptoms referable to a syphilitic involvement of the nervous system; namely, marked headache and malaise. The headaches of the secondary period are frequently the result of meningeal involvement.

TABOPARETIC NEUROSYPHILIS (" taboparesis "); death from TYPHOID MENINGITIS.
Autopsy.

Case 82. Frederick Estabrook was a salesman, who, be it
noted, had never had typhoid fever or any disease remotely
resembling typhoid fever. He had acquired syphilis at 19;
had married at 22; was the father of two healthy children
(no miscarriages); had had a certain disturbance of bladder
and rectum, but remained a successful salesman to the age of
28, when advancing tabes confined him to bed for a time.
At 30, mental signs of PARETIC NEUROSYPHILIS developed,
and death followed at 32, after an acute illness of a week.

The details of the history after the first symptoms at 28
are as follows:

At twenty-eight patient lost control of limbs and was confined to the house about two months, under medical care.
Three months later he had regained partial control of his
limbs but had lost all control of his sphincters. After another
month he had returned to work, but did not work steadily
and seemed to have lost ambition. In the summer of 1905,
his mind became obviously altered. He grew indolent and
extravagant and given to buying expensive and useless articles. Loss of interest in things followed, together with loss
of memory for recent events, lack of insight into illness, delusions of persecution by wife, irascibility followed quickly by
crying. Before admission to hospital, he was euphoric, drawling and tremulous in speech, sprawling in penmanship, alternately depressed and exalted in manner. Knee-jerks were
absent, gait ataxic, pupils stiff to light.

The family history was negative with respect to insanity.
All the family were reported as nervous. A brother died of
peritonitis at twenty-eight, a sister of pneumonia under twenty.
Another brother and sister are living. Father and mother died
of heart trouble at about sixty-seven and sixty respectively.

The patient was at high school one year and was a fair

student.   Considerable tobacco was used, and some alcohol.
Intoxication denied.   There was no history of typhoid fever
or other acute disease.

The patient on admission was sallow, poorly nourished, and
flat-chested, with a slight lateral curvature.   There was
slight dulness over right apex in front and in right upper
back.   Voice sounds were increased over right apex in front
and over whole right back.   The right chest showed bronchial
respiration throughout.   The respiration in front of right chest
was of an interrupted character.   The liver seemed moderately enlarged.   The urine showed a very faint trace of
albumin.   There were a few small nodes in right groin and a
scar on dorsum of penis.

Neurological Examination.   Slight swaying in Romberg
position.   Slight tremor of protruded tongue and extended
fingers.   Pupils irregular, left slightly larger than right.   Left
pupil reacted to light consensually, but not directly.   Right
pupil reacted very slightly to direct light, not consensually.
Knee-jerks and Achilles jerks absent.   Ankle clonus absent,
abdominal and cremasteric reflexes brisk.   Sharp and dull
points were recognized in the legs with numerous mistakes.
Vocal and facial tremor.   Speech slow and drawling.   Test
phrases repeated well if care was taken.   Consciousness clear.
Orientation perfect.   Calculating ability preserved.   Many
words omitted in writing.   Penmanship clear but shaky.

Hallucinations absent.   Memory of recent events poor.
Associations of a logical or defining type.   Patient denied
various statements in commitment papers and had little or no
insight into the mental side of his disease — slight euphoria.

After a month's observation the patient was removed to a
quiet ward and set to work a few days in the scullery.   One
night he began to yell as if assaulted and said later that he
had an idea that he was going to die.   Before three months
had passed he had become untidy, disorderly, and imperfectly
oriented.

The general degeneration continued rapidly.   One week
before death the temperature rose to 103 degrees F., and the
patient succumbed to what seemed clinically like a bronchopneumonia.   Unconsciousness two days before death.

Note with respect to history of typhoid. — Inquiries of his physicians, wife, employer, and brother tend to show conclusively that the patient never had a disease even remotely resembling typhoid fever.

The **autopsy** findings were as follows:

Acute conditions:

Hypostatic pneumonia, with early serofibrinous pleuritis and without lymph node swelling; **enlargement of mesenteric lymph nodes; acute cerebrospinal leptomeningitis;** multiple small hemorrhages of spleen.

Other findings:

Scar of penis; sclerosis of aortic arch (Heller's type?) and slight coronary arteriosclerosis; **calvarium** thin and **dense; dura mater thickened** and adherent to calvarium; calcified arachnoidal villi; **chronic** cerebral and cerebellar **leptomeningitis; atrophy of frontal lobes; granular ependymitis; sclerosis of posterior columns** of spinal cord; emaciation; unequal pupils; slight parietal fibrous endocarditis, slight mitral sclerosis; gastrointestinal atrophy; chronic cystitis; chronic abscess of prostate.

The description of the head findings is as follows:

Skin exceedingly loose, and the whole skull cap thinned. The diploë are absent. Adhesion with dura easily separated. The dura somewhat thickened, but not distended. Along the longitudinal sinus extensive calcareous granulations adhere to it. The longitudinal sinus does not contain blood, and the inner surface is normal in color. The pia is extensively thickened and opaque and a general subpial exudate exists which is more marked over the vertex where it lifts the pia from the brain surface to the extent of three centimeters in Rolandic, superior frontal, intraparietal, and mesial precentral sulci on each side. The arteries at base are free from atheroma. The temporal lobes are much bound down by adhesions, as is the cerebellum. Post-mortem softening is evident. The hemispheres show no asymmetry, but the frontal convolutions are markedly atrophic. The corpus callosum is united to the cortex by old adhesions and has to be dissected away from it. Lateral ventricles contain some slight amount of cloudy fluid, and the pia along the vessels is opaque. Some granulations in ependyma. Brain weight, 1305 grams. Pons and cerebellum, 195 grams.

Cord. — Dura much thickened, and the pia corresponds to its appearance in brain with a like exudate. Cross-sections of cord show sclerosis of posterior columns.

Bacteriologically the *typhoid bacillus* was cultivated *from the meninges and from the swollen mesenteric lymph nodes*. The blood was negative; the intestines were negative so far as lesions were concerned.

The microscopic examination confirmed the clinical diagnosis of GENERAL PARESIS and of TABES, since there was not only an extensive chronic encephalitis, with the usual lymphocytic and plasma-cell deposit and irregular gliosis, but also a well-marked posterior column sclerosis, not unusual save in its extreme degree.

It might be surmised that some difficulty would arise in distinguishing the effects of paretic meningoencephalitis from those of the more recent typhoidal process. The well-known tendency of typhoidal processes to escape polynuclear exudation, at least until frank necrosis has set in, gave rise to the idea that the two mononuclear pictures — that of general paresis and that of typhoidal processes — might be confusing.

The picture presented by the meninges was scarcely what might be expected. Although numerous mononuclear phagocytic cells are everywhere found, yet the predominant picture is that of a polynuclear exudation.

The polynuclear leucocytes occur in greatest numbers in the tissue spaces, especially in the meshes of the lumbar arachnoid and in the spaces of the frontal and paracentral pia mater. In the lumbar region of the spinal arachnoid wide fields occur in which the cells are almost one hundred per cent polynuclear leucocytes. In places phagocytic cells occur, and in a few fields, even in the open tissue spaces, the number of phagocytic cells may arise to fifty per cent. Edema is a considerable feature in the meninges. Fibrin is found chiefly in the cerebral meninges and appears in numerous delicate strands in the tissue spaces.

Moloch, horrid king, besmeared with blood
Of human sacrifice, and parents' tears;
Though, for the noise of drums and timbrels loud,
Their children's cries unheard that passed through fire
To his grim idol.

Paradise Lost, Book I, lines 392–396

IV. MEDICOLEGAL AND SOCIAL.

Neurosyphilis in a public character: eloquence, reformatory efforts, notoriety.

Case 83. Major Isaac Thompson, M.D., was a character. He had been regarded as eccentric for many years prior to his death at 63. In fact, it seems that there had been more or less definite symptoms and signs about his fortieth year. The doctor himself had a ready explanation for his Argyll-Robertson pupils; he explained that he had had a peculiarly heavy smallpox at about the age of 27 (which would be about 1872).

The doctor had a good secondary education, he had gone through the Civil War as a hospital steward, went into business after the war, married, and then went to the medical school, graduating at the age of 34. He continued in practice for a dozen years, and then gave it up. For years he had been especially interested in certain literary lines and he had published any number of pamphlets, all of a somewhat striking description, often with a political color and intended to stir up reform measures. The doctor never bore a very good reputation, and years later it was recalled that certain books disappeared from libraries and their loss was almost certainly traced to Dr. Thompson. In general, however, he was considered to be a rather worthy local figure.

It is possible that a fall on the ice in his 61st year actually started the fatal process, since after that time the patient had difficulty in walking, and a few months later developed periods of excitement with peremptory insistence on obedience to his wishes. Whereas formerly the doctor had finished up one literary piece of work after another, he now began to do very scattering work. He appeared in public

289

to denounce certain financial schemes with great force and unusual eloquence. His eloquence was greatly complimented, and these compliments induced the doctor to a remarkable crusade against a certain corporation; there was so much truth mixed with the fiction of his eloquence that he obtained a considerable following in his campaign. He wanted to start a bureau of information for the instruction of the public on these matters, and he planned to put up a building adjoining his own home for the accommodation of the various clerks and writers in this bureau. However, before the building had been actually started, an outbreak occurred.

One morning the doctor was very excitable and noisy over the telephone, ordering typewriters and giving directions to mechanics. He repaired to Boston in connection with certain resources that he supposed (and gave others reason to believe) had been supplied by the Government and by a large newspaper. One evening he returned very late. It appeared that he had had a fracas at a hotel and had knocked down one or two colored porters, acting as though drunk. Upon being put to bed, the doctor talked incessantly of religious matters, proposing to undertake a Sunday School class. His interlocutor did not exhibit a particular interest in this scheme, whereupon Dr. Thompson threatened him with violence. Police and doctors were called in and a constant stream of conversation lasted for hours. The patient was finally brought to Danvers Hospital upon representation by physicians, to whom he told that his luck had turned, that he was about to be made senator from the district, and that he and Roosevelt were going to break up the trusts, and that, as a matter of fact, he was a relative of Mr. Roosevelt.

Upon admission, the patient was a well preserved and well groomed man with gray hair and beard. He was somewhat pallid but his teeth were well preserved and well cared for, and there was little or no physical change except a slight hypertension. He claimed that he had suffered from kidney disease for some years, and there was in fact a trace of albumin in the urine.

Neurologically, the plantar and Achilles reactions could not be obtained, but there were no other reflex disorders except the bilateral Argyll-Robertson pupil. The doctor's explanation for these stiff pupils, which he described as existing for many years, was frank and circumstantial, so that the unlikelihood of Argyll-Robertson pupils due to small-pox was rather frowned upon by him. Without entering upon a detailed description of the clinical symptoms and course of the disease which led to death a little over a year after admission, it may be said that the differential diagnosis lay between the expansive form of general paresis and a maniacal condition, presumably the maniacal phase of manic-depressive psychosis. From the data of a special staff meeting held upon the case, we learn that the diagnosis of manic-depressive psychosis was entertained more strongly than that of general paresis. Thus, for general paresis alone was the somewhat gradual onset with increasing excitement, accompanied by expansive delusions concerning unlimited finance, personal over-importance, and Argyll-Robertson pupils. Dismissing the Argyll-Robertson pupils from consideration, the diagnosticians were led to see in the constant motor activity displayed in conveying an enormous number of thoughts on paper, inconsistent talking with digressions, a manic-depressive psychosis. There was no amnesia and no other sign of mental deterioration. There was a certain improvement early in the hospital stay of the patient. Consciousness was clear and orientation perfect. The delusions themselves, though extravagant, were not inconsistent or fantastic. The hallucinatory disorder was hardly characteristic either of manic-depressive psychosis or of paresis.

The patient might be described as "interesting." A good preliminary training with years of travel and variety of occupation, furnished him with a fund of knowledge. An excellent memory, prompt replies and repartee, endless digressions with voluntary return to the original topic, caused him to be an amusing and even instructive interlocutor. However, his commitment and confinement in the institution seemed always entirely wrong, and he expressed mixed feelings about the family, now being bitter against them, and again condoning their mistakes. The patient's conduct was good and he was tidy in habits, and tried as far as possible to conform to the requirements of the hospital. The doctor showed a marked antipathy toward a certain male attendant, who had removed articles from his clothing upon admission and had reclaimed a book on rules and regulations. The doctor prepared a list of 327 different acts of abuse, lack of care, and insubordination which he said he had observed in the hospital.

In the last weeks of the patient's illness, his ideas became more expansive and extravagant, dealing with a grapevine system of wireless communication and delusions of unlimited wealth. He would at times keep his room flooded with urine and water for the purpose of keeping down the plague which he said was infecting the hospital. Later he mixed food with urine and other ingredients, claiming that he was constructing an elixir of life.

The **autopsy** showed few changes of the calvarium or of the dura mater, nor was the pia mater more than slightly thickened and milky over the frontal poles, along the longitudinal fissure and over the sulci. There were fairly firm adhesions of the pia mater to the dura mater along the longitudinal fissure and over the frontal poles and at the temporal tips. The hemispheres were firmly interadherent, and the cerebello-pontine tissues were covered with a firm leptomeningitis. The floors of the ventricles were smooth and the basal vessels showed little beyond a few spots of sclerosis. There was a generalized increase of consistence. The frontal gyri were rather prominent with wide sulci, but upon section no very marked atrophy of the gray matter could be shown. The rest of the brain failed to show any flaring of sulci or any special evidence of cortical atrophy. The brain weighed 1250 grams; a possible diminution of 100 grams, considering the patient's body length. However, it must be remembered that he was at this time 63 years of age.

Microscopically, the diagnosis of GENERAL PARESIS was confirmed on the basis of plasmocytosis, lymphocytosis, gliotic changes and nerve-cell destruction. There was an unusual variation in the degree of the destructive process, which picked out, for example, certain regions of the right side for maximal lesion (cornu ammonis, gyrus rectus, and superior frontal gyrus).

If the patient's own estimate of 35 years' duration for his Argyll-Robertson pupils can be trusted (and in general his memory was extremely good), we may well conceive an unusual duration for the process in his case. There was, however, in the body at large no very marked degree of changes. There was a slight old tuberculosis. There was a slight interstitial nephritis, with cardiac hypertrophy and fibrous myocarditis. There was also a sclerosis of the mitral and aortic valves; there were chronic changes in the spleen, liver, and bladder; there was generalized arteriosclerosis of mild degree; there were two round gastric ulcers near the pylorus. The liver weighed but 800 grams, and its left lobe was somewhat rough.

This case is placed among the medicolegal and social cases because the phenomena that ushered in his last illness were mistaken by the local public for meritorious social reform measures. They were regarded as not markedly different from the variety of steps taken by the very active doctor in previous years; indeed the public eloquence that he displayed a year before his death was quite in line with previous habits, despite the suspicious over-brilliance of language. It is an important question, how far the eccentricity and literary overactivity of the latter half of the doctor's total life can be explained on the basis of a mild syphilitic irritation of the nervous system. In this connection we are tempted to recall the suggestions of Mœbius concerning a portion of the literary products of Nietzsche. Our doctor was by no means so brilliant an exemplar of syphilitic literature as was Nietzsche, if we grant the hypothesis of Mœbius to cover our doctor's case as well as that of Nietzsche. In the future, important studies of character change under the influence of syphilis will doubtless be made. With modern diagnostic methods, of course, the diagnosis would have been rendered almost at once in the case of Major Isaac Thompson, M.D., and much of his past life would have been brought under special review in connection with the syphilis which doubtless the blood serum or at any rate the cerebrospinal fluid would have shown.

This case illustrates but one of the many social complications arising as the result of paresis. When one recalls that the onset is often insidious and not correctly understood for a period of time, it is readily seen that many unfortunate acts may be committed by a patient. As hypersexual desire is not an infrequent early symptom and as judgment is early disturbed, loose morals may ruin the patient's reputation. The poor judgment and expansive delusions often lead to foolish business deals wherein the patient's family is left destitute. At other times the onset is sudden and then the danger of false commands or acts by a person in a responsible position, as a steamship captain, an engineer or chauffeur, may lead to loss of life and property.

Sudden grandiosity: debts. PARETIC NEURO-
SYPHILIS ("general paresis"): Question of liability.

Case 84. Lester Smith was a salesman, 31 years of age,
who, while on a business trip, accompanied by his wife,
suddenly developed grandiose ideas. He originated a scheme
of cornering the phonograph market. His prospects seemed
so certain to him, that he hired an expensive suite of rooms
in a hotel at something over $35 a day. As at the first
presentation of his bill it was found that he had no money
to meet these charges, he was taken into custody and at
once transferred to a hospital for the insane, where it was
discovered that he was suffering from GENERAL PARESIS.

1. What is the patient's responsibility for these debts?
Legally the patient or his estate is responsible for
debts accruing from services rendered or goods received. As he is adjudged *non compos mentis* con-
tracts entered into would not hold, and he would not
be considered liable for criminal acts.

Note: This case shows how dangerous paresis may be
not only to the life and usefulness of a patient, but further
how it may ruin a family financially. Mr. Smith's little
escapade used up all the money that he had been able to
save in his life and when he was taken to a hospital his wife
was left destitute.

Suicidal attempt (?) by a neurosyphilitic.

Case 85. At first Mrs. Annie Monks, a widowed seamstress, 50 years of age, did not particularly suggest syphilis. Mrs. Monks was sent to us from a general hospital. She had been found unconscious in her room, with gas turned on, and a diagnosis of gas poisoning was made. Mrs. Monks remained unconscious for 24 hours, and her apparent suicidal attempt seemed to warrant her being sent to the Psychopathic Hospital. Mrs. M., however, scoffed at the idea of any attempt at suicide, and claimed to have had no recollection of any such affair. On the contrary, she had gone to mass the morning of the day on which she was taken to the hospital, remembered well enough returning to her room but nothing of what followed until she woke up.

Mrs. Monks was not cooperative and would reveal few facts about her history. For years, she had had edema of the feet and palpitation of the heart (the heart was somewhat enlarged, with a double murmur in the aortic area, systolic louder, and a blood pressure of 160 systolic and 85 diastolic; clubbed fingers; palpable liver). She had been treated in the out-patient department of a general hospital for a number of months. We could obtain no evidence of mental impairment, particularly none of memory.

Aside from the heart lesions above indicated, the patient was fairly well nourished, with a slight enlargement of superficial glands, and was otherwise normal.

Neurologically, the slightly irregular pupils reacted poorly to light; the right knee-jerk could not be obtained, whereas the left knee-jerk was very active. Systematic examination revealed no other disorder except that the abdominal reflexes could not be obtained.

Here we have, in a cardiac patient, a possibly or probably accidental gas poisoning, and little to go upon for a profounder diagnosis than the sluggish irregular pupils and unilateral absence of knee-jerk.

The routine serum W. R. came through as positive. Following custom, we examined the spinal fluid, finding the W. R. here again to be moderately positive (strongly positive to 1 cc., moderately to 0.7 cc., and negative to 0.5, 0.3, and 0.1 cc.). The gold sol index was 1 2 2 1 0 0 0 0 0 0, which must be interpreted as syphilitic. There were 16 cells to the cmm., the albumin was 1+, and the globulin stood at 2+.

Here, then, we seem to have evidence of an inflammatory process of the central nervous system, and it is natural forthwith to be sceptical as to the accidental nature of the gas poisoning. Perhaps there was an attempt at suicide based upon a passing impulse, or perhaps there was a period of confusion in which the cock was not turned off.

In any event, we feel justified in making the diagnosis of cerebrospinal syphilis on the basis of the neurological and laboratory findings. On the whole, we are inclined to make a diagnosis of VASCULAR NEUROSYPHILIS with a moderate involvement of the MENINGES.

1. What is the outcome in such cases as that of Annie Monks? The case somewhat resembled that of Martha Bartlett, who still survives. The case of Annie Monks illustrates another outcome. A few days after her admission, she became unconscious once more, and upon recovery remained very much confused and aphasic, moaning, and unable to handle herself well, although without definite paralysis. Three weeks later the patient died, although in the meantime strenuous antisyphilitic therapy was practised. Death was sudden. We thought death due to cerebral embolism.

Early delinquency and neurosyphilis in a juvenile.

Case 86. Frank Johnson was 21 years of age when he was taken up by the police for threatening his sister with a revolver. The police thought he deserved an examination at the Psychopathic Hospital. The patient protested that he had threatened his sister only to frighten her because, he said, she nagged him and made him nervous. In fact, they had always had trouble as she had always nagged him and they had always fought together. Moreover, their mother always took the sister's part. They had been troubling him for days, and at last Frank could stand it no longer. His sister had complained of the way he treated her dog. Moreover, Frank said he had not been feeling well; there had been some trouble with his stomach; and after one of the nagging attacks, he had taken out an old empty pistol to scare his mother and sister.

In these cases, it is good practice to consult the sister also. She said that Frank had always been very difficult to manage, unwilling to work, preferring to loaf about, spending every obtainable cent; he was once in a reformatory for several years, but not reformed thereby; recently given to drinking; at times acting somewhat peculiarly (sitting at the window with his hat on, refusing to move).

Further **mental examination** of Frank showed that he was properly oriented and in possession of a good memory, although he was quite obviously a liar. He lay about in bed at the hospital, saying that he was too weak to be up. He was a bit dull, at times not readily grasping ordinary questions.

Physically, Johnson was rather thin; the teeth were somewhat peg-shaped although far from typically Hutchinsonian. The pupils were unequal and irregular, and failed to react to light or even to accommodation when tested. The deep reflexes of arms and legs could not be obtained, though the superficial reflexes were present. For the rest systematic examination proved negative. Serum W. R. negative.

The first thought in such a case would be that the crimi-
nological diagnosis of delinquency would be sufficient.   However, the pupillary disorder and the areflexia are suggestive
despite the negative serum W. R.   Resort was naturally had
to lumbar puncture, whereupon a positive W. R. was found,
a characteristically " paretic " gold sol reaction, globulin, excess albumin, and 134 cells per cmm.   In short, it would appear that we must consider a diagnosis of JUVENILE PARESIS,
and, in point of fact, the patient deteriorated rapidly from
this time, becoming demented at the end of a few months.

1. How far are the early difficulties of management (leading to a reformatory) due to syphilis?   We should not
   dogmatically say that there is a relation between the
   early delinquency and syphilis.   Still, it is not unusual
   to find emotional disorder and instability as well as
   delinquency in congenital syphilitics.
2. What suggestion, if any, should be made to the patient's
   intelligent and seemingly normal sister, two years
   older?   We prevailed upon Miss Johnson to submit
   to the W. R. of the serum, which was found, as in the
   case of Frank, to be negative.   Frank's sister should
   undoubtedly submit to a lumbar puncture; but in
   the present phase of mental hygiene, she would be
   difficult to persuade.
3. How is it possible to find such a marked evidence of
   congenital syphilis in a younger sibling with no evidence of syphilis in the elder?   In the first place, there
   may be a history of entrance of syphilis into the lives
   of the parents between the pregnancies.   However, in
   other instances, there is no evidence of such intercurrent syphilis, and contrary to the prevailing opinion
   it is not so infrequent to find congenital syphilis in
   the younger brother or sister of a normal person.
4. What can be said of treatment in such cases?   In the
   first place it is clear that delinquent cases should be
   tested far earlier for the possibility of syphilis.   Had
   this case been examined by a neurologist or alienist
   many years earlier, it is probable that the same pupillary signs and the peg-shaped teeth would have been
   found, and that the hypothesis of syphilis might have
   been raised.   There is no good evidence as yet that
   these cases can be markedly benefited by treatment.

```
Neurosyphilis in a " defective delinquent."
```

Case 87. Vivian Walker, 22 years of age, was arrested on the streets of Boston for drunkenness. Upon arrival at the jail, she developed a series of convulsions, each lasting a very brief time, with loss of consciousness, frothing at the mouth, and jerky movements of the arms and legs.

The Walker family was known to the police, since there were police records in two generations on the maternal side. The father was regarded as of rather low-grade mentality; a sister had committed suicide. Vivian herself had been irregular at school, was regarded as vicious, and had been hysterical. She had been committed to a reformatory at the age of 15 years. In the reformatory she had a number of excited outbreaks, with resentment of discipline, and these outbreaks presented hysterical traits. After each outbreak Vivian was depressed. It was during her stay at the reformatory that her sister committed suicide. Vivian attended the funeral, and the idea of suicide appears to have taken hold of her mind, as she constantly spoke of suicide, threatened suicide, and made several attempts. She claimed at this time to see visions and to hear her sister's voice. On that ground she had been committed to a hospital for the insane at 16.

At the hospital there were many fluctuations in mental condition. Vivian professed discouragement on account of poor home influences, telling how her mother had often been in prison, allowing Vivian to come under the influence of bad girls. Now and then Vivian had outbreaks of profanity and glass-breaking, and she also made at the hospital for the insane several half-hearted attempts at suicide. At the age of 19 she was returned to the reformatory, whence she was placed out on probation and allowed to return home.

However, she was shortly re-committed to the insane hospital in a phase of excitement, talking continuously of men and sex relations, and also of imaginary illicit sex relations with any man whom she happened to see. Again from time to time she made attempts at suicide. However, she was allowed to go out on visit, returned to her habits, and at the time of her arrest was living as a prostitute.

After her convulsions in jail, she was admitted to the Psychopathic Hospital. At first obstinate and stubborn, later she became tractable. Special mental tests left her in the subnormal class, but we could hardly class her as feebleminded. We were able to observe her in a number of seizures, during which she would drop to the floor, apparently lose consciousness, writhe about, and assume the position of opisthotonos, the whole attack lasting but a minute or two.

There was pelvic tenderness, with gonococci in the urethral smear. Salpingectomy had to be performed, but after the operation Vivian insisted upon getting up and running about on the second day, tearing the bandages from her abdomen, and infecting the wound. Outbreaks of excitement also followed the operation.

In the diagnosis of this case, we must probably separate the convulsive phase from the remainder of the phenomena. The conduct disturbance, emotional outbreaks, and suicidal attempts date from early youth, and no doubt the diagnosis defective delinquent would fit Vivian from the beginning. The hereditary taint is characteristic enough. The sundry phenomena in the insane hospital, and particularly the hallucinations, lead one to wonder whether Vivian is not possibly even suffering from dementia praecox.

As to the convulsions, it would hardly appear that they are typically epileptic, although certainly epileptoid. Their onset at 22 is somewhat unusual. Several features of the seizures together with the opisthotonos and the previous history of hysteria, lead one to think of making the diagnosis hysteria.

1. Can cerebrospinal syphilis cause the symptoms? We found the serum W. R. to be positive though Vivian denied syphilitic infection. (She also denied gonorrhœal infection despite the clinical and laboratory findings.) We found that the spinal fluid yielded a

gold reaction of a typical syphilitic nature, showed an excess of albumin, a slight amount of globulin, and 130 cells per cmm. Even these findings, however, would perhaps not justify stating that the convulsive seizures are of syphilitic nature. The seizures disappeared under the administration of antisyphilitic remedies. It would seem, therefore, that the seizures should be regarded as of syphilitic nature. In any event, the diagnosis of cerebrospinal syphilis is justifiable. This syphilis, however, is of an active nature and probably of recent production. We should be at a loss to explain the earlier mental features in Vivian as syphilitic and are therefore fain to associate the two psychoses, PSYCHOPATHIC PERSONALITY and DIFFUSE CEREBROSPINAL SYPHILIS.

NEUROSYPHILIS ("paresis sine paresi") in an habitual criminal, a forger.

Case 88.* ———— was brought to the hospital by the police. He was charged with having forged a check, and on account of the crudeness of the work his mental condition was suspected.

Family History. The paternal grandfather was considered fast, drank a great deal and was said to be a thief. The father is said to have been forced to leave the State when a young man in order to avoid the reformatory. Paternal cousin murdered a man; the sisters of this cousin said to have been wild and one brother married a prostitute. Nothing known of maternal relatives.

Past History. Medical history is unimportant. He denies syphilis. His early childhood is of little significance. He was somewhat dull in school. At about the age of twelve he began to lie and steal, and has continued this ever since. His attempts have all been very crude, it is said, and when confronted he would strenuously deny his deeds, even when the evidence was overwhelming. He forged checks, borrowed money from all his friends, and charged things at stores to the family. The family paid the bills for a time, and then later had him sent to a reform school. He was married at nineteen, but wife has left him and obtained a divorce. He has been excessively alcoholic for years, and is suspected also of taking drugs. He was discharged from the navy dishonorably. He later joined the army and was discharged therefrom on account of "rheumatism," according to his account, but in reality deserted. He had finished a jail sentence of thirteen months for forgery a little over a year before entrance.

Physical examination shows a well-developed and nourished man. The general physical examination is negative.

---

* Reprinted from article by Southard and Solomon: "Latent Neurosyphilis, the Question of *Paresis sine paresi*," *Boston Medical and Surgical Journal*, XXIV, 1.

The lungs show nothing abnormal. The heart is not enlarged, there are no murmurs or irregularities; blood pressure, 145 systolic. The alimentary system is negative. No palpable lymph glands. **Neurological examination:** pupils equal and react to light and accommodation. Extraocular movements well performed. Tongue projects in the median line, with no tremor. There is no evidence of facial paresis or weakness of the muscles. The biceps, triceps, knee-jerks and ankle-jerks are present and equal on the two sides. There is no Gordon, Babinski or Oppenheim; no ankle clonus. There is no tremor of the extended hands. No Romberg sign. There is a little difficulty in the finger-to-finger test. There is no sensory disturbance either subjective or objective. No tenderness over nerve trunks.

Mental examination shows nothing of a psychotic nature. Patient is well oriented; memory for remote and recent events is well preserved, school knowledge well retained, grasp on current events good; no delusions or hallucinations elicited. Patient is not feeble-minded, according to the intelligence tests of Binet and Simon and Yerkes-Bridges, but shows poor attention and gives evidence of weakness in volitional spheres; is very suggestible.

To summarize the case, then, we have a man of thirty years of age who has shown criminalistic and anti-social tendencies since childhood, whose general physical and neurological examination is negative (excepting the laboratory tests), whose mental examination shows no psychotic symptoms, and who seems not feeble-minded. In other words, with the exception of the serological and chemical findings in the blood and cerebrospinal fluid, there is nothing to suggest that he is more than a " criminal type."

Wassermann reaction in blood serum positive.

Wassermann reaction in cerebrospinal fluid positive. Examination of cerebrospinal fluid: globulin ++, albumin ++, cells 55 per cubic millimeter; large lymphocytes, 9.1 per cent; small lymphocytes, 90 per cent; plasma, 90 per cent. Gold sol reaction, 3321000000.

1. Can the criminalistic tendencies be condoned in this case on the ground of neurosyphilis? As a matter of fact the delinquencies in this patient reach back to early childhood and as there is no evidence of congenital syphilis it cannot be held that syphilis had any bearing in the causation of symptoms. Even were the delinquencies only of recent date it is doubtful if the court would take cognizance of the laboratory findings in the absence of definite mental symptoms. In this connection it may be stated that the court takes cognizance only of the acts of a patient at time of examination, and not of the history or laboratory findings, in committing a person. We have had several patients who from history, physical signs and laboratory tests made the diagnosis of paretic neurosyphilis easy and yet who could not be committed because they were mentally clear at the time. Such patients may be of grave potential danger to themselves and families, and present numerous social problems. See case of Joseph Wilson (95).

JUVENILE PARETIC NEUROSYPHILIS ("juvenile paresis ") with initial trauma.

Case 89. Margaret Tennyson was a small girl of six years, described as having been normal until run down by a double-runner sled about 13 months before her arrival at the hospital. The change was stated to be remarkable. " She was as unlike her own self as darkness and daylight." Once fat and sunny, talkative and demonstrative with her toys, now Margaret had become silent, sullen, worried, and of a violent temper, stubborn and unmanageable. It does not appear that the patient was seriously injured by the double-runner, as she was able to walk a short distance home. Shortly, however, she began to have trouble with her feet (diagnosed at the time as flat-foot), and thereafter her whole character and disposition changed. Upon arrival at the hospital, the patient walked with a typical scissors gait of spastic paraplegia.

Physical examination was very difficult through lack of coöperation and a screaming and kicking resistance upon every attempt. There was a suggestion of hydrocephalus in the protrusion of the forehead. The pupils reacted readily to light and accommodation. The knee-jerks were active, but there was otherwise no disorder of reflexes. The patient had great difficulty in getting up from the floor, and for the most part insisted upon lying in ventral decubitus on the floor, crying when attempt was made to raise her. An attempt was made to test her by the Binet scale, by which she was found to rate at 2⅘ years although a portion of this low-rating was thought to be due to a failure of coöperation.

The **family history** threw little or no light upon the case. The parents were living and well; a brother of 16 years was at work in the market district; two of the other siblings are in the first and second grades at school and regarded as exceptionally bright by their teachers. The fourth was the patient, Margaret; a fifth had died at 9 weeks of heart trouble;

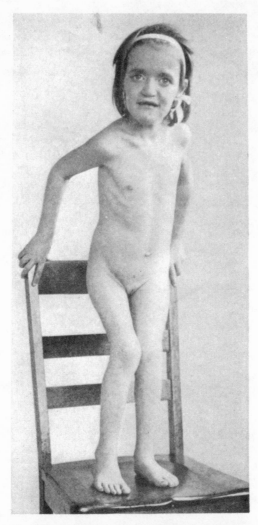

Juvenile paresis — spastic paraplegia.   5 years.

the sixth, seventh, and eighth, of 3, 1½ years and 3 months respectively, appeared entirely well. There were no miscarriages or stillbirths.

The scissors gait and spasticity seem to point undoubtedly to organic disease of the nervous system, along with which the mental deterioration seemed to suggest an active progressive involvement of the cerebrum. The history seemed to be convincing that the child was not an instance of congenital feeblemindedness.

A neurologist's clinical diagnosis would naturally be syphilis. In point of fact, this diagnosis was borne out by the laboratory tests, which showed a positive W. R. in the serum and spinal fluid, positive globulin, a slight excess of albumin, and a syphilitic gold sol reaction.

1. What is the significance of the trauma in the case of Margaret Tennyson? The trauma seemed to the family the precipitating cause. We find cases of general paresis in adults very definitely following trauma, yet neurosyphilis, both in adults and in younger patients, mainly occurs without trauma. On the whole, in this case, it is perhaps safer to regard the trauma as mere coincidence. A sister older than Margaret was found upon examination to have a positive W. R. The other children could not be examined.

Traumatic form of PARETIC NEUROSYPHILIS
(" general paresis ").

Case 90. The point about Joseph O'Hearn was his entire
mental soundness up to the time of an injury at work, when
he was blown through a double window in an explosion,
badly bruising his head.   Shortly after the accident, although
not immediately, the patient began to show signs of mental
disorder, doing very foolish things, losing his memory, and
becoming unable to work.

It was eight months after the explosion when O'Hearn, at
the age of 36, was admitted to the hospital with general mental
impairment.   O'Hearn was confused and disoriented for
time and place, although he seemed to understand that he
was in a hospital.   He was given to foolish laughter and a
silly manner.   There was considerable emotional disorder;
judgment was clearly impaired, and memory was poor.

Physically, there was little to be found except upon **neurological examination.**   The right knee-jerk was greater than
the left; the tongue and fingers showed marked tremor, there
was a speech defect and writing disorder.

On the whole, it seemed impossible not to make the diagnosis GENERAL PARESIS, especially in view of the laboratory
tests, with positive W. R. in both serum and fluid, a " paretic" type of gold reaction, 59 cells per cmm., excess albumin,
and a large amount of globulin.

I.   What is the relation of the trauma to the paresis?
     Trauma is regarded as a precipitating cause, and In-
     dustrial Accident Commissions have been known to
     allow damages in such cases.   Mott believes that the
     symptoms of a post-traumatic paresis must not develop
     until after a week's interval of freedom from symptoms,
     since he believes that time is required to destroy or
     irritate the brain to the point of producing the paretic
     picture.   Our data are in agreement with those of
     Mott.   Mott also points out that gumma sometimes
     occurs at the site of the trauma.

False claim for compensation in neurosyphilis.

Case 91. The facts in the case of Levi Sussman can be brought out by the following extracts from a report to the Industrial Board: A claim was made to the Board that the symptoms had developed after a fall from a building, some *nine months before hospital observation.* No connection could be found between this accident and the PARETIC NEUROSYPHILIS found. We introduce the case to emphasize the possibility that irrelevant accidents may be regarded by ignorant or unscrupulous persons as setting up a mental disorder for which damages are claimed. If symptoms are already in existence before the accident and are not especially increased thereafter, naturally no damages should be recovered. Unscrupulous persons may falsify about the pre-traumatic history and claim the development of symptoms immediately after the accident. Such claims are beyond question to be viewed with the greatest suspicion. Some days or weeks should elapse before definite symptoms in post-traumatic paresis appear. Just how long an interval may elapse between trauma and paretic symptoms and shall entitle the case to be regarded as one of traumatic paresis, is perhaps a matter of doubt. It would seem, however, on general grounds that three months is the longest period in which the post-traumatic effects are likely to be delayed.

The question of traumatic paresis is of great interest on account of the war. The great strain under which the men at the front live and the physical injury due to being " buried " is probably responsible for an increasing number of cases of neurosyphilis. Such at least is the impression of Canadian medical officers with whom we have spoken. See Section VI, Neurosyphilis and the War.

Traumatic exacerbation(?) in PARETIC NEURO-SYPHILIS (" general paresis ").

Case 92. The case of Joseph Larkin was of note from the point of view of the Industrial Accident Board. This Irish teamster was said to have been injured in his head two or three months before coming up for examination at the age of 45. For a week Larkin had had frontal headaches, had been sleeping poorly, and had been somewhat worried. In fact, he had stopped work. The W. R. of the serum was positive and a diagnosis of PARESIS could be made. The case did not come up for consideration by the Industrial Board until two years after his initial appearance.

The **physical examination** showed irregular pupils, sluggish pupillary reactions, Achilles absent, swaying in the Romberg position, enlargement of the heart to the left, positive W. R. of the blood and of the spinal fluid.

Mentally, the patient's orientation for place was poor and his memory defective. Emotionally he was depressed or apathetic and was apprehensive. His flow of thought was slow, and his insight into his condition poor.

It is interesting that a variety of causes have been assigned in this case for the condition: such as, his work, anemia, unhygienic surroundings, and arteriosclerosis.

This case is not a sharply-defined case of post-traumatic general paresis, since there had undoubtedly been a variety of mental changes before the accident. Accordingly, recovery of damages to a full amount could hardly be expected as in certain cases in which the phenomena of paresis appear only after the trauma.

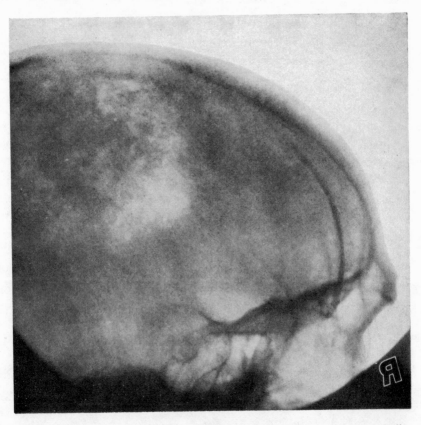

Post-traumatic cranial gumma — developing 13 months after local injury of skull.

Trauma : syphilitic lesion of skull at site of injury.

Case 93. The medicolegal interest of Richard Marshall
is extreme, as may be seen from the following brief report by
the Psychopathic Hospital to the Industrial Board.

" As to the case of Richard Marshall, a patient under
the provisions of the temporary care act from December
1 to December 10, inclusive, this case has proved unusually interesting in that the patient has proved to be
syphilitic by the Wassermann reaction of the blood.
There is no evidence of syphilis in the examination of
the cerebrospinal fluid. The X-ray examination of the
skull, taken in connection with the Wassermann reaction of the blood, warrants the diagnosis of syphilitic
osteitis of the skull at the site of the old injury. We
regard his present condition as shown by the X-ray
as a syphilitic bone condition predisposed to by the
injury. We do not find that the patient has any features of traumatic neurosis.

" Mentally, having an actual age of 30, patient grades
at 11.2 years. It may be that patient has always been
a moron. He has earned about $8.30 a week.

" We regard the patient as deserving treatment and
feel that responsible parties in the case would do well to
have such treatment instituted."

The principal symptom of which Marshall complained
was headache chiefly felt in the region of the osteitis.
There was marked sensitiveness to percussion in this area.
It is of course difficult to decide whether the headache
was entirely due to the gummatous lesions or whether the
trauma had caused contusions of the brain as well. It is
also possible that the dura underlying this area was involved.

OCCUPATION-NEUROSIS in a granite-cutter: SYPHILITIC NEURITIS?

Case 94. David Fitzpatrick was a case referred to the Psychopathic Hospital by the Industrial Accident Board. He was a granite-cutter of 52 years of age, and had begun to complain of pain in the forearm, extending back from the elbow, about six months before admission. It seems that the patient had been growing progressively worse and had thought he would have to quit work because of difficulty in grasping the hammer. A physician had told him that he must stop his work at granite-cutting or else he would entirely lose the use of his arm. He was in point of fact laid off because of slackness of work and had been unable to get work again. The pain in the arm, however, had continued and at times was very severe. Sometimes the pain and the worry led to insomnia. Fitzpatrick wanted the insurance company to pay certain accumulated bills, and maintained that he would be able to do work at $15 a week if work could be found for him. The general situation in this case can be gathered from the following abstract from the report to the Industrial Accident Board.

" Secretary Industrial Accident Board,
    " Dear Sir:
      " *In re* David Fitzpatrick
referred to us with a copy of an impartial report filed by the Massachusetts General Hospital, — we concur with said impartial report that there is now no evidence of paralysis of the arm. We do not find that the positive Wassermann reaction, although it indicates a history of syphilis, has affected the patient other than possibly to have reduced his general mental capacity. Our special tests yielded a percentage of 62% of what a patient of his age and station should possess. There seems, however, to be no connection between this reduction of mental capacity and the difficulty with the arm. We cannot connect the history of alcoholism with the arm trouble.

"There is some evidence that other stone workers have at times shown such effects.

"The patient's fairly circumstantial account of his difficulty seems to point to a degree of myalgia or muscular pain in the region of the forearm when held in a certain position and a feeling of numbness in the third and fourth fingers. Whether these phenomena are due to local pressure upon nerves in the upper part of the forearm due to neuritis, or whether we are dealing with a functional neuralgic phenomenon is a question.

"We have applied some special tests for faradic sensibility to all the fingers of both hands and have found that the fingers of the right hand are still less sensitive than those of the left, particularly the thumb and the little finger. This test has not yet been applied in a sufficiently large number of cases to prove any difficult point, nevertheless the findings are in line with the patient's own circumstantial account of former feelings of numbness in the third and fourth fingers of the right hand.

"Obviously, then, our opinion is that there is still to be found some effect of the disease, whatever it was, which caused the patient to knock off work. If we had more experience with such cases and more data with the new test which we have applied, we should perhaps be inclined to admit the diagnosis of *occupation neuritis* and to suppose structural alterations in the nerve trunks corresponding with the location of the muscular pain and the anesthesia of fingers and the dulling of electric sense, but in the present stage of our experience, it is probably wiser to call the case one of *occupation neurosis.*"

It is clear that the W. R. in this case was of peculiar value in at least partially clearing up the findings, yet it must be remembered that it is a principle of the modern administration of industrial accident boards and similar organizations that it is the employer's lookout whether the employee has syphilis. Recovery can be made as if the injury were due wholly to an accident. It was not possible however definitely to prove or disprove a relation of syphilis in the form of a syphilitic neuritis to the condition in this case.

The special tests above referred to are the electric sensory threshold tests of E. G. Martin.

Character change : neurosyphilis.

Case 95. Joseph Wilson offered a very serious social problem. He was the father of two children, and his wife was pregnant at the time of his admission to the Psychopathic Hospital. He was a husky-looking man of 33 years of age, but for the past four years he had been deteriorating in his work; he had been drinking heavily, and finally had stolen to obtain money for liquor. It was on account of his alcoholism and delinquency, which were taken as an indication of change of character, that he was sent to the hospital.

Examination on his arrival disclosed at once that there was more to the case than alcoholism, for the **neurological examination** showed that the pupils were irregular, the right being larger than the left, both reacting sluggishly to light, and there was an inequality in the reaction of the two eyes, the left being better than the right. The tendon reflexes were exaggerated, with ankle clonus on both sides, more marked on the right. There was also a marked speech defect. Otherwise the **physical examination** showed nothing of importance.

The W. R. of the blood and spinal fluid was strongly positive. The globulin test was strongly positive, the albumin was markedly increased, there were 74 cells per cmm., and a gold sol reaction of the " paretic " type.

A formal **mental examination** did not show very much of consequence; his memory showed no marked impairment, he was not deluded or hallucinated, and he had a pretty good insight into his failings. However, he was somewhat childish, and his irritability was quite marked. Were one to rely upon the mental signs alone, it is probable that a diagnosis of chronic alcoholism with deterioration would be made; but in the presence of the physical findings and the laboratory tests, the diagnosis of neurosyphilis had to be given. It is obvious that, while the patient was suffering from a progressive **brain disease**, and while he did show mental symptoms, there was not sufficient ground on which to commit him, and therefore he had to be turned out into the community. As a matter of fact, he was not prosecuted on account of his theft, because, although legally responsible, it was felt that his disease was at the basis of the character change which had led him into difficulties. Further developments of his relations with society had to be considered, however. It was possible to get him to discontinue the use of alcohol altogether, and for nearly a year he has taken no alcoholic liquor and has been self-supporting. However, his irritability has been very great, making it very difficult for his wife to live with him, and causing his sister to break off all relations with him.

Here, then, is a man with a marked CHARACTER CHANGE as the result of neurosyphilis, so that it is difficult for him to maintain the usual social relations. It does not seem possible to remove him from the community.

1. May one speak of general paresis without mental symptoms? If one considers general paresis a mental disease, of course it cannot exist without mental symptoms. However, if one considers the disease as a chronic syphilitic meningoencephalitis characterized by its pathological anatomy, then one may readily speak of general paresis although no real evidence of mental symptoms can be discovered. It would seem that we must take this attitude with our present conception of brain localization, for it is easy to conceive of a general paretic process affecting areas which do not definitely relate to psychic function. And further, such a process may exist but not be of such a grade as to cause mental symptoms.

> The neurosyphilitic's family should not be forgotten in diagnosis and treatment.

Case 96. The Bornstein family is remarkable. Let us hang the story on Becky, the mother, an Austrian woman of 43 years, who appears to have been perfectly well up to within a year. About a year ago, Mrs. Bornstein began to suffer from severe headaches, which were treated with apparent success by an osteopath: at all events, Mrs. Bornstein recovered therefrom in about six months. However, two months later, she had a convulsion, with foaming at the mouth, blueness of face, and general muscular stiffening. The convulsion lasted for several minutes. Again, a fortnight before admission, the patient had five convulsions of an identical nature in a single night.

Moreover, since the first convulsion, Mrs. Bornstein's **mental condition** has altered and become variable, so that at times she is excited, at times depressed. She would assert inaccurately that there was some one in the house, and that she had at different times committed crimes of a heinous nature. Now and then she would seem to see moving pictures. Her memory was poor and she seemed to believe that events of five or six years ago had just happened.

The pupils were sluggish, the knee-jerks and ankle-jerks were absent, there was slight ataxia, and there was speech defect. The suspicion of neurosyphilis was so strong that it seemed surprising that the W. R. of the blood serum, even after repeated tests and after the provocative injection of salvarsan, proved negative. However, the spinal fluid yielded a positive W. R., and a gold sol reaction of the " paretic " type, together with 12 cells per cmm., and a marked increase of albumin, with positive globulin. It would seem warrantable to make a diagnosis at least of syphilis of the nervous system in this case, but it is a question whether we should be warranted in making the diagnosis general paresis.

That the diagnosis is doubtful may perhaps be seen from

the variety of diagnoses in the rest of the family. In the first place, Mrs. Bornstein's husband admits syphilitic infection many years before. He states also that his wife after marriage showed signs of syphilis and received some treatment, although limited. It is stated also that the husband himself at this time has a positive W. R. and has stiff pupils and petit mal attacks. The oldest son, 22 years of age, is confined in an institution with juvenile paresis. The second son has recently died at the age of 20 years, receiving a diagnosis of rupture of the aorta. A third son, 19 years of age, has the appearance of having achondroplasia, although the proportions of his limbs do not quite correspond with those of an achondroplast. The fourth son, 17 years of age, is suffering from caries of the spine. A fifth son, 14 years old, is neurotic and has the so-called Olympic forehead. The sixth and last son died shortly after birth of unknown cause.

Neurosyphilitic's normal-looking family proved syphilitic.

Case 97. Walter Heinmas was a draughtsman 33 years of age when he was brought to the Psychopathic Hospital suffering from mental disease. This was diagnosed as general paresis, both on account of the clinical symptomatology and on account of the laboratory findings. In fact, it was a case of the classical type with marked euphoria and grandiosity.

As is the routine procedure at the Psychopathic Hospital, in the case of all syphilitic patients, the family was sent for. This consisted of the wife and two daughters, aged 9 and 7 respectively. The patient denied any knowledge of a syphilitic infection. The wife, also, gave no history of any primary, secondary, or tertiary symptoms; there had been no abortions, miscarriages, or stillbirths; both children had been born at term and had been entirely healthy. Examination showed that the mother had no signs referable to syphilis, and that both the children were mentally well endowed, with good physique and showing no stigmata of congenital syphilis. Still the W. R. of all three (the mother and the two children) was positive in the blood serum. These tests were repeated several times on the children, with and without injections of salvarsan, and they remained consistently positive.

1. Are these children to be considered congenital syphilitics despite the absence of stigmata or symptoms? We must consider these children as congenital syphilitics and candidates for the group frequently spoken of as *syphilitis hereditaria tarda*.
2. What is the frequency of syphilitic involvement in the mate and children of paretics? In our series, we have found that about 15% of the marriages where one member develops paresis, result in sterility; that in 18% abortions, miscarriages and stillbirths occur; and that in 15% positive W. R. is obtained. We have adopted the motto: **"The families of paretics are the families of syphilitics."**

Neurosyphilis: question of marriage.

Case 98. Mr. Jacobs' wife was admitted to the hospital with a diagnosis of general paresis. A few weeks after her admission, she died as a result of her disease. According to our routine, her husband and the children were examined for evidences of syphilis.

Mr. Jacobs' blood serum was found on repeated tests to be positive. He resolutely denied any knowledge of a syphilitic involvement, but it was later learned from his brother that about two years before his marriage — that is, more than 25 years before we saw him — he had acquired syphilis and had had a very small amount of treatment.

Mr. Jacobs' was put upon antisyphilitic treatment in the form of injections of .3 gram of salvarsan every two weeks with occasional intramuscular injections of mercury salicylate. After seven months of treatment, the blood serum still remained positive. At about this time, the patient came to us to ask about getting married again. He said that he was living with his sister, who kept telling him that he was the cause of his wife's death, and this was so unpleasant that he desired to start a home for himself again!

1. What advice should be given? It is a general opinion that the longer the period after the initial infection, the less the chances of infecting a partner. This chance is further reduced under antisyphilitic treatment, of which a considerable amount had been given in the case of Mr. Jacobs. However, when one considers the trickiness of syphilis and the fact that there is some chance of infection, which we would apparently overlook if we gave him permission to marry at this time, the only possible course was to tell the patient that he should not consider marriage until his Wassermann had become negative and remained so for some time. The children in this case were negative.

2. What is the physician's duty to the family of a syphilitic patient? It is our firm conviction that it is the duty of

every physician to his syphilitic patient, to the patient's family, and to the community, to examine the mate and the children for evidence of syphilis acquired or congenital and to offer treatment if it is found to be needed. This is one of the chief means at our disposal today to prevent the late disasters of syphilis, acquired or congenital, for by such examinations the syphilitic condition is discovered before lesions have occurred which are irreparable. We know that the mate and children of a syphilitic patient have been exposed to syphilitic involvement, and it is our duty as physicians in possession of such knowledge, and as guardians of the public health, to investigate such cases, so that if they be found to have syphilis, steps may be taken to treat them early.

3. How much danger is there of causing unhappiness and breaking up families by this procedure? This question offers a chance for many theoretical answers. The facts are, however, that in doing this as a routine for nearly three years and examining several hundred families, there has been no instance to our knowledge in which a family has been broken up or grave difficulties have been encountered by this procedure.

4. In what percentage are the mates or children of neurosyphilitics found to show definite symptoms of syphilis? It is our opinion that the situation in regard to neurosyphilitics is the same as for syphilitics in general: That the same laws of attenuation of virus, and of chance occur here as elsewhere.

Just as this book is going to press, we have learned that the distraught Mr. Jacobs, still desirous of starting a home for himself and feeling entirely well, consulted a physician. This physician took a sample of blood and had it tested at a competent laboratory, which reported the blood negative.

On the strength of this test, the physician felt himself warranted in recommending, or at least not advising against, Mr. Jacobs' marriage, which has probably now taken place.

Although there is some doubt what ethical relation a state institution shall maintain with physicians in private practice, we took occasion to call the attention of our patient's new counsellor to the fact of the patient's neurosyphilis. We noted that the man's serum had been constantly positive

(Massachusetts State Board of Health findings) in a score or more of observations. We called attention to the fact that lumbar puncture had shown positive signs of neurosyphilis, including a positive W. R., globulin, excess albumin, pleocytosis, and positive gold sol. These facts, according to a letter received from the private practitioner in question, have not altered his opinion in the slightest to the effect that our patient is completely normal and entirely suitable for marriage. It is clear that he regards the patient as not a victim of General Paresis.

5. What is the significance of the negative observation eventually obtained in Jacobs' serum? One's first thought is to impugn the accuracy of the laboratory work, but against this suspicion is the excellent reputation of the laboratory in question, and the agreement in the majority of its findings with those of the State Board of Health. It is more likely, as we assured the private practitioner at whose request the observation was made, that this negative test was an exceptional and isolated observation such as is not infrequent in long series of observations, particularly those made under therapeutic conditions. In so important a matter, we are inclined to feel that the physician in question should have resorted to two more observations at intervals before running counter to the position taken by the hospital.

— many a hard assay
Of dangers, and adversities, and pains.

Paradise Regained, Book IV, lines 478–479.

V. SOME RESULTS OF TREATMENT

Cases 99–103 show the Variety of Structural Lesions that Treatment has to face.

SPASTIC HEMIPLEGIA in PARETIC NEURO-SYPHILIS ("general paresis"), showing marked degenerative changes, a condition in which therapy could be theoretically of very little avail. Autopsy.

Case 99. James McDevitt arrived at the Danvers Hospital, July 20, 1906 (saying that he came to be "thawed out"), and died less than six months later: January 12, 1907. He was 34 years of age. He had been a shoe-worker after leaving school, had worked eight years with the General Electric Co., and had then become a bartender. He had, however, stopped work in September, 1905, and we may safely say that mental symptoms had begun insidiously at about that time. His symptoms, if there were any, had been masked by a heavy alcoholism, but an obvious change had appeared in November, 1905. The patient lost ambition, smoked and loafed about his room, and developed speech disorder. He denied venereal disease, nor was there any superficial evidence of such.

Physically, the patient showed little or no disorder except acne of the trunk, patches of eczema on the left lower chest, and numerous brownish scars along both tibiae.

Neurologically, the Romberg position was maintained, but the gait was very unsteady on attempts to walk a straight line; fingers, tongue, and face were tremulous, and finer movements were performed with marked incoördination. No direct or consensual light reactions could be obtained in the pupils, which were dilated and irregular.

The condition of the reflexes is important on account of the autopsy findings. The abdominal and cremasteric reflexes were prompt, and the knee-jerks equal and very lively.

323

COMMON THERAPEUTIC CONCEPTION

[M]VP = TYPICAL PARESIS

MV[P] = TYPICAL CEREBROSPINAL SYPHILIS

[M]V[P] = TYPICAL SYPHILITIC ARTERIOSCLEROSIS

(M = Membranes,   V = Vessels,
P = Parenchyma,   [ ] = not involved)

CHART 21

Achilles and normal plantar reactions were present; there was no clonus; the arm reflexes were very brisk.

The **mental symptoms** need not detain us. Consciousness was clear; orientation for time, place, and to some extent for persons, was imperfect. Arithmetic had been largely forgotten. Handwriting was irregular and scrawling, and in places unintelligible. Although the patient claimed that his memory was intact, it was decidedly imperfect. He remarked that John D. Rockefeller, a Chicago king, was President; the General Electric Works had almost 50,000 people at work; and in fact Lynn was one of the largest cities in the state, having over 12,000 people. The height of patient's room was estimated at 25 feet. There was a slight euphoria. There was never any doubt of the **diagnosis** of PARETIC NEUROSYPHILIS (" general paresis ").

Five months after admission, slight convulsions developed, after which the patient was more dull and demented; he became bedridden. More convulsions followed, leaving the right arm and hand useless. There were clonic spasms of the muscles of both lower legs. Decubitus developed and death occurred.

We may set the total duration of symptoms in the case of James McDevitt at a little over a year; nor is there any evidence of previous or prodromal symptoms beyond a total period of about 15 months, unless we may regard his leaving the General Electric Works to become a bartender some nine years before death, as a symptomatic change of character. In any event, it is of note that the **autopsy** showed singularly few lesions. Death was due doubtless to complications following decubitus, and there was a slight acute splenitis. The kidneys showed some parenchymal change. The aorta showed many patches of sclerosis, with calcification or ulceration throughout its length. These changes were not characteristic of syphilitic disease. There was considerable coronary arteriosclerosis and a slight mitral valvular sclerosis. There was a brown atrophy of the heart muscle, somewhat surprising in a man of 34 years. The **brain** was practically normal, weighed 1200 grams, and showed convolutions normal in size, relation, and arrangement. There was no sclerosis grossly evident in the blood vessels. The pia mater appeared to contain a considerable excess of clear fluid. The calvarium was of normal thickness and showed diploë and the dura mater failed to show adhesions. There were no macroscopic signs of lesion in the spinal cord.

Microscopically, the lymphocytosis, plasmocytosis, and phagocytosis of the perivascular spaces, (relative?) increase in blood vessels, the gliosis, and evidence of nerve-cell destruction, taken together warranted the diagnosis of PARETIC NEUROSYPHILIS. It was plain that the nerve-cell destruction was best marked in the *inner layers of the cortex*. The microscopic study of the spinal cord showed that there was very possibly a slight sclerosis of the posterior columns in the lumbar region, but this was so slight that it could hardly be noted in the myelin sheath stains (Weigert). Very sharply marked, on the other hand, were the *bilateral pyramidal tract lesions* in the lumbar and thoracic regions, less marked at the cervical levels.

Without attempting to analyze carefully all these findings, it is interesting to note in this case a foil to the usual spinal cord picture of paretic neurosyphilis. The spinal cord, ordinarily normal, or perhaps more usually affected by a degree of posterior column sclerosis, in this case showed such well-marked pyramidal tract sclerosis that we may perhaps place the case in a subordinate group of SPASTIC PARETIC cases of NEUROSYPHILIS. The source of the pyramidal tract disease lodges, however, in the cortex cerebri itself, being part and parcel of the lesions mentioned above as affecting more directly the inner layers of the cortex. Many of the so-called giant, or Betz, cells had undergone a complete destruction. It will be remembered that clonic spasms of the muscles of the legs appeared in the fortnight preceding death, and that there had been convulsions for about six weeks before death. There was no evidence at the autopsy why the right arm and hand should have become useless, whereas the left upper extremity remained normal. This case, then, forms an exception to the ordinary paretic neurosyphilis group in that the brunt of the microscopic process was borne by the inner layers of the cortex. The cells of origin of the pyramidal

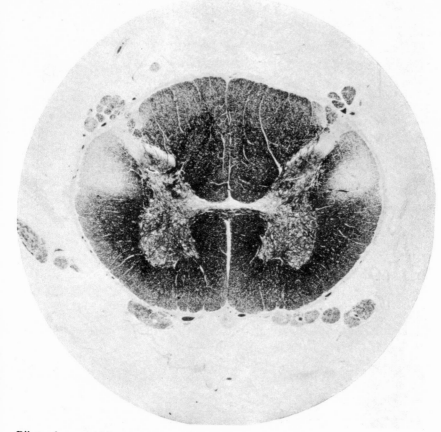

Bilateral pyramidal tract sclerosis, secondary to destruction of large motor (Betz) cells of motor (precentral) cerebral cortex — paretic neurosyphilis.

tract fibres had been cut in this lesion, and had become subject to partial or complete destruction. Note, however, that the lesion remained a microscopic one and that the marked convulsions were not related to gross lesions, thereby following the rule for paretic seizures.

From the standpoint of possible treatment, it is of course true that few organs of the body showed grave lesions save in the calcified and ulcerated aorta, which conceivably might have become quiescent under appropriate treatment. But, although the brain was almost if not quite normal in the gross, and although its membranes showed practically no lesion, treatment would not have been very promising. To be sure, the exudate might have been cleared away if the spirochetes responsible therefor had been destroyed by treatment. Yet the destruction of the giant cells of origin of the pyramidal tract fibres to such an extent as in this case could hardly have been compensated for by any known process. So far as we are aware, the destruction of considerable numbers of the smaller association elements of the brain is subject to the compensation of other elements of the nervous system, which conceivably might be re-educated or newly educated to perform certain processes. The histological picture in a case like that of McDevitt accordingly leads to the hypothesis that so well marked a spastic paresis, even in the presence of otherwise favorable signs, would be of especially baneful portent therapeutically.

NEUROSYPHILIS with total duration of symptoms twenty-two days. The comparatively MILD BRAIN LESIONS, INFLAMMATORY AND NOT DEGENERATIVE in type, suggest the possibility that therapy might have been successful. Autopsy.

Case 100. Jacob Methuen, 35, was a carpenter from Newfoundland. He was working upon a certain Thursday with his brother, who noticed that Jacob was lifting the tools about in an unusual manner and talking strangely to his fellow workmen. He fell asleep, going home in the street car, and said afterward that he felt dazed and peculiar. He talked all kinds of nonsense to his wife upon arrival. Methuen remained in bed next day, fancying he was going to die, calling his family together, and saying good-bye to them. He remained in bed all through the next day, but on Sunday appeared better, — more active, and in fact quite natural. He slept only an hour Sunday night, calling to his wife that it was time to get up. On Monday he began to be irritable to his wife, and accused her of flirting with his brother and intending to elope with him. He struck his wife several times, and when two brothers came to watch him, accused them both of trying to steal his wife, and struck them. Tuesday he remained in bed until late at night, when he arose and tried to assault the family.

It seems that another brother of the patient had died but eleven days before his admission to the hospital and five days before the onset of Jacob's symptoms. Since his brother's death he had been dwelling upon religious matters, and in fact the day after his brother's death, he waked up during the night, saying that he was too happy to sleep, that he heard the Master's voice, and at times the devil's voice; that there was to be a modern miracle and his spiritual life from now on would be different.

Eleven days after admission to the hospital, Methuen died, making a total duration of symptoms, beginning at his brother's death, of 22 days.

NEUROSYPHILITIC LESIONS

LESIONS OF THE SECONDARY PERIOD

(1) INTERSTITIAL ENCEPHALITIS OR MYELITIS
  ("meningitis")

(2) PARENCHYMATOUS ENCEPHALITIS OR MYELITIS
  ("encephalitis," "myelitis")

LESIONS OF THE TERTIARY PERIOD

(1) CHRONIC INTERSTITIAL ENCEPHALITIS OR MYELITIS
  ("gummatous meningitis")

(2) CHRONIC PARENCHYMATOUS ENCEPHALITIS
  ("dementia paralytica")

(3) CHRONIC PARENCHYMATOUS MYELITIS
  ("tabes dorsalis")

"We have shown that the central nervous system is affected by syphilis at the same periods and in the same manner as are other internal organs. In addition the 'parasyphilitic' lesions are also of a typically syphilitic nature, being directly comparable to the parenchymatous affections found elsewhere in the body. They are 'tertiary' lesions differing only from the so-called 'gummatous' processes in the central nervous system in that their localization is in the parenchyma while that of the latter is in the interstitial tissues."

MCINTOSH AND FILDES, 1914

CHART 22

Physical examination showed a man 5' 9" tall, weighing 149 pounds, rather pale and poorly nourished, with a somewhat enlarged heart and no evidence of venereal disease.

Neurologically there was a slight facial and digital tremor, but otherwise no symptom or reflex disorder except that the tendon reflexes were generally increased; the knee-jerks especially were very vigorous. There was no speech defect. His handwriting was fairly legible.

The patient was very noisy and uncontrollable, tearing clothing and biting, striking the attendants, refusing food, talking rapidly, loudly, and incoherently. His manner suggested auditory hallucinations but no positive evidence of these was obtained. His clothes could not be kept on him. The following is a sample of his reactions: As the examiner entered, the patient stood stark naked and glaring. He started to talk as follows: " Methuen, — I, Saviour, come to life and ought to die ——— Now I lay me ——— Now I die ——— The heart beats ——— No, I ain't going to die ——— I am going out soon. I want my clothes ——— You can't hold me; I am strong." (Struggles violently with the attendants.) "I am God. God. I know you, you can't fool me. ——— I am here ——— I can do you all. How many doctors are there here?" (Struggles violently. Looks at examiner.) "He is writing something. Sir, you can't fool me in a million years. Do you understand that, doctor? You can't fool me. Write all the prescriptions you want to. Ten thousand years; you hear that, doctor? Ten thousand years. You can't fool me; ten thousand years. Ten thousand years are but a day for the spirit of the Lord," etc., etc.

The excitement continued unabated. The patient became entirely disoriented, and finally almost unable to move. He lay in bed trying to talk and muttering broken gibberish, still attempting to struggle to the extent of his limited strength.

The **autopsy** showed no sign of lesion (brain weight 1380 grams), unless, perhaps, the occipital regions were slightly firmer than the rest of the brain. Death was apparently due to a bilateral pneumonia, bronchial type. There was an acute splenitis. The only chronic lesions of the body

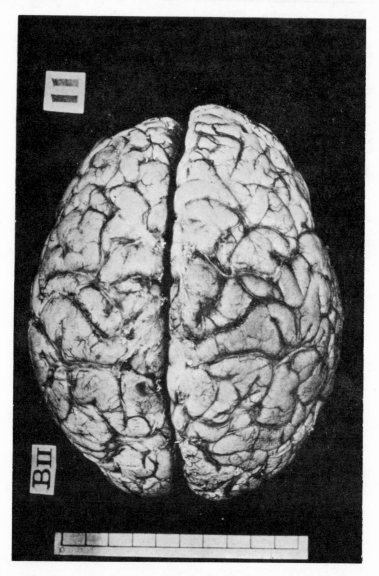

Paretic neurosyphilis ("general paresis") macroscopically normal, microscopically characteristic. Treatment does not have to face massive destructive processes already complete.

were a bilateral chronic adhesive pleuritis and a slight sclerosis of the arch of the aorta.

Microscopically there was a distinct though mild degree of lymphocytosis of the perivascular spaces in many regions. Somewhat extended *search failed to reveal plasma cells,* and it is certain that if plasma cells existed, they must have occurred in very small numbers.

Here, then, was a case of DIFFUSE NEUROSYPHILIS (with brain picture consistent) with symptoms lasting but 22 days and with an appearance of acute mania. It is to be noted that this case arrived at the hospital on the eleventh day of his symptoms. The case occurred long before the development of the temporary care system in Massachusetts. It is probable, or at any rate possible, that he would have been brought to the hospital far earlier, say, upon the sixth day, had the modern temporary care system been installed at that time. The routine W. R. examination would then have been made. With more effective hydrotherapy, it is possible that the patient's life might have been prolonged and that treatment might have been effective. So far as we can see, the case would have been a singularly good one for treatment despite the practical unmanageability of the case under ordinary home treatment, and even under hospital conditions where modern hydrotherapeutic appliances are not available.

PARETIC   NEUROSYPHILIS   showing   very
MARKED MENINGITIS, suggesting that therapy
might have produced improvement. Autopsy.

Case 101. We report the case of John Baxter, a boat
tender of 48 years, because this particular victim of PARETIC
NEUROSYPHILIS seems to have had the most markedly thickened and altered meninges in our whole series. Of course, the
therapeutic theory upon which we now proceed in the treatment of non-paretic and possibly even of paretic neurosyphilis is that, other things being equal, the meningitis
can be removed by treatment, or in the course of treatment,
so that the degree of ultimate recovery rather depends upon
the condition of the brain substance itself than upon the
condition of the meninges.   Here, at all events, is an example
of the most highly meningitic neurosyphilis that we have
seen.

Curiously enough, two of Baxter's brothers were also
patients at the hospital at which Baxter died, and a number
of the other members of the family are reported as "nervous."
It seems that at 35 Baxter began to drink heavily and had
never given over the habit of alcoholism.

Upon admission to the hospital, in fact, he showed a sufficiently typical picture of delirium tremens.   His consciousness was clouded, he had vivid visual hallucinations and was
very apprehensive.

His heart was enlarged to the left; the pulse, 120, was of
increased tension and irregular; there was peripheral arteriosclerosis; the teeth were poor; the tongue coated; and
the mouth foul.   The urine showed a trace of albumin and
rare hyalin casts.

Neurologically, the gait was somewhat unsteady, there
was an extreme tremor of the whole body, including the
tongue and fingers.   The Romberg sign was negative although
there was marked swaying.   The pupils were equal and reacted
normally; the knee-jerks were markedly exaggerated, the

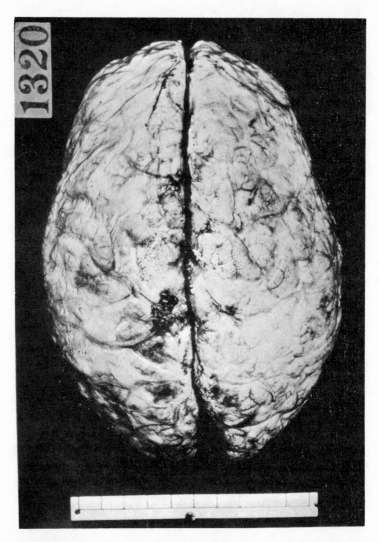

A high degree of chronic leptomeningitis. Pia mater thick, opaque, concealing brain. In paretic neurosyphilis ("general paresis").

arm reflexes somewhat exaggerated. The remainder of the reflexes upon systematic examination were negative.

Upon arrival, Baxter was put to bed, but he barricaded his door and fought with the attendants. The tremor increased, the hallucinations were both visual and auditory. After a few days, Baxter became so weak that he could not move. He refused to eat for a period of two days, explaining in whispers that he did not wish to be poisoned; a voice had told him the food was to be poisoned. The voice was of agreeable tones, probably belonging to a lady; it did not speak, but sang to him. The clouding of consciousness failed to clear up, as in delirium tremens, so that, though patient was admitted March 3d, it was hardly possible to speak freely with him until more than a month later, April 9th. A goodnatured conversation would run as follows·

"What is your name?"	" Baxter."
"First name?"	After long pause, "Don't know."
"John?"	Pause of 7 seconds, " Yes, I think it is."
"How old are you?"	" There are legs —— there is a body —— up to here —— "
"Say the alphabet."	Term not understood.
"Say the *a*, *b*, *c*."	"Oh yes; a, b, c, d (long pause), e, f; I cannot say it, I did not have much education; I am not intelligent." (In point of fact, the patient had a good grammar-school education, and had long worked as a clerk in a grocery store, with good wages.)

There was some speech defect.

Soon the hallucinatory phase passed, and the patient remained in a cloudy and disoriented state, inaccessible, rarely speaking, and gradually failing physically. Death occurred about three months after admission (pulmonary symptoms).

In estimating the duration of the process in John Baxter, we must take into account that he left the grocery business and became a hard-working but poorly-paid boat tender at

about 35 years, at the same time that the alcoholic habit
began.

The **autopsy** showed that death was due to bronchopneumonia with pleurisy. There were in the body a variety
of chronic lesions, such as gastritis, colitis, epididymitis,
splenitis, parietal and valvular endocarditis, prostatitis, chronic
appendicitis, and some mesenteric lymphnoditis. The heart
was somewhat hypertrophied. There was a slight diffuse
nephritis with cysts, emaciation, and decubitus. The calvarium was thick and somewhat dense. The dura was
thickened and adherent, and the pia mater, — as above
stated, the most thickened and altered pia mater in our
series, — is described as everywhere thickened, of a brownish
gray and white color, especially over the vascular lines, and
as showing small white areas of deeper thickening scattered
over the surface, but most markedly over the sulci, and not
as a rule over the crowns of the gyri. There were also yellowish brown spots with a suggestion of fibrin over the lateral
aspects of both hemispheres. The vessels at the base were
not remarkable in the gross. The brain weighed 1220 grams,
and appeared to be of darker color than usual.

Some cases of PARETIC NEUROSYPHILIS ("general paresis") have so much BRAIN ATROPHY that it is not possible to expect much improvement through antisyphilitic therapy.

Case 102. Theodosia Jewett, dead at 58 years, showed the most remarkably wasted brain in a long series of victims of paretic neurosyphilis. We present her case to emphasize what therapy must face in certain instances, but would recall the fact that exceedingly few such wasted brains have come to our attention in cases dying in the institutions of Massachusetts.

Mrs. Jewett, a housewife, whose parents died of shock, and one of whose two brothers also died of shock, was a normal child and schoolgirl, and worked as dressmaker until she was married, at 24, to a grocer, by whom she had two children. At the age of 46, Mrs. Jewett began to suffer from so-called "nervous prostration." The attack lasted some two years, but there were no psychotic symptoms beyond worry and insomnia. The menopause occurred at 52, at which time the first signs of psychosis appeared, namely, a forgetfulness concerning familiar matters, such as sewing, cooking, and the like. At 55, this amnesia had become so marked that Mrs. Jewett could neither write nor tell time. She, however, was a perfectly quiet and easily manageable patient, often subject to drowziness in the day.

Six months before her admission to the hospital, she began to suffer from insomnia, failed to recognize her surroundings, and had a number of crying spells. Restlessness had begun a month before admission; auditory hallucinations developed in the form of imaginary conversations with dead persons. A certain loquacity set in, and for a week before admission, Mrs. Jewett became somewhat resistive.

Physically, the patient was sallow, poorly nourished, with pale mucous membranes, peripheral arteriosclerosis, no teeth, muscular feebleness, tremor of hands and tongue, and active knee-jerks. **Mentally,** the patient was depressed, talked to herself, assumed a supplicating position, suddenly altered her attitude, and was very tremulous. Her talk was low, mumbling, and incoherent, for the most part composed of answers to her own questions. Sometimes there was a curious difficulty in speaking, such that the lips moved but no sound emerged; but for the most part there was no difficulty in uttering words. The patient either could or would not write. Only when the attention was secured by speaking to her sharply was she apparently able to understand questions, and the answers to these sharp questions came spasmodically and as if interrrupting her own thoughts. Nor was it ever possible to obtain a repetition of the same answer.

The patient died in exhaustion, with pulmonary symptoms three weeks after admission.

The **autopsy** which was performed $3\frac{1}{2}$ hours after death showed the following points of interest:

The heart weighed 210 grams. There was marked thickening of the aortic valve. The coronaries were slightly thickened.

The lungs were slightly adherent to the chest wall at the apices and posteriorly. The right lung was consolidated in the lower two lobes posteriorly and the bronchi exuded pus; the left lung was not remarkable. There was a chronic splenitis.

The liver showed fibrous changes, was a brownish-red in color, mottled with yellow.

Combined weight of the kidneys 195 grams. The capsules were adherent, tearing the cortex when stripped.

The diploë were well marked. The dura was not adherent. The pia was slightly thickened and raised from the cortex by a large amount of subpial fluid (showing atrophy of the cortex). The pial vessels were injected, more markedly so on the left side. The arachnoid villi were reported as moderately developed, especially along the longitudinal fissure.

The brain was rather soft in all regions. The weight was 1045 grams. According to Tigges' formula the weight of the brain should be approximately 8 times the body length in centimeters. The length in this case was 158 cm., therefore,

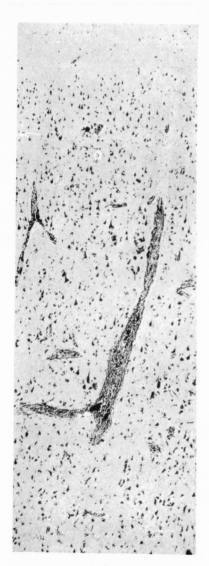

Perivascular exudate (low power) in atrophic cortex from case of general paresis.

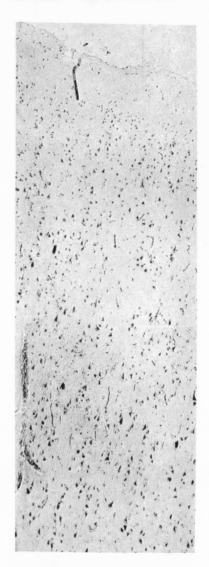

Markedly atrophic cortex, but without local perivascular exudate.

according to this formula the weight of the brain should have been 1464 grams. The difference of more than 400 grams is evidently a loss to be accounted for by atrophy, a very heavy loss.

1. Was the "nervous prostration" at 46 of syphilitic origin? One cannot give a categorical answer to this question. The high incidence of shock in the family suggests poor stock in which a psychoneurosis is not an unusual phenomenon. The presence of syphilis might act as a debilitating factor or *agent provocateur*, if it were not to cause any demonstrable brain lesion. As pointed out in the case of Harrison (9), however, it is not unusual in neurosyphilis to find a history of symptoms occurring years before the final breakdown and symptoms frequently not recognized as of neurosyphilitic nature.

2. Does the fairly long duration of the psychosis (at least 3 years) explain the marked atrophy? Cases having symptoms even much longer than three years at times show relatively very little atrophy, so that this factor in itself cannot be said to explain the tremendous destruction of tissue.

The **THERAPY OF NEUROSYPHILIS** has to face not merely variations in the degree of brain wasting and in the degree of meningitis, but also variations in the topographical distribution of lesions. Autopsy.

Case 103. To bring out this point we may instance the case of Alfred Weed, a victim of PARETIC NEUROSYPHILIS, dying at the age of 48 years after a course of about seven years. The following is an abstract of the clinical history:

A. W. suffered from lues some 24 years before his death at Danvers Insane Hospital in 1907. There is no account of insanity in his family. The patient had been undergoing mental changes for six years before death. At the age of 42 began to take interest in socialism and spiritualism. Would become excited at times and was observed to talk to himself. At times it seemed that he was reacting to visual hallucinations. After eight months he became depressed and apprehensive and developed delusions of poisoning.

On admission to the Danvers Insane Hospital in June, 1902, the subject was found to be ataxic, falling in the Romberg position. Pupils were equal but of pin-point size. There was tremor of the facial muscles. The knee-jerks were absent. Speech was ataxic. Memory defective. Depressed. Thought he was to be punished. Refused to eat.

Later in the year of admission, patient became more negativistic. He refused to have his clothes brushed. His answers were slow. Mental arithmetic was correctly but slowly done. During January, 1903, the patient was apt to be active and talkative for a time, and then his attitude would suddenly change to one of silence, resistiveness and untidiness. From time to time he would be querulous and sulky. In August, 1903, the patient became weaker and could walk with assistance only. Paralysis developed in the left facialis region and in the left external rectus. Pupils were still small, but the left had become smaller than

the right.   Light reaction tests unsatisfactory.   Knee-jerks
could not be obtained.

In December, 1903, the patient was untidy and helpless,
lying with his thighs and legs flexed.   The limbs were spastic
on passive motion.   In 1905, the pain sense of the legs was
found lost and the pupils were small and stiff.   The protruded tongue was deflected to the right.   The right labial
fold was more prominent than the left.   Knee-jerks remained
absent.   Ataxia was extreme.

The **Neurological Findings** may be summed up as follows:

1. Ataxia of the legs.
2. (Probable) Diminished sensibility in the legs.
3. Pupils small and stiff. Left smaller than the right.
4. Paralysis of left facialis.
5. Paralysis of left external rectus.
6. Tongue protruded to right.
7. Right elbow jerk greater than left.
8. Knee-jerks absent.

The cause of death was bronchopneumonia.   The walls
and valves of the heart showed a few chronic changes.   There
was a marked splenitis and an atrophy of the liver.   The
kidneys showed numerous depressed scars.   The arch of the
aorta was somewhat sclerotic.   The following is a full description of the head findings which we present by way of
comparison with other cases.   Note especially the cerebellar,
dentate, and olivary changes.   Note also the fact that palpable sclerosis is demonstrable over a far larger area than
atrophy, so that we may almost safely conclude that the process of induration sometimes precedes that of atrophy.   One
gets the impression from the extent of visible atrophy and
tangible induration in this case, that a possible therapy would
have not merely to clear the perivascular spaces of cells and
spirochetes, but would also need to arrest the indurating and
wasting process.   Nor could any therapy deal effectively with
the superior frontal and upper central atrophy of the cerebrum
of this case, or with the olivary and cerebellar lesions.

Head: Hair thin at vertex.   Scalp normal.   Calvarium

thin and dense. Dura mater slightly adherent to calvarium at vertex. Sinuses normal. Arachnoidal villi well developed. Pia mater of anterior and central regions contains an excess of fluid. The pial veins well injected.

The **pia mater** exhibits one unusual lesion: Faintly yellowish brown spots of miliary and slightly larger size are scattered irregularly in clusters over the vertex. These miliary pial macules are observed especially over the posterior third of the left superior frontal gyrus (a group of twelve or more). Two are seen in the pia mater of the right superior frontal gyrus. One is seen in the upper part of the left post central gyrus. The upper end of the right postcentral gyrus contains three macules.

Besides these brownish macules, the pia mater also shows focal white thickenings which resemble the more frequent appearances of chronic fibrous leptomeningitis. The white thickenings are of irregular size but are, as a rule, larger than the macules above mentioned. They occur, as a rule, over the sulcal veins and are most frequent in the anterior region.

The vessels at the base are normal. There is no evidence of pial thickening at the base of the brain. **Brain** weight, 1265 grams. There is visible atrophy of both superior frontal gyri and of the upper two-thirds of both central gyri. The extent of palpable sclerosis surpasses that of visible atrophy. Palpable increase of consistence is shown by the prefrontal, orbital (more marked on left side), frontal, central, hippocampal and occipital regions. The temporal cortex is of normal or slightly reduced consistence.

Section of the cerebral cortex shows everywhere preservation of the cortical markings. The sclerosed areas show a diminution in depth of the cortex, which is more marked in the left prefrontal region. The white matter of the centrum semiovale of the prefrontal and occipital regions on both sides shows an increase of consistence. The cerebellar cortex also shows variations in consistence. The clivus and lobus cacuminis and the posterior half of the inferior surfaces of both cerebellar hemispheres are firmer than normal. The laminæ of the left clivus are a trifle narrower than those of the right. There is visible extensive atrophy of the laminæ

on both sides of a fissure in the middle of the left lobus cacuminis.   In the coordinate portion of the right cacumen there
is a similar process which is less marked.   The dentate nuclei
are firm.   The olives show an increase of consistence, equal
on both sides.   The left olive shows on section a crowding
together of its folds in the middle part of the upper limb.

Spinal cord was not remarkable.

Summary:

Adhesive pachymeningitis
Chronic fibrous leptomeningitis
Miliary pial macules
Cerebral atrophy
Cerebral sclerosis
Cerebellar atrophy and sclerosis
Bronchopneumonia
Chronic splenitis
Nephritis
Aortitis

> It is generally recognized that DIFFUSE NEURO-
> SYPHILIS ("cerebrospinal syphilis") frequently
> is cured through antisyphilitic therapy. Example.
> Mental improvement, in one month; recovery from
> paralysis, ten months.

Case 104. John Edwards, a man of 28 years, well developed and nourished, with general enlargement of glands
and skin lesions, came to the hospital in a stuporous condition, with evidences of a complete hemiplegia.

According to the wife, Edwards had had a chancre of
the lip about a year before, for which he had been treated
with an intravenous injection, presumably of salvarsan, and
also presumably with mercury. The lip lesion had then
disappeared. For a month before admission, Edwards had
had headache and dizziness, for which he was given pills
and drugs. There had also been difficulty with speech and
numbness of the left arm as far up as the elbow, but this
paresthesia had quickly disappeared. The hemiplegia was
of only a few days' duration. After a feeling of nausea and
vomiting, the patient had fallen with left-sided paralysis.
Afterwards, he had shown mental peculiarities, eventually
becoming noisy, hard to manage, and appropriate for hospital care.

The **physical examination** showed a variety of increased
reflexes, including ankle-clonus on the left side.

The question might arise whether this case was one of
hemorrhage or thrombosis, and the facts about the onset
of the hemiplegia are inadequate for a decision. However,
at so early an age, the probability of syphilis is large and the
history of labial chancre was quite suggestive. If we may
conclude neurosyphilis, the diagnosis of thrombosis rather
than rupture of blood vessel is likely. The laboratory tests
bore out the diagnosis since the W. R. of serum and fluid
both proved positive; the gold sol reaction was syphilitic;

NON-PARETIC NEUROSYPHILIS

DIFFUSE NEUROSYPHILIS, MENINGOVASCULAR PAREN-CHYMATOUS, CEREBROSPINAL SYPHILIS

CASES SYSTEMATICALLY TREATED   13

CLINICAL RECOVERY, C.S.F. NEGATIVE   11

UNIMPROVED   1

UNIMPROVED, BUT C.S.F. NEGATIVE   1

MASSACHUSETTS COMMISSION ON MENTAL DISEASES,
November, 1916

CHART 23

there were 176 cells per cmm.; there was excess albumin, and a positive globulin reaction.

The outcome in such a case is dubious. If death does not occur soon, recovery is not impossible under treatment. At all events, a considerable improvement is likely.

Edwards was given bi-weekly injections of salvarsan, intramuscular injections of mercury salicylate, and doses of potassium iodid, averaging 100 grains, three times a day. Under this treatment, he slowly recovered and became mentally clear after a few weeks. The paralysis seemed complete and permanent. Even after three or four months, there was absolutely no change in the condition, and Edwards was quite unable to move either arm or leg. Meanwhile, the spinal fluid had become practically negative to all tests.

Treatment was somewhat optimistically continued and was *rewarded at the end of ten months* with marked improvement such that the patient was able to stand on the paralyzed leg and move the arm to a certain degree. This improvement is still continuing. The spinal fluid and the serum have remained negative to laboratory tests.

Note: A period of six months is commonly regarded as that period in which improvement in paralysis is to occur if there is to be any improvement. There was certainly not the slightest improvement in the paralysis of this case before eight or nine months of treatment had elapsed, and it took ten months to secure the marked improvement mentioned.

1. What is the significance of the prodromal symptoms? The headache and dizziness should have been viewed with great gravity. They are characteristic in MENINGOVASCULAR NEUROSYPHILIS.

   Moreover in this case there had also been difficulties with speech and other transient symptoms which should have called attention far earlier to the possibility of neurosyphilis.

2. What is the significance of the high cell count: 176 per cubic millimeter? Such high cell counts are frequent enough in diffuse neurosyphilis, but low cell counts are frequent also. But although the high cell count taken alone is of lesser significance, the fact that the high

cell count in this case is associated with a " syphilitic " gold sol reaction is of far greater significance for diagnosis. These associated findings are characteristic of meningovascular neurosyphilis.

3. What kind of recovery may be expected in successful examples of treatment in meningovascular cases? Recovery with defect. It will be noted that ten months elapsed before any marked improvement occurred on the paralyzed side. We could not expect a complete recovery from this paralysis.

4. Was inadequacy of treatment following the chancre responsible for the early cerebrospinal involvement? In this connection one must remember that such neural involvements occur occasionally even during active treatment (neurorecidives). The discontinuance of treatment after a short period, in this case less than a year, is always a risk to say the least. And this is true even though the W. R. becomes negative, for trouble of a neurosyphilitic nature may occur later; this when both blood and spinal fluid have previously been found negative. The old rule of following and treating a syphilitic for several years despite the disappearance of symptoms is still a good rule.

The results of systematic, intensive, intravenous
salvarsan therapy in atypical neurosyphilis (cases
not certainly paretic, tabetic or the common types
of meningovascular neurosyphilis) may be in our
experience as good as the results of treatment in
common meningovascular cases: example.

Case 105. Henri Lepère, a machinist, 48 years of age,
came voluntarily to the Psychopathic Hospital for a gradually failing memory and inability to work. He had had
indigestion for four years (epigastric distress, nausea, no
vomiting). He was still suffering from epigastric distress
and from headaches. At times he had had difficulty in
walking.

Physically, Lepère looked older than he was; he was very
poorly developed and nourished, and seemed very weak.
There was a slight visceroptosis.

Neurologically, there was considerable speech defect, particularly well marked in test phrases. The pupils were
contracted and gave the Argyll-Robertson reaction. Neurologically there were no other signs.

Mentally, there was a depression with worry; but it was
a question whether these phenomena were not entirely
natural. The special complaint was of failing memory.

The Argyll-Robertson pupil also *prima facie* signifies
neurosyphilis. Lepère, in fact, admitted syphilitic infection
at 23. The gastric symptoms at once suggested tabes. The
knee-jerks and ankle-jerks were, to be sure, preserved; however, this is not very unusual in tabes. The amnesia and
aphasia naturally suggested paresis. Without resort to
laboratory findings, accordingly, the diagnosis of taboparetic neurosyphilis ("taboparesis") was suggested.

The serum W. R. proved positive, but the spinal fluid W. R.
very slightly so (yielding only moderate reaction with 1 cc.,
0.7 and 0.5 cc., and a negative reaction with 0.3 and 0.1 cc.).

EFFECT OF EARLY TREATMENT ON THE DEVELOPMENT OF NEUROSYPHILIS

TOTAL CASES.................................. 4134

DEVELOPED GENERAL PARESIS............ 198 = 4.8%

DEVELOPED TABES DORSALIS............. 113 = 2.7%

DEVELOPED CEREBROSPINAL SYPHILIS.... 132 = 3.2%
$$\overline{}$$
443 = 10.5%

EFFECT OF TREATMENT

	None	1 course	Repeated energetic
NUMBER OF CASES...100		134	924
DEVELOPED G.P......	25 = 25%	31 = 23.1%	30 = 3.2%
DEVELOPED TABES...	11 = 11%	16 = 11.9%	25 = 2.7%
DEVELOPED C.S.S......	3 = 3%	21 = 15.6%	71 = 7.6%

	Poorly treated 1880–84	Better treated 1895–99
NUMBER OF CASES...617		1139
DEVELOPED G.P......	60 = 9.7%	37 = 3.2%
DEVELOPED TABES...	22 = 3.5%	16 = 1.4%
DEVELOPED C.S.S.....	15 = 2.4%	28 = 2.4%

MATTAUSCHEK AND PILCZ

CHART 24

Globulin was moderate, and albumin was found in only moderate excess. There were 21 cells per cmm. in the spinal fluid. The gold sol reaction was that which we regard as typical of syphilis or tabes. If we were to rely upon the weakness of the fluid W. R. and the nature of the gold sol reaction, we should be inclined to favor the diagnosis of DIFFUSE NEUROSYPHILIS ("cerebrospinal syphilis") rather than resort to the diagnosis of paretic neurosyphilis.

Salvarsan treatment was attended by the rapid disappearance of headaches and gastric symptoms and by a rapid gain in weight and feeling of well-being. Salvarsan was continued twice a week for two months, whereupon Lepère returned to work. He has been successfully at work now for seven months without return of symptoms. Four months after beginning of treatment, the spinal fluid was examined and found entirely negative. Nevertheless, the serum W. R. has remained positive despite eight months of salvarsan treatment.

1. What is the meaning of the titrations in the spinal fluid Wassermann reaction? When Plaut originally applied the Wassermann reaction to spinal fluids, he used 0.2 of a cc. of spinal fluid. With this amount of fluid he found that cases of general paresis gave a positive reaction in about 100% of the cases while this positive reaction was only given by 40 to 60% of the cases of cerebrospinal syphilis and tabes dorsalis, hence he promulgated a differential point that a negative reaction in spinal fluid indicated that the case was not general paresis. Hauptmann later showed that if 1 cc. of spinal fluid were used, a positive reaction would occur in practically 100% of the cases of general paresis, cerebrospinal syphilis and tabes. Therefore, at present, we use the different titers of spinal fluid from which we draw the following conclusions: If the reaction in the untreated case is negative with 0.1 and 0.3 of a cc. and positive with the 0.5, 0.7 and 1 cc. dilutions as in the case of Lepère, we are probably dealing with non-paretic neurosyphilis. With this method of titration we are also better able to watch the progress of treatment as the dilutions of 0.1 and 0.3 cc. become negative first.

2. How soon can one expect improvement after commencement of salvarsan therapy in cases of diffuse neurosyphilis? The time relation of results in treatment varies with each individual case. In the case of Lepère gastric symptoms that had been present for a number of months disappeared as if by magic after the first injection of salvarsan. As a rule, it is true that the more acute the symptoms the quicker their disappearance but this does not hold for all cases, as in this particular instance the long standing symptoms disappeared very rapidly. The symptoms often disappear very much more rapidly than the laboratory tests change.

3. How can the mental symptoms (depression and failing memory) of which patient complained be explained? In the first place, as has been stated, it is doubtful if these are more than subjective and the result of the patient's feeling of discomfort and pain. However, it is also possible that there may be intracranial involvement of the meninges or of the brain itself. And, if such were the case, the improvement might be the result of the treatment.

The Argyll-Robertson pupil should not be used as a basis for a necessarily bad prognosis if treatment can be given.

Case 106. Frederick Stone was a business man of large interests. He had been in the hands of physicians for several years for a variety of disorders such as renal, respiratory, cardio-vascular, and so on. No suspicion of syphilis had apparently been uttered by the physicians despite the fact that Mr. Stone readily stated that he had had a chancre thirty years before, and that he had received several years' treatment of mercury and potassium iodid by mouth.

It appeared that a few years ago he had begun to have trouble with his nose, which was cauterized and operatively interfered with without satisfactory results. This nasal condition had later been diagnosticated as gummatous, and had improved considerably under a mild antisyphilitic treatment. However, this nasal condition had been considered and treated quite separately from the remainder of Mr. Stone's troubles.

What brought him to attention was a sudden diplopia with ptosis. There was a paralysis of the external rectus of the left eye, as well as a drooping of the lid on this side. The left eye was much inflamed. The diplopia greatly bothered the patient, and there was also considerable pain in the left frontal region, confined chiefly to the distribution of the first division of the trigeminal nerve. According to the patient this headache was periodic. There was considerable tenderness to pinprick over the area and a diminution of sensory discrimination of fine touch. Both the pupils failed to react to light.

The remainder of the neurological symptomatic examination was surprisingly clear of disorder, nor was there anything in the history suggestive of tabes. There was ozena as well as evidence of the operative work upon nares and throat. Possibly the arteries were slightly hardened; blood pressure

PARETIC NEUROSYPHILIS

(GENERAL PARESIS)

Cases systematically treated   50

CLINICAL REMISSIONS   34   68%

C.S.F. ALTERED TO NEGATIVE   4   8%

C.S.F. ALTERED TO WEAKER   16   32%

C.S.F. UNALTERED   14   28%

CLINICALLY UNIMPROVED   16   32%

C.S.F. WEAKER   7   14%

C.S.F. UNALTERED   9   18%

MASSACHUSETTS COMMISSION ON MENTAL DISEASES
November, 1916

CHART 25

was 165 systolic. There was a large trace of albumin, and there were numerous hyalin casts in the urine.

Mentally, there was a degree of depression and worry hardly out of keeping with the general situation. Despite the preservation of memory, Mr. Stone failed to do rather simple arithmetical calculations; this was the more remarkable as in his business he had to handle figures a great deal and had been doing so until recently. There was a slight tremor in his writing, as well as a certain difficulty in enunciating test phrases. Insomnia, irritability, and a feeling of nervousness and of being tired out, completed the picture.

A suggestion for diagnosis would be classically offered by the Argyll-Robertson pupils. Should not a patient with the Argyll-Robertson pupils have either tabes or paresis? However, in favor of tabes, besides the pupil, are to be counted merely the troubles with the eyes. In the direction of paresis we have to consider speech defect, to say nothing of less definite symptoms such as insomnia and increased irritability.

We are inclined to think, however, that the disease in this case is meningovascular. This diagnosis is suggested by the cranial nerve palsies and by the headache. Headache is much more rarely a phenomenon in the paretic type of neurosyphilis than in the meningovascular type.

In point of fact, the spinal fluid phenomena bore out the diagnosis of MENINGOVASCULAR NEUROSYPHILIS inasmuch as the globulin, albumin, cellular content, gold sol, and W. R.'s were all weakly positive.

1. How far can we regard the cardiorenal defects as syphilitic? Perhaps we may do so on the general principle of parsimony in scientific interpretation.

The diagnostic lumbar puncture led to an extremely severe exacerbation of the pains on the left side of the head. In fact, these pains could not be held in check by the exhibition of pyramidon. Mr. Stone regarded the pain as due to the lumbar puncture. However, there was no improvement in the pain in the prone position, — a feature characteristic of lumbar puncture pains. Upon administration of salvarsan, this local pain rapidly disappeared. In fact, there was a startling improvement; the ocular palsies disappeared in a few weeks, although these palsies had been present for several months before the administration of salvarsan. The blood pressure was reduced; the urine became negative. Perhaps the most startling feature of all (although of this we are not sure) was that the patient states he was accepted by a life insurance company although he had been twice refused previously.

Note in this case the 30-year interval between infection and generalized neurosyphilitic involvement. Note also the amenability of the process despite this duration. We are perhaps entitled also to note that a neurological examination careful enough to detect an Argyll-Robertson pupil should have been made by a number of examiners long before the particular crisis which we have sketched. It is also permissible to note that the rhinological work should not have been carried out independently of all other medical work.

2. What are the untoward results of lumbar puncture? It is true that there is always a possibility of setting up a septic meningitis by lumbar puncture, but this is a very remote possibility and with any reasonable care it is not to be considered. Lumbar puncture also has a considerable danger in cases of increased intracranial pressure. In cases of brain tumor where the tumor is located in the posterior fossa, sudden death may occur from withdrawal of spinal fluid. This is supposed to be due to the medulla being pressed down into the foramen magnum and causing paralysis of respiration. Therefore lumbar puncture should never be performed except with the greatest caution in a case in which brain tumor is suspected.

However, aside from these remote serious consequences which play very little rôle in the ordinary procedure of lumbar puncture, certain unpleasant symptoms do frequently arise. These symptoms are chiefly headache and nausea, but, however, may go as far as vomiting. These symptoms occur almost entirely in the cases in which there is no abnormal condition producing increased spinal fluid pressure. Such unpleasant symptoms may last as long as four or five days; as a rule, however, last only for a period of a day o two.

3. What is the treatment of discomfort following lumbar puncture? It is a rule well worth observing that the patient after lumbar puncture should remain flat on his back without a pillow for 24 hours in order to avoid any unpleasant symptoms. If any symptoms do occur, it will be almost certainly when the patient arises, and in nearly every instance they will be overcome if the patient again assumes the prone position. Raising the foot of the bed so as to lower the head also helps. Veronal or bromides may be given but as a rule are not very satisfactory.

4. How permanent is the improvement obtained in the case of Mr. Stone likely to be? As a matter of fact, the patient discontinued treatment as soon as he felt well again, but after two months the pain returned to be again quickly dispelled by salvarsan. This improvement must be considered as only temporary. Under continued treatment there may be no further relapse. There is, however, evidence that much damage has been done to the body by the spirochetes, much of which is irreparable. It is even possible that further disintegration might occur even while undergoing treatment. Still treatment offers much in such a case and is to be highly recommended.

In DIFFUSE NEUROSYPHILIS, rendering the
spinal fluid negative by treatment may mean
neither cure nor disappearance of symptoms.

Case 107. Greta Meyer, a widow, 51 years of age, came
voluntarily to the hospital, seeking medical aid for a marked
depression. She was also suffering from a right hemiplegia.
It appeared, according to Mrs. Meyer, that she was married
at 16, and lived with her husband until 29, whereupon she
left him on account of his alcoholism, his abuse of her, and
the discovery through his physician that he was suffering from
venereal disease. She had had two healthy children and
there never had been miscarriages or stillbirths. Six years
after the separation, namely at 35 years of age, and 16 years
before resort to the Psychopathic Hospital, Mrs. Meyer
developed certain red areas on her hand, and learned at a
hospital that these were due to syphilis. She kept up
treatment for these lesions for a year, until she seemed perfectly well.

She had, in fact, remained perfectly well for some 14 years,
until at 49, a small tumor had appeared on the right side of
the forehead, near the hair line. This tumor was firm and
not sore. Medical treatment reduced it, leaving, however,
a depression in the bone. One day, about a month after the
appearance of the tumor, the patient lay down for a nap,
and upon awaking found she could only with difficulty move
her right arm and leg. Her face was not affected; she was
not in pain; and there was no disorder of speech. In a few
days she got much better and she had been improving
for some time past through the administration of further
medicine.

However, since the onset of the hemiplegia Mrs. Meyer
had been very despondent. There had been ups and downs
but she had rarely felt well. The depression was a mild one
and in point of fact may perhaps be regarded as non-psychopathic, since at her age with her disability, there might well be

METHODS OF TREATMENT

I. BY MOUTH.

    1. MERCURY

    2. IODIDES

    3. ARSENIC

II. INTRAMUSCULAR INJECTIONS

    1. MERCURY

    2. SALVARSAN, NEOSALVARSAN, OTHER ARSENIC PREPARATIONS

    3. SODIUM NUCLEINATE

    4. ANTIMONY

III. INTRAVENOUS

    1. MERCURY

    2. MERCURIALIZED SERUM

    3. SALVARSAN, NEOSALVARSAN, ARSENIC

    4. IODIDES

IV. SPINAL INTRADURAL

    1. SALVARSANIZED SERUM (IN VIVO — SWIFT-ELLIS)

    2. SALVARSANIZED SERUM (IN VITRO — MARINESCO-OGILVIE)

    3. MERCURIALIZED SERUM (BYRNES)

V. CEREBRAL SUBDURAL AND INTRAVENTRICULAR

    1. SALVARSANIZED SERUM (IN VIVO)

    2. SALVARSANIZED SERUM (IN VITRO)

    3. MERCURIALIZED SERUM

CHART 26

a degree of sadness and unhappiness concerning the future. **Mentally,** there was no other disorder of note, and in particular no disorder of memory.

Physically, the patient showed a right-sided hemiplegia with excessive right knee-jerk, but without Babinski or other abnormal reflex phenomena. The extra-ocular movements were somewhat restricted in range but there was neither strabismus nor nystagmus.

The question arose whether the hemiplegia was of hemorrhagic or thrombotic origin. After all, at 51 years, hemiplegia is rather unlikely to be of a non-syphilitic arteriosclerotic origin; moreover, we had a clear history of syphilis. The serum W. R. proved positive as well as the spinal fluid W. R. The finding of 77 cells per cmm., excess albumin, and positive globulin test, taken in connection with the entire picture seems to warrant a diagnosis of CEREBROSPINAL SYPHILIS. If we proceed on statistical grounds, it might be regarded as more probable that the hemiplegia is THROMBOTIC in origin rather than hemorrhagic. It appears that syphilitic cerebral thrombosis rather characteristically occurs without preliminary symptoms, despite the fact that many cases do show headache, dizziness, and restlessness as prodromal symptoms.

1. What is the treatment indicated in the case of Mrs. Meyer?

    It would appear that little or nothing can be done for the hemiplegia unless the claims of Franz with respect to reëstablishment of a degree of function in certain hemiplegics are substantiated. However, the indication of meningitic process as shown by the spinal fluid, suggests that the case is not a purely vascular one but may be regarded as meningovascular. (Possibly, also, we should regard the left frontal depression and scar as indicative of a non-parenchymatous and non-vascular process.) Accordingly, antisyphilitic treatment should be theoretically of some value.

    In point of fact, the patient was given injections of mercury salicylate, mercury by mouth, and potassium iodid. Her psychopathic depression under this treatment, supported by proper hygiene and rest, diminished. However, six months later, the patient slipped on a wet floor and fell. Though the impact seemed hardly sufficient to cause a fracture, the pelvis was somewhat severely fractured. Very probably there was a syphilitic rarefaction of the bone. Six months later the patient's depression was still in evidence, though somewhat less than upon admission. The blood serum remained positive but the spinal fluid had become entirely negative, both in respect to the W. R. and in respect to the other findings.

2. How may one explain the continuance of the depression after the spinal fluid had become entirely negative under treatment? It may be that while the active process had been stopped, as seems probable from the negative spinal fluid, that a permanent destruction of brain tissue may account for the depression. We recognize this readily in instances of vascular disturbance where (as also in this case) the active process being stopped, a residual defect remains.

3. Should treatment have been discontinued on reduction of the gumma? It cannot be too often emphasized that the disappearance of symptoms in cases of syphilis can not be considered as evidence of cure. The neurologist and psychiatrist see only too often cases of neurosyphilis occurring in patients who have been declared cured at some time previous because the symptoms then present had cleared up and remain in abeyance for years.

Contrary to various warnings, arteriosclerosis by
no means absolutely contraindicates intensive
salvarsan therapy.

Case 108. Victor Friedberg, 42 years of age, gave the following history. He acquired syphilis at 22 years. He had "adequate" medical treatment for two years with inunctions of mercury and mercury by mouth and potassium iodid. The only secondary symptoms were skin lesions of the legs; these disappeared upon treatment. Married, Friedberg has one child, apparently normal. There had been no miscarriages or stillbirths.

At about 34 years, there began to be shooting pains in the legs, occurring at first about once in three months, but later much more frequently. These pains were severe, lightning in character, lasting several days at a time, at which period his head would feel heavy; but there were no disturbances, crises, or difficulty in locomotion.

At 36 years of age, Friedberg waked up with pain one night, and found he was unable to move his left leg or hand, and he felt his mouth drawn to the left. Upon trying to get out of bed, he fell to the floor. In five hours, however, he was entirely recovered, able to get up and walk about, and to use his left arm quite normally. He went to sleep, but upon waking up after an hour, discovered that his left side was again paralyzed. After two weeks in a hospital, he was able to walk with a crutch. The arm remained helpless for about a year. Both arm and leg improved slowly for two years, after which time his condition had remained stationary. For four years past, there had been no more pain, but at 42 — about two years before admission — the pains returned in his legs, back, and side. At that time he received four injections of salvarsan, mercury tablets, and potassium iodid. Three weeks before admission to the hospital, Friedberg again began having headaches, very much worse than formerly. At first these headaches were frontal, then occipital, and there was a feeling as if something were growling inside of the head. There was a feeling of pressure in front on the head and at the base of the nose.

Physically, Friedberg appeared somewhat older than his assigned age. There was a degree of general peripheral arteriosclerosis, but in general the physical examination was negative. **Neurologically,** there was a left hemiplegia with appropriate increase of the reflexes on that side, spasticity, Babinski reflex, and an Oppenheim; the pupils reacted properly; there was no Romberg reaction.

Mentally, Friedberg was entirely negative.

The W. R. of the blood serum was doubtful, as was that of the spinal fluid. There were but two cells per cmm. and there was neither globulin nor excess albumin in the spinal fluid.

The **differential diagnosis** might lie between cerebral hemorrhage and syphilitic thrombosis. Thrombosis is much more common as a result of syphilis than is hemorrhage. The occurrence of the thrombosis during sleep without premonitory symptoms is also characteristic in syphilis. Possibly there was a low-grade spinal meningitis at the bottom of the lancinating pains. Whether the headache is an arteriosclerotic effect or due to a meningitis not shown in the cerebrospinal fluid is doubtful. However, the absence of inflammatory products in the cerebrospinal fluid rather indicates that the headache is of arteriosclerotic origin. Autopsies, however, warn us that we may have a localized meningitis in various parts of the cranial cavity without the determination of any inflammatory products in the spinal fluid.

1. How shall we explain the doubtful (slightly positive) W. R. in the spinal fluid if the case is one of VASCULAR BRAIN SYPHILIS? The finding is not unusual in these cases. The W. R. producing body is recognized to be of a separate nature from the globulin and albumin bodies, and is probably also separate from the gold sol reaction producing bodies.

Treatment: The theory of treatment is that any spirochetes that may be still active in the body should be destroyed. Accordingly, although salvarsan can certainly have no effect in reproducing nerve tissue, it nevertheless seems indicated. It is frequently stated, however, that salvarsan is dangerous in cases of this group. We have not found this statement correct. In this case, there was a symptomatic improvement, as far as pain and discomfort went, under salvarsan and iodids.

2. What precautions should be taken in intensive salvarsan treatment of syphilitic arteriosclerosis? Treatment should be begun with very small doses of salvarsan, that is, about 0.1 of a gram and then the amount slowly increased. The injection should be given slowly so as not to put too great a load upon the cardiovascular system.

3. What rôle does the mental attitude of the patient play in a case like that of Friedberg? It was quite evident that Friedberg was neurotic and that he had a syphilophobia. Consequently some of the symptomatic improvement may have been more results of assurances offered by the physician and knowledge that he was being treated, than results of salvarsan. In some cases mental anguish suffered by the patient is of more importance than the actual symptoms of the disease and this point must be always borne in mind in handling syphilitic patients.

Symptoms of intracranial pressure cured by anti-syphilitic treatment.

Case 109. Mrs. Annie Rivers, a housewife 36 years of age, sought advice and treatment for severe convulsions which she had had during a period of several weeks. She left the hospital before being properly examined, and had several more convulsions, after which she was brought back in a state of marked confusion. The confusion shortly disappeared almost completely, and a good history was obtained.

It appears that the patient led a normal life and had had six children, the last of whom was born about four months before her coming to the hospital. The first symptoms appeared about a month after the birth of the child, when, one afternoon, Mrs. Rivers suddenly fell unconscious while ironing. She remained unconscious for nearly three hours. During this attack there were no convulsive movements or tongue biting; and after the spell, she felt neither lame nor sore, but merely tired. This was Mrs. Rivers' statement; but her daughter stated that the patient really did have convulsive movements. A week later came a second convulsion, followed by daze and stupor. This second attack lasted two hours.

About a week before entrance, the patient had remained in bed on account of dull grinding pain in the left side of the head, below the ear, and upon this day the patient vomited twice. In addition to the dull grinding pain, there were pains referred to the ear itself and to the left side of the head, especially over the left eye; there were no pains on the right side of the head. The next day the patient was better, but the day thereafter again remained in bed. The only other symptoms were cold feelings at times and bright spots in the field of vision.

No **mental symptoms** were observed in Mrs. Rivers except a bit of depression after her hasty retreat from the hospital the first time. Upon her second admission, however, after

UNTOWARD SYMPTOMS OF THERAPEUTIC AGENTS

A. SALVARSAN

CYANOSIS   MALAISE
RAPID PULSE
PERSPIRATION
RESPIRATORY DIFFICULTIES
FEVER
NAUSEA, VOMITING, DIARRHOEA
DERMATOSES
EDEMA
KIDNEY IRRITATION
LIVER IRRITATION
INTENSIFICATION OF SYMPTOMS
COLLAPSE

B. MERCURY

SALIVATION
    FETID BREATH
    EXCESS FLOW OF SALIVA
    TENDERNESS OF TEETH — LOOSENING AND FALL-
      ING OUT
    SPONGY GUMS — EROSION
    METALLIC TASTE
    NECROSIS OF BONES OF JAW
    SORENESS OF PAROTIC AND MAXILLARY GLANDS
    SWELLING AND EROSION OF TONGUE AND MUCOUS
      MEMBRANES
GASTRO-INTESTINAL SYMPTOMS
ANEMIA
PAIN IN JOINTS
NEPHRITIS

C. IODINE

SKIN LESIONS
METALLIC TASTE
SALIVATION
CORYZA
URTICARIA (EVEN TO GRADE OF ANGIONEUROTIC EDEMA)
PAINS
CONSTIPATION
INVOLVEMENT OF JOINTS
FEVER
SOFTENING AND BLEEDING OF GUMS
EROSION OF MUCOUS MEMBRANES
GASTRO-INTESTINAL SYMPTOMS
ANOREXIA
WEAKNESS

CHART 27

a week or ten days' residence, apathy developed together with considerable amnesia for the same facts she had quite readily remembered a few days previously. Along with the apathy and amnesia developed considerable headache; and there were attacks of vomiting.

On the **physical** side, it is interesting to note that the ophthalmoscopic examination upon Mrs. Rivers' first admission to the hospital was entirely negative, whereas a week later, pronounced difficulty with vision appeared so that in a few days she was able to make out only very large type. The fundi now showed hazy and indistinct disc outlines, with small yellowish areas of fatty degeneration above the disc, reduction of arterial calibre, and dilated and somewhat tortuous veins (no projection of papillæ), so that the ophthalmological diagnosis was chronic neuritis.

The physical examination otherwise was mostly negative. The skin presented irregular areas covered with silvery scales over the arms and chest, back, abdomen, and legs (the patient had had psoriasis several years before). Both pupils reacted to light and distance, though the right was slightly larger than the left and somewhat irregular. There was a slight tremor of the tongue and extended fingers. The reflexes were active, especially the knee-jerks; no abdominal reflexes could be obtained. The serum W. R. was positive, but the spinal fluid W. R. was negative. The spinal fluid showed but 3 cells per cmm., but there was a positive globulin test and an excess of albumin.

Diagnosis: After the symptoms had fully developed, it became clear from the optic neuritis, headaches, and vomiting that a condition of intracranial pressure existed. In view of the positive serum W. R., it is natural to conceive that the agent producing the intracranial pressure was a gumma.

It is, of course, possible that a marked degree of meningitis might be so localized as to produce the same symptoms. The diagnostician would crave a pleocytosis of the spinal fluid if a diagnosis of meningitis is to be made; and there was no such pleocytosis. On the whole, we do not feel that it is possible to make a diagnosis either of MENINGITIS or of GUMMA.

Treatment: Treatment, however, caused a disappearance of all symptoms. The treatment consisted of but one injection of 0.3 gram of salvarsan, followed by a few injections of mercury; whereupon Mrs. Rivers became much brighter, recovered her vision, lost her headaches, ceased to have convulsions or vomiting spells.

1. Is salvarsan contraindicated in cases with involvement of the optic or auditory nerves? Such a contraindication exists according to prevailing opinion. In this particular case, a hemorrhagic retinitis occurred after the injection of salvarsan, but this retinitis disappeared along with the other symptoms. On the whole we believe that in many cases of optic or auditory nerve involvement salvarsan should be used. However, one should never lose sight of the possibility of untoward results and should advise such treatment only when other treatment seems inefficient.

TABETIC NEUROSYPHILIS ("tabes dorsalis")
may show very marked improvement as a result
of intraspinous therapy.

Case 110. Mr. McKenzie* was a retired merchant of 42
years whose complaint was that he tired very easily, could not
make his legs go where he wished, was unsteady and felt a
numbness in his legs. These symptoms had been in progress for a few months only when the examination was made.
This disclosed Argyll-Robertson pupils, absent knee-jerks
and ankle-jerks, Romberg sign, unsteady gait, moderate
ataxia and dysmetria. The W. R. was negative in the
blood serum but positive in the spinal fluid with 0.2 cc., and
there were 107 cells per cmm. With the symptoms and signs
it was therefore easy to make the diagnosis of TABETIC
NEUROSYPHILIS ("tabes dorsalis").

The patient was given five intraspinous injections of mer-
curic chloride in blood serum (mercurialized serum) according
to the method of Byrnes. The dose was 0.001 gm. of mercury.
Two weeks after the first injection the cell count was 58 cells
per cmm., the Wassermann was positive only with 0.4 cc.
After the fourth injection there were but 18 cells and the
Wassermann reaction was negative even with $1\frac{1}{2}$ cc. of spinal
fluids. The symptoms had improved to such a degree that the
patient had no complaint whatsoever and considered himself
cured.

1. What are the unpleasant results of intraspinous therapy?
    Frequently there is an exacerbation of symptoms and
    pain may be quite severe after intraspinous injections.
    This, however, lasts only a short period, that is, as a
    rule less than 24 hours. There may be other symp-
    toms of cord irritation as retention of urine or lack of
    sphincter control. A rise of temperature is not unusual.

---

* (This case was furnished by Dr. D. A. Haller from the
Peter Bent Brigham Hospital series.)

Treatment may alter the W. R. to negative in
blood and spinal fluid in TABES DORSALIS.

Case 111. Ivan Rokicki was a baker, 43 years of age, who
came complaining of exceedingly severe attacks of abdominal
pain with vomiting. He described these attacks as having
occurred periodically for a number of years, lasting sometimes
as long as a week, during which time Rokicki could not eat or
get relief short of large doses of morphine.

Upon his arrival, Rokicki was seen in one of his attacks;
he was curled up with excruciating pain, and the abdomen
was rigid, though it was impossible to produce additional
pain by external pressure. There was spasmodic vomiting,
frequently followed by slight relief from the pain, which
however shortly recurred and caused the patient to cry out in
his suffering. The condition was controlled by opiates but
lasted a full week. The leucocytes remained normal and
there was no rise of temperature. The attack ceased spontaneously.

Save for the pain, Rokicki's **mental examination** proved
entirely negative. **Physically,** Rokicki was fairly well developed and nourished. His pupils were slightly irregular: the
left markedly larger than the right; both pupils failed to
react to light, and the left pupil also failed to react in accommodation. There were no other reflex disorders evident
to systematic examination, nor was there sensory disturbance or speech defect. The heart seemed somewhat enlarged but there were no murmurs; blood pressure: systolic
150; diastolic 110.

The correct symptomatic diagnosis in Rokicki's case proved
to be gastric crises, and this diagnosis must perforce be the
first to entertain in view of the chronicity, the periodicity,
the non-relation to diet, and the spontaneous cessation of
the seizures. The observation of Argyll-Robertson pupils
was naturally held to substantiate the diagnosis of TABES
DORSALIS.

The possibility of abdominal inflammation could be shortly
dismissed on account of the absence of tenderness (the rigidity in this case was not accompanied by tenderness), fever,
and other characteristic signs.   There was no diarrhoea, such
as is found in lead colic, and there was no other sign of
plumbism.   Jaundice was absent and there was no special
radiation of pain from the abdomen.   One had to think of
gastric ulcer and hyperchlorhydia, and possibly malaria or
gastroenteritis.

The pupillary reactions pointed to a syphilitic condition
despite the fact that the lack of reaction to accommodation
(over and above the Argyll-Robertson phenomenon) in the
right pupil is not entirely typical.   Accordingly, although
there was no areflexia, Romberg sign, or ataxia, resort was
had to the W. R.   This however proved negative, in blood
and spinal fluid; nor was there any globulin or excess albumin; there were 5 cells to the cmm., in the spinal fluid.

We are left, accordingly, with characteristic gastric crises;
Argyll-Robertson pupils, slightly irregular; and a somewhat
enlarged heart.

Upon investigation, it appeared, however, that a year
before the attack above described, the patient had been
examined and both blood and spinal fluid found positive to
the W. R.   At that time, treatment, consisting of intravenous
injections of salvarsan and intraspinous injections of salvarsanized serum (Swift-Ellis), had been instituted.   Whereupon
the laboratory tests had become negative, as above stated,
and there had been no alleviation of the symptoms.

1.   How can Rokicki's normal deep leg reflexes be explained?
     The abolition of the deep reflexes is of course due to
     lesions properly localized.   It is probable that this
     particular case of tabes dorsalis is more truly " dorsal "
     than most cases; for most cases exhibit lesions involving
     regions lower than the dorsal.   Both in these dorsal
     cases and in certain rare cases of cervical tabes, the
     deep leg reflexes are preserved.   (See cases Green (30)
     and Halleck (31).)
2.   What is the mechanism by which a characteristic gastric
     crisis is produced?   The mechanism is unknown.   Some
     endeavors have been made to meet gastric crises by

surgery of the posterior roots, on the assumption that the irritation causing the pain was located either in the posterior ganglion or in the passage of the nerve through the meninges. In only a few instances, however, has the result been what was desired. In many instances the gastric crises and pain continued uninterrupted and in addition came discomfort due to the lack of sensation in the part supplied by the severed nerve. At present this treatment is seldom carried out.

3. Should antisyphilitic treatment be continued in such a case? As far as our present knowledge of syphilis goes one would hesitate to suggest further antisyphilitic treatment, feeling that the active process had been entirely stopped as suggested by the absence of any positive findings either in the blood serum or in the spinal fluid. We should perhaps conclude that there was no more activity in this case and that the crises were due to the changes that had already taken place in the nerve tissue and which could no longer be changed.

The literature is in doubt concerning (in fact is preponderantly against) the success of treatment in PARETIC NEUROSYPHILIS ("general paresis"). Our experience has yielded a number of apparently successful results through systematic intensive intravenous salvarsan therapy. Example.

Case 112. Albert Forest had always been a successful salesman, but in the middle of March, in his 46th year, he was arrested for grabbing a purse from a woman in front of a theatre and running down the street with it. In court, Forest acted strangely and he was sent to the Psychopathic Hospital for observation. Upon investigation, it appeared that his wife thought he had been showing mental changes for about a year. For example, he would embrace his wife on a street car, or refuse to pay her fare. He once attempted to hit his son on the head with a red-hot poker. Now and then he would become sleepy and stupid. He looked rather older than his age and had a coarse tremor of the hands. Otherwise, no change could be detected in the physical examination, either neurologically or otherwise. As for the manual tremor, Forest's wife gave a history of considerable alcoholic indulgence on his part.

For several days, nothing abnormal could be detected in the man; and in particular, his memory for both remote and recent events was very good and his knowledge of current events was good. Simple arithmetic was easy to him.

One evening his temperature was found to be 104° F. and no cause could be discerned for this. The next morning, Forest was discovered in a stupor, with a complete right hemiplegia. The Babinski reflex, the Oppenheim reflex, and ankle clonus had appeared on the right side, and the right arm was spastic.

However, all symptoms of this paralysis had disappeared by four o'clock in the afternoon, and the paralytic phenomena were replaced with violence. The patient fought with the attendants and for some time remained extremely difficult to manage, being confused and subject to outbreaks of violence with destruction of furniture and other property about the ward.

Diagnosis. At first we were naturally inclined to dismiss the case with a diagnosis of alcoholism. The transient hemiplegia at once raised a considerable question of brain syphilis or of brain tumor.

The W. R. of the serum was doubtful. The spinal fluid yielded, besides marked excess of albumin and much globulin, also a " paretic " gold sol reaction and 75 cells per cmm. The W. R. was positive.

Treatment. The patient was given injections of salvarsan, 0.6 gram, twice a week, with potassium iodid. After a few weeks improvement followed, and after several months all the laboratory tests became negative, the patient was apparently perfectly normal mentally and was discharged from the hospital, and has remained well for 18 months without further treatment. The serum W. R. has continued to be negative.

1. What is the significance of the so-called " doubtful " W. R.? Where there is not a complete uniformity the results of the strong and weak antigens (see appendix on technique of Wassermann reaction) the result is reported as doubtful. In the majority of instances repetitions will give a strong positive reaction.

2. Is the case of Forest to be regarded as one of general paresis? Sometimes such cases are termed in the literature *syphilitic pseudoparesis* (see case Burkhardt (58)). The differential diagnosis of this group is entirely therapeutic. There are, unhappily, no laboratory tests which will suffice in the present stage of knowledge to differentiate a case of so-called pseudoparesis from general paresis. We are inclined to term the case one of GENERAL PARESIS, with recovery, or, at all events, with remission.

The literature is in doubt concerning (in fact is preponderantly against) the success of treatment in PARETIC NEUROSYPHILIS (" general paresis "). Our experience has yielded a number of apparently successful results through systematic intensive intravenous salvarsan therapy. Example.

Case 113. We present the case of Gussie Silverman, a housewife, 35 years of age, among other reasons, for its social interest. The case is, on the whole, sufficiently typical of GENERAL PARESIS. **Physically,** for example, the pupils failed to react to light and accommodation and were unequal, the right being larger than the left. The knee-jerks were sluggish though equal. The ankle-jerks could not be obtained. The abdominal reflexes were not obtained. Otherwise, there was no reflex disorder.

From the **laboratory** point of view, the W. R. was positive in the blood and in the spinal fluid. There were 80 cells per cmm. and there were an appropriate globulin and albumin reactions. Mrs. Silverman was rather poorly nourished and had a slight edema of the ankles.

Mentally, she was found on admission to be markedly depressed. It appeared that during a recent pregnancy, terminated by the birth of a 7-months child, she had fainted several times a day, that since the confinement she had been very nervous, that she had been asking her husband not to send her away, that she had refused to leave the house, that she had become excited even to the point of injuring herself, especially at night, and that she would go so far as to scratch her husband, shortly afterward being very sorry for her performances. Before this last pregnancy there had been four others and the resulting children were all apparently in good health. Except for the fainting spells during the pregnancy, it would not appear that the story just told is at all characteristic of paresis.

However, in the hospital Mrs. Silverman could hardly be got to answer questions, continually saying, " You know what it is; I don't have to tell you." She claimed so marked a degree of confusion as not to know where she was and what she was doing. She would beg despondently that something be done for her, and iterate and re-iterate these claims. There appeared to be a marked degree of amnesia. Some one, she felt, had controlled her thoughts and made her do things she did not want to do and say things she did not want to say, things she did not know she was about to say. She said, " I feel like jumping around. I couldn't believe myself as if I am me. Some one is making me jump around. I used to hear him talking. I don't know who it is. I used to keep my eyes open and I couldn't move. I feel only I would like to talk, and talk, and talk, and talk all the time. It seems to me that some one talks in me. I couldn't sleep for five minutes. My God, I wish I could sleep! I used to feel something in my heart. I used to faint. It seems to me I used to see a funny thing. What it was I can't tell. It used to talk to me, make me get out of bed, throw me about, make me do things. O, I don't know what it was."

These not entirely characteristic mental symptoms, together with the suggestive physical signs and the laboratory examination, caused treatment to be instituted; under which treatment (intravenous injections of salvarsan) she improved rapidly. Mental symptoms disappeared under the administration of 12 injections of salvarsan within two months. Moreover, the spinal fluid became entirely negative. Two and a half years have now elapsed since her discharge and she has shown no return of symptoms. The serum W. R. has always remained negative although there has been no treatment since leaving the hospital. There has, however, been no change in the reflexes, which remain as on admission. The 7-months baby has continued to be perfectly healthy. Its W. R. is negative, as are the W. R.'s of the husband and the other three children. It must seem surprising that a healthy child could have been born from a mother with generalized syphilis as in this case. However, perhaps there are more instances than we imagine like the case of baby Silverman.

1. May a patient be considered permanently cured although there has been no recurrence of symptoms for 2½ years and although the Wassermann has remained negative? One would hesitate to give a definite statement that the patient was cured until more time had elapsed. It is quite possible that spirochetes may be lurking in some portion of the body without causing the production of symptoms or Wassermann bodies and yet ready to break out at any time. This hypothesis has added weight from the recent work of Warthin already quoted. We advise examination of this patient at intervals of not longer than six months for a good many years.

2. Should the course under treatment cause us to change the diagnosis? It has often been stated that a differential point between cerebrospinal syphilis and general paresis is the reaction to treatment, that is, that a case which recovers could not be general paresis. Head and Fearnsides state that if six months after beginning of treatment the spinal fluid has become negative, the case should be considered as one of cerebrospinal syphilis and not general paresis. We do not feel ready to concur in this view as we know of no similar logic in medicine. We have many cases in which a spinal fluid has remained positive for six months and later become negative, so that where the symptoms shown are those of paretic neurosyphilis, we are inclined to consider the case such until such time as more definite evidence checked by post mortem examination causes us to change this point of view.

3. Do the reflexes change under treatment? The signs of spasticity often do disappear under treatment and also when there is no treatment. A few instances have been reported in the literature where Argyll-Robertson pupils are said to have altered to normal. It has never been our good fortune to see such a change nor have we seen an absent knee-jerk become normal, as has also been reported, except where it is the result of pyramidal tract disease superimposed upon the posterior column sclerosis causing a return of reflex. This, of course, is not to be considered as a return of the normal. (See Case I.)

Some RESULTS of systematic intravenous salvarsan therapy are PARTIAL (*e.g.*, clinical recovery and persistence of positive laboratory tests).

Case 114. Walter Henry was an undertaker in a small town. He was married and the father of two healthy children. In May, 1914, he began to lose his appetite. He felt restless and seemed to be losing his grip, and in August he repaired to a sanatorium, where he remained for two months. Shortly after leaving the sanatorium, he fainted one day, while digging a grave, during a spell of great heat. Since that time there had been numerous "weak spells," with headaches and general debility, insomnia, and loss of weight.

In February, 1916, Mr. Henry came to the hospital for advice, but the trip from a distant part of the state was apparently such a strain for him that shortly after admission he collapsed. There were no convulsive movements in this collapse, but the patient was confused and his breathing was rapid and stertorous. The semi-stupor lasted for about 48 hours. Upon recovery from the stupor, Henry was found entirely disoriented, much confused, and laboring under the belief that he was digging a grave. After a time he again fell into a stupor and his temperature rose to 103° F.

The emaciation of this man was striking and unusual, but systematic **physical examination** showed no special disease. **Neurologically,** there were marked tremors, and there were purposeless movements of the arms. There was a marked speech defect. The pupils were dilated, regular, and equal, and reacted, though slightly, to light. Nothing abnormal was noted upon systematic examination of the reflexes.

The W. R. was strongly positive in the blood and in the spinal fluid; the gold sol reaction was typically "paretic"; there were 16 cells per cmm., globulin was present, and albumin was greatly increased.

The **diagnosis** GENERAL PARESIS was accordingly made, and treatment instituted. Intravenous injections of arsenobenzol, at first, and later of diarsenol, were given, as a rule twice a week (usual dose, 0.6 of a gram). Mercurial injections and potassium iodid were also given. This treatment was continued as the patient began to improve. The improvement was of such a degree that at the end of four months, Mr. Henry returned to his home and his work. He had had 30 intravenous injections of salvarsan substitutes. Despite the treatment and the clinical improvement, the laboratory tests remained essentially unchanged. The W. R.'s of the blood and spinal fluid remained strongly positive, as well as also the globulin and albumin; the gold sol reaction was still "paretic"; the cells stood at one per cmm. The patient has continued antisyphilitic treatment since leaving the hospital, and has remained apparently well, with good insight into his condition.

1. What is the significance of a temperature of 103° in a paretic without signs of infection and a normal leucocyte count? Temperatures of this type are not infrequent in the course of general paresis. They are usually spoken of as " paretic temperatures." Their meaning is not understood, but they are often stated to be due to a disturbance of the heat-regulating mechanism. Such temperatures may remain elevated for a considerable period of time, but the elevation may be very transitory. At times they vary, like septic temperatures.

2. What can be argued from the fact that the cell count became normal? If thorough antisyphilitic treatment is vigorously given, it will be found that in the vast majority of cases of neurosyphilis the cell count will return to normal. It matters not whether the treatment be intravenous or subdural. It is very difficult, however, to obtain this result in general paresis by the use of mercury alone. It cannot, however, be urged that this finding has any great prognostic significance as it occurs in the cases which do poorly as well as in those which recover symptomatically.

3. Is it safe to give large doses of salvarsan to a patient in a stupor? It is not a good plan to give a large dose to such a patient on account of the danger of sudden death. This is probably due as much to the strain put on the heart as it is to any effect on the nervous system, or specific arsenic effect. In this particular instance, a dose of 0.15 gm. was the initial injection and this was increased five centigrams per injection.

IMPROVEMENT IN PARETIC NEUROSYPH-
ILIS (" general paresis ") may become evident
only after several months of intensive treatment.

Case 115. Henry Ryan was a shipping clerk, 54 years of
age, who was brought to the hospital following a convulsion. For a few months preceding this period, Mr. Ryan
had been failing in his abilities. He had been very forgetful,
showed no energy, and had become very irritable. He also
complained of insomnia and of feeling nervous.

On admission to the hospital, the most striking feature in
the mental situation was that he claimed that he had not
slept a wink for three months, and each day he would solemnly
affirm that he had not slept at all the preceding night, although
the records might show that he had slept eight hours. Argument was of no avail against this conviction. In addition,
his memory was very poor; he showed little knowledge of
current events, and had no ability with arithmetical problems.

Neurologically viewed, the points of chief significance were
contracted immobile pupils and a speech defect, especially
noticeable on the repetition of test phrases. The whole
picture was suggestive of general paresis, and this diagnosis
was confirmed by the laboratory findings. It was found that
the W. R. was positive in the blood and spinal fluid, that
there was a pleocytosis, positive globulin reaction, excess of
albumin, and a "paretic" gold sol reaction. Consequently,
the diagnosis of GENERAL PARESIS seemed justified, although
the patient denied any knowledge of a syphilitic infection.

Treatment in this case consisted of intravenous injections
of salvarsan, diarsenol, or arsenobenzol, whichever drug was
most easily obtainable, given twice a week in doses of 0.6
gram each. In addition, he was given occasional injections
of mercury salicylate as well as potassium iodid by mouth.
Once or twice a week, 40 to 60 cc. of spinal fluid were withdrawn. Under this treatment for a period of three months,
the patient showed no improvement whatsoever, either in

his mental condition or in the laboratory findings. However, treatment was faithfully persevered in, and shortly after the three months, improvement began to be noticed. At first, the patient began to admit that possibly he may have slept a few winks some time during the previous six months, for he said he realized it was not possible for a man to live without sleep for that period. Then he began to admit that he might have slept a few hours during the night, and later that he was sleeping pretty fairly. His memory also showed improvement. His general attitude showed alertness, and he began to interest himself in his surroundings and in the events of the world, and finally he gained complete insight into his condition.

In the meantime, that is after three months of treatment, the laboratory findings began to grow weaker. The gold sol reaction was the first to decrease in strength, and after four months of treatment, it vacillated between negative and a mildly positive "syphilitic" reaction. Then the globulin and albumin became less in amount, and the W. R. began dropping off in the 0.1 and 0.3 cc. dilutions. As is usually true in those cases of neurosyphilis that receive adequate treatment, the cell count early dropped to normal. The W. R. in the blood serum, however, remained positive.

As the patient's condition seemed so much better, he was allowed to leave the hospital at the end of five months. He took things easily for the following seven months, and then, after being out of employment for the period of a year, as his health continued good, he decided to return to work. Before doing so, he entered the hospital again for a lumbar puncture. At this time, it was found that the cell count was normal, there was a very faint trace of globulin, possibly a slight increase above normal albumin content, and a very mild gold reaction. The W. R. in the spinal fluid was negative including the 1.0 cc. dilution; the blood serum remained positive.

The patient then returned to his old position and has done satisfactorily for the past six months. During this entire time, he has been coming to the hospital for treatment: during the major portion of the time, about once in two weeks; of late, once in four weeks.

The significant point in this case is that improvement did not show itself until after more than three months of intensive treatment, and then the improvement was synchronous with a weakening of the spinal fluid tests.

It is further significant that his mental and physical condition was good before the tests had reached anything like normal; and that under treatment, these tests continued to grow weaker and weaker, until at the end of a year, they were practically negative.

The case further illustrates the enormous number of injections of salvarsan preparations that may be given to a patient without causing any appreciable damage to the general health or to the kidney function. Mr. Ryan has had more than 60 injections.

1. How soon after treatment is instituted does improvement usually occur in paretic neurosyphilis? In our experience improvement usually shows itself in from two or three months of treatment. Occasionally the improvement may be very marked shortly after treatment is commenced, that is, after three or four injections of salvarsan. This is not, however, the rule and as in the case of Ryan, it may be only after more than three months that improvement is seen. This means that in the treatment of these cases patience must be exercised and much work done.

2. What is the point of withdrawing large amounts of spinal fluid as in the case of Henry Ryan? It has been stated that the withdrawal of 40 or more cc., of spinal fluid while the patient is under treatment has the effect of reducing the intraspinous and intracranial pressure and thereby allowing the drug to diffuse into the nervous tissue better than it would do under ordinary conditions. How much truth there is in this contention it is difficult to say and there is as yet no experimental evidence to confirm this contention. As a matter of fact, the spinal fluid in cases of paresis is usually under increased pressure and it is at least plausible to conceive that a reduction of this pressure may give some symptomatic relief.

Evidence of the activity of syphilis outside the
central nervous system may be seen in cases of
neurosyphilis despite intensive treatment.

Case 116. William Rossetti was a speculator, 43 years of
age, when he was brought to the Psychopathic Hospital on
account of an outbreak in which he smashed a showcase at
the store where his sweetheart was employed; he caused so
much commotion that he was arrested.

On admission, he was very excited, talking loudly and at
length. For some days it was very difficult to manage him,
he was so active. At any moment, he would insist upon
undressing and taking physical culture exercises. He was
very euphoric and expansive, and had no insight into his
condition.

Physically, he was a powerfully-built man and in very good
physical condition except for an iritis and moderate thickening
of the peripheral arteries. The **neurological signs** of importance were Argyll-Robertson pupils, and absent knee-jerks
and ankle-jerks. With these findings in mind, a tentative
diagnosis of GENERAL PARESIS was made, and this was substantiated by the laboratory tests, which gave positive W.
R.'s in blood and spinal fluid, globulin, excessive albumin,
slight pleocytosis, and a " paretic " gold sol reaction.

When the patient's mental condition was somewhat better,
he gave a history of syphilitic infection 15 years before, for
which he had had almost continuous treatment. As a matter
of fact, treatment had been pretty strenuous because he had
recurring skin lesions and iritis. It was practically impossible to get the skin lesions to heal with mercury, and it was
not until salvarsan was introduced that a good result was
obtained in this respect. After one or two injections of this
drug, the skin lesion disappeared and has never returned.
However, at least once a year, he has had attacks of iritis,
and for this reason was still being treated for syphilis at the
outbreak of his psychosis.

He was at once placed on more strenuous antisyphilitic treatment in the form of diarsenol, semi-weekly, aided by mercury injections. After a few months of this treatment, his mental condition improved so much that he seemed to be entirely normal. Treatment was continued, however, without any abatement, and it was of great interest to note at the end of five months of such treatment that, although mentally he seemed entirely well, he had an attack of iritis, which was considered as a sign of active syphilis. This would appear to indicate the great difficulty of getting results in certain cases of syphilis with any drugs at our command at present, as in the iritis we are dealing with a condition which as a rule reacts fairly readily to antisyphilitic remedies.

1. Are there different strains of spirochetes showing various degrees of malignancy? This question has been discussed at length in the literature but there is no satisfactory answer at the present time. We must always consider the reaction of the organism and the host; and it is true in syphilis, as in every other disease, that in some individuals it is more difficult to get any therapeutic results than in others.

2. Was the failure to obtain results by long years of treatment due to "drug fastness" of the spirochetes? It has been held that the organism of syphilis will develop an immunity after a time to mercury and arsenic preparations. This led Fournier to recommend intermittent treatment as more efficient than continuous treatment. Noguchi has shown that in test-tube experiments, the spirochetes develop a tolerance to increasing doses of arsenic. It must be emphasized, however, that this finding has not been established for the conditions *in vivo*. Another explanation of the failure of treatment in certain instances has been offered by McDonagh, who describes a life cycle of the organism of syphilis under the name of *cytorrhyctes luis*, of which he believes the spirochete to be merely one form, the other forms not being affected by arsenic or mercury.

Some results of systematic intravenous salvarsan therapy in PARETIC NEUROSYPHILIS (" general paresis ") are partial in the sense that with clinical recovery the laboratory tests remain partially or less strongly positive.

Case 117. Annie Martin was a charwoman, 37 years of age. She had applied for relief at a general hospital, to which she was admitted on the suspicion of nephritis; but upon admission she became markedly excited and noisy, and spoke of seeing angels and hearing God speak to her. As the attendants were unable to quiet her, she was promptly transferred to the Psychopathic Hospital. She maintained that she had been sent to the Psychopathic Hospital through the spite of the general hospital doctors, and she claimed that other people were also attempting to work her harm for the purpose of taking her children from her. Visual and auditory hallucinations were marked, as was the patient's loquacity, irritability, and flight of ideas. However, she seemed entirely oriented and her memory appeared to be intact. She was able to explain somewhat clearly her supposed condition. The voices told her that somebody was after her and that her soul belonged to the devil; that she was to be married but that her soul was to be damned. These voices probably belonged to priests. She was under the impression that she was going to be sent to an electric chair and said, " I think I am coming to the end and I want a pair of rosary beads before the end comes."

This patient's pupils were markedly unequal and entirely stiff to light and accommodation. **Neurologically,** however, there were no other symptoms. There was a slight trace of albumin in the urine and there were no casts.

The psychiatric **diagnosis** in this case would off-hand undoubtedly be dementia praecox. Yet the stiff pupils are almost proof positive of neurosyphilis. If further proof were necessary, it is found in the laboratory tests, which

showed a positive W. R. of the serum and fluid, with a
" paretic " gold sol reaction; there were 22 cells per cmm.,
there was excess albumin, and a positive globulin reaction.

Under intensive antisyphilitic treatment, there was a slow
improvement. After several months, the patient was entirely free from mental symptoms; the spinal fluid tests
became entirely negative except that the gold sol reaction
has remained strongly positive.

1. Should treatment be continued in the case of Annie
Martin in spite of the clinical recovery and the negative
tests except the gold sol? We would again emphasize
that it is unreasonable to suppose that a long standing
case of syphilis can be cured in a period of a few months
of treatment and while the tests may become negative,
it would seem foolhardy to stop treatment on this
account. We do know that in many cases a Wassermann reaction remaining negative for many months
may again become positive, indicating that the negative reaction did not mean cure but rather the absence
of the Wassermann bodies in the circulation at the time
the test was made.

2. What is the significance of the paretic gold sol reaction
when the other tests have become negative? As
previously stated, the gold reducing substance in the
spinal fluid seems to be different from the substances
which give the other pathological reactions. We
should feel in this case that the process which was
producing these gold reducing bodies had not been
stopped, in other words, cure was not complete.

3. Should one make a diagnosis on the " paretic " gold sol
reaction alone? The so-called paretic gold sol curve
is not always indicative of general paresis or even of
syphilis but may occur in non-syphilitic conditions as
brain tumor, multiple sclerosis, etc. In our experience
we have seen no case of *untreated* neurosyphilis in
which the gold sol alone was positive, that is, in cases
in which therapy has not changed the findings in the
spinal fluid. In our experience the gold sol reaction
has been fortified by one or several of the other tests
as the W. R., globulin test, pleocytosis.

Some effects of systematic intravenous salvarsan therapy in PARETIC NEUROSYPHILIS (" general paresis ") are limited to the laboratory findings without clinical improvement.

Two examples of such limitation are offered: William Roberts (118) and John Silver (119).

Case 118. A bank teller, William Roberts, 39, was sent to the Psychopathic Hospital for a depression so marked that he had become entirely unable to work or care for himself. The story was that some money had been left him by his uncle, that Roberts could not prove his right to the money, and that depression, insomnia, and occasional periods of confusion had followed during a period of about five months.

On admission, Roberts appeared wholly disoriented and unable even to give his correct age. Attention could not be held, and the patient would slide off into statements like: " Oh, I made a mistake, I fooled a lot of people, I have a terrible disease, they are going to get it, they are going to get me," etc., etc. There was great difficulty in thinking, and a marked reaction of fear. This cluster of phenomena certainly suggested very strongly the diagnosis of manic-depressive psychosis.

Neurologically, Roberts proved quite negative except that the tendon reflexes were very active and the pupils reacted somewhat sluggishly to light. The blood serum W. R. was negative. No history of syphilis could be obtained; nevertheless, Roberts kept dropping remarks about the terrible disease from which he was suffering. It seemed best to proceed to lumbar puncture, and the spinal fluid disclosed a positive W. R., globulin, increased albumin, pleocytosis, and " paretic " gold sol reaction.

The **diagnosis** of GENERAL PARESIS was accordingly made. During the next year and a half, no improvement was made; a slight speech defect was developed, and tremors of the hand and tongue appeared.

The effect of treatment is particularly instructive. Only after 18 months in the hospital was intensive antisyphilitic treatment instituted; but after a few months of this treatment the W. R. of the spinal fluid had become negative, the cells normal in number, globulin absent, albumin present only in normal amount. Only the gold sol reaction remained positive. It is still of a paretic type. Treatment, however, did not succeed in altering the patient's mental condition in the slightest. At the end of many months of treatment, we still confront a man showing marked psychic symptoms and a " paretic " gold sol reaction without other laboratory signs.

1. What is the significance of the practically negative tests in this case without clinical improvement? One must believe that the tests became negative as the result of treatment, and that this change in the tests was due to the clearing up of some inflammatory reactions which were present. This may mean that the syphilis had been reduced to inactivity or latency if not cured, or at least that there was no activity sufficient to cause a positive W. R. in the blood serum, whereas whatever activity was present in the brain was in such a region that it did not cause any reacting substances to be cast into the spinal fluid. This would not mean that there would necessarily be any return of function already lost, because this may be considered as a permanent loss which cannot be compensated for. As to these tests, we now feel that the case should remain stationary; that is, that no new symptoms will be added. However, we believe that it is somewhat premature with our present knowledge to make this claim very forcibly, and would rather suggest that this case be considered as demonstrating an interesting fact, the meaning of which can be learned only after a period of years.

2. Why does the gold sol reaction remain strongly positive when all the other tests become negative? As already pointed out, above (Case Martin (117)) there is no known rule about the disappearance of one or other of the abnormal findings in spinal fluid under treatment, and we can at present offer no explanation of this phenomenon. It does, however, illustrate how careful we must be in drawing any conclusions from tests in cases that are being treated.

Diminution in the spinal fluid tests may occur
in treated cases of neurosyphilis without clinical
improvement.

Case 119. John Silver, a man 29 years of age, presented
classical symptoms of GENERAL PARESIS: He had a convulsion shortly before his admission to the Psychopathic Hospital,
his memory was poor, he was only partially oriented, he was
very euphoric and expansive — thought he had millions,
that he was the Czar of Russia, and so on. His tendon reflexes were very much increased and there was a marked
speech defect. The W. R. of both blood and spinal fluid
were strongly positive; the spinal fluid showed globulin,
increased albumin, pleocytosis, and a " paretic " gold sol
reaction. There was, therefore, no question about the
diagnosis, and the patient was at once put under antisyphilitic treatment. This was continued for five months; slowly
the intensity of the reactions in the spinal fluid diminished.
At the end of the five months, there was the very slightest
possible trace of globulin, with a doubtful increase in albumin,
one cell per cmm., and a mild syphilitic gold sol reaction.
The W. R.'s in the blood and spinal fluid, however, remained
strongly positive. There was no mental improvement coincident with the weakening of the spinal fluid tests, and at
the end of the five months, the patient had a series of convulsions in which he died.

This case is given as a contrast to Case Henry (114) in which
clinical improvement occurred without diminution in laboratory tests; in the case of John Silver, marked diminution
in the intensity of these tests had no prognostic significance. This was in keeping with the condition as shown in
Case Roberts (118) where, while the gold sol was the only test
to remain positive, the patient did not improve mentally.

1. What is the explanation of the lessening of the patho-
     logical elements in the spinal fluid under treatment?
     We have seen that the various findings may occur in-

dependently of one another, and we must admit that we do not know definitely what it signifies, or why one may be present or absent. It has been held by Head and Fearnsides that the findings in the spinal fluid represent conditions in the spinal cord and spinal meninges, or at the base of the brain only, and not conditions elsewhere. This is in keeping with our finding that the gold sol reaction in the spinal fluid post mortem very often differs from that in the ventricular fluids or cerebral, subdural, and subpial fluids. And further, we have found that during life the findings in paresis in the spinal fluid may differ markedly from those in the third ventricle, and that the change in the fluid in these two areas under treatment may not occur simultaneously.

Systematic intensive treatment of PARETIC
NEUROSYPHILIS ("general paresis"), including
intraventricular injections of salvarsan, may entirely fail.

Case 120. James McGinnis, aged 39, came to the hospital
on a stretcher, semi-conscious, moaning, unable to reply to
questions; there were signs of a right hemiplegia.

The next day, McGinnis cleared a little and became able
to utter a few words. His wife said that he had been entirely well up to four years ago. At that time he was struck
in the eye by the head of a hammer that flew off the handle.
Diplopia had developed, but disappeared.

Only two years later did a marked change appear. McGinnis became careless as to personal appearance. Seemed
absent-minded, apathetic and drowsy; he would fall asleep
in his chair or while at work. He lost his position and became apprehensive, making not very strenuous efforts to
find work, and finally consulted a physician. The physician
told him that he had a sluggish liver and gave him calomel.

Six months later, McGinnis was restored to his position
as foreman, and his work remained satisfactory for some six
months. Then (about six months before coming to hospital),
his speech became slow and somewhat unintelligible. He
quit work, saying that his speech was going from him and
that he might be considered to be drunk. His memory
grew rapidly worse. There was improvement after a vacation
and he returned to work, but continued to be ataxic, complained of vertigo, and fell down several times, though
without loss of consciousness. On the very day of his admission to the hospital, in attempting to get out of bed, he
fell, and psychotic symptoms at once appeared. There
was slight improvement again with entire disappearance of
all paralysis after a few days, a slow clearing up of the speech
disturbance, and a certain return of memory.

Physically, there was little to note. **Neurologically,** the left pupil failed to react to light. The tendon reflexes were all very active, and more active on the left side. Other abnormal reflexes were absent. Improvement continued for a number of weeks, but the patient never recovered from his speech defect, and his memory remained impaired. Irritable at times, McGinnis was for the most part very happy and sure he would get well. The W. R. of the blood serum was negative, but the spinal fluid reaction was strongly positive, even down to 0.1 cc. The globulin and albumin amounts were excessive. There was a "paretic" gold sol reaction. There were 7 cells per cmm. The diagnosis of GENERAL PARESIS was made.

Intravenous injections of salvarsan, arsenobenzol or diarsenol were made, and intramuscular injections of mercury, and potassium iodid by mouth were given. No real improvement occurred after a certain initial betterment; the spinal fluid yielded no changes. Diarsenolized serum according to the Swift-Ellis technique was then injected into the third ventricle. Under this treatment also there was no change for the better over a period of several months. The patient died suddenly after a series of convulsions, apparently from paralysis of respiration.

1. What are the causes of hemiplegia and confusion or unconsciousness? We must consider epilepsy, brain tumor, cerebral thrombosis, cerebral hemorrhage, multiple sclerosis, cerebral spinal syphilis, and general paresis.

MILD TREATMENT, often thought "adequate,"
MAY FAIL, WHEN INTENSIVE TREATMENT
PROVES SUCCESSFUL.

Case 121. Arthur Bright, a printer, had acquired syphilis
in his 49th year, some six months before examination. He
had been treated during these six months by three injections
of salvarsan, injections of mercury, and mercury by mouth.
He had been apparently cured until about a month before
admission. He had fallen without warning from his chair
in a convulsion accompanied by unconsciousness, which lasted
about two hours. The patient had since been feeling rather
peculiar. For instance, time seemed to flow too rapidly.
Sometimes the patient had had difficulty in talking.

Physically, nothing abnormal could be found either in
general condition or **neurologically.** The patient was, however, incontinent. **Mentally,** he was apathetic and unalert,
even paying no attention to his outside physician when he
came to visit him.

The **diagnosis** of cerebrospinal syphilis already suggested
by his history was confirmed by the laboratory tests, which
showed a positive serum and spinal fluid W. R., paretic
gold sol reaction, 41 cells per cmm., an excess of albumin,
and a positive globulin test.

1. What is the prognosis in cerebrospinal syphilis in the
    early secondary stage? The prognosis appears very
    good provided that intensive treatment be given and
    provided that no vascular insult or other focal destruc-
    tive lesion occurs before treatment has had time to do
    its work.
2. Why did not the "effective" (?) treatment for the syphilis,
    dating from the primary lesion, succeed in staving off
    the cerebrospinal syphilis? It remains a question
    whether the treatment by three injections of salvarsan
    was efficient in this particular case. Of course, it may
    prove true that no treatment whatever in the present
    stage of knowledge will stave off cerebrospinal symp-
    toms in certain cases.

Treatment: Bright was given intravenous injections of diarsenol twice a week, with occasional injections of mercury salicylate. After two weeks, the patient seemed markedly improved, and continued to improve rapidly. He was symptomatically well at six weeks. The spinal fluid had then become negative, although the serum W. R. had remained positive.

After discharge from the hospital, Bright returned to his work, but continued to take the diarsenol treatment weekly, and two months later the serum W. R. became negative.

Small injections of diarsenol at intervals of a month were continued, and Bright remained perfectly well for four months, when a peculiar seizure developed and lasted for several hours. This seizure consisted in a sort of somnambulism in which Bright stood up at a table, making marks on paper, and could not be persuaded to desist. After this seizure, Bright re-entered the hospital, again showed no mental or physical symptoms and no abnormalities of blood or spinal fluid.

3. What is the explanation of this seizure? It is possibly due to a small vascular insult, for which potassium iodid may be suggested with precautions as to hygiene and continued observation. He has since remained entirely well.

Another example where MILD MEASURES (though conceived to be "adequate") SEEMED TO BE LEADING TO FAILURE; INTENSIVE THERAPY SUCCESSFUL.

Case 122. Levi Morovitz, a waiter, 39 years of age, came to the hospital with evidences of an old left hemiplegia, including the left side of the face (there was a left-sided Babinski, Gordon, and Oppenheim, and all the reflexes were fairly active; sluggish pupil reactions, Rombergism, and speech defect). Morovitz was much depressed, very slow in thinking processes, had a marked memory disturbance in general and apparently much deterioration mentally.

A history was obtained to the effect that Morovitz had acquired syphilis at about 33, but that he had received practically continuous treatment ever since at a dispensary. He had, in fact, received four injections of salvarsan a year before coming to the hospital. Of late, Morovitz had become much more cheerful and talkative, imagining he could do great things if he had money. He had begun to eat very rapidly and to be very nervous. His feet had begun to drag; a distinct speech defect developed, but from this he had recovered. About six weeks before entrance, Morovitz had a shock, which left him with the left hemiplegia above mentioned and with considerable headache.

Even while the preliminary examination was being performed, Morovitz developed a minor seizure without loss of consciousness. First came severe pain over the frontal region, which grew in severity so that the patient held his head in his hands. A bit later, twitching movements began in the thumb and in the fingers of the left hand, and the small muscles of the extensor group of the thumb and third finger showed contractions. These contractions grew more general and the excursions of the fingers greater, until finally every finger of the left hand became involved, whereupon movements of the same sort, though of smaller amplitude,

began in the other hand. Finally the left arm began to jerk
with alternate contractions of the biceps and triceps. The
whole seizure lasted more than five minutes. During the
seizure there was dizziness and pain in the head, chiefly on
the right side.

Diagnosis: The attention is at once arrested by the data
of the seizures described. It appeared that we had to assume an irritation of the right side of the brain, possibly due
to vascular disease, or to brain tumor, or perhaps to syphilis.
The shock with residual hemiplegia would be consistent
enough with any of these diagnoses. However, the history
seemed somewhat long for brain tumor. Nor were there
any definite symptoms of intracranial pressure. "Adequate"
treatment unfortunately does not rule out syphilis. The
comparatively early age (39) of the patient makes it difficult
to explain the vascular disease except on the basis of syphilis.
Add to the hemiplegia the euphoria and grandiose ideas of a
year's duration, and we arrive at a diagnosis of neurosyphilis,
probably PARETIC NEUROSYPHILIS.

The laboratory tests showed the W. R. of the serum and
spinal fluid positive, 80 cells per cmm. in the fluid, large
amounts of globulin and albumin, and a " paretic " type of
gold sol reaction.

To be sure the Jacksonian seizure is not especially characteristic of paretic neurosyphilis, and even suggests a local
irritation in the motor area, such as a localized meningitis,
possibly of a diffuse gummatous nature.

This patient was put on intensive antisyphilitic treatment, namely, salvarsan twice a week and injections of
mercury. He recovered rapidly. After a few months he
left the hospital, and after treatment had continued for a
year, he resumed his work by which time both blood and
spinal fluid had become negative.

It must be recalled that this patient had from the time of
his infection what has been considered good antisyphilitic
therapy, in spite of which he developed after a period of
years, the symptoms and signs of neurosyphilis in its most
dangerous form. The conclusion must be drawn that
however good such treatment is for the majority of cases, it

was insufficient for Morovitz. That the early failure to cure was not due to any "drug-fastness" of the spirochete or to any peculiarity of strain is proved by the result of more vigorous antisyphilitic treatment which caused an apparent if not a real cure. With our modern methods of treatment checked by Wassermann reactions and spinal fluid examinations, treatment is given according to the *needs of the individual patient* rather than according to general preconceptions. We have reason to believe that under these conditions there will be fewer cases developing late symptoms on account of insufficient treatment given even to patients who are willing to co-operate to the last degree.

The fact that Morovitz had no apparent symptoms for several years led to rather desultory treatment chiefly in the form of mercury by mouth. Previous to the time when the W. R. and lumbar puncture were available, the physician had no exact means of determining cure except the non-appearance of symptoms. But a period of years of quiescence before the outbreak of symptoms referrable to the involvement of the nervous system is characteristic of syphilis. With this knowledge in mind it is evident that today the care of a syphilitic patient must be guided, in part at least, by examinations of the spinal fluid and W. R.

Salvarsan treatment may even occasionally be of value in simple FEEBLEMINDEDNESS due to congenital syphilis.

Case 123. The somewhat unattractive Robert Matthews was brought, at 5 years of age, to the hospital for backwardness of mind. It appears that the patient was born at term, with instruments, that he began to talk at a year, and to walk at 13 months, but that in point of fact, he had not talked intelligibly to date. Robert had never played with other children and is regarded by his parents as backward. In fact, Robert's sister — a year his junior — is much brighter. Robert had had scarlet fever but without sequelae.

Examination by the Binet scale showed that, although he is actually $5\frac{1}{2}$ years, he graded by the Binet scale at 4 and was regarded as feebleminded.

The **physical examination** showed a general adenopathy and prominent frontal bosses. In the study of the family history in the search for an etiology for the evident feeblemindedness, little or none could be found. There were no miscarriages or stillbirths; the parents were living and well. There was only the one sister above-mentioned, who is brighter than Robert.

The advantage of a routine W. R. is here well shown, for the W. R. in the serum was positive.

1. What is the prognosis of cases of syphilitic feeblemindedness? It would appear that every case is an individual problem.
2. What is the effect of treatment? Robert Matthews was given mercury protoiodid $\frac{1}{8}$ gr., three times a day, by mouth, for three months. The protoiodid was followed by ten injections of salvarsan, average: 0.15 gram, during six months. At the end of this period, the W. R. in the blood had become negative. A re-examination by the Binet scale, when Robert was $6\frac{5}{12}$ years of age, showed him to grade at $5\frac{2}{5}$, so that one might conclude that Robert had shown more mental progress in a year than he had previously.

Note: The patient's sister, 4 years of age, is attractive and bright, measuring beyond her actual age according to the intelligence tests. However, the girl was found to have a positive W. R. It may be that Robert and his sister illustrate the hypothesis of Mott: that the syphilitic virus becomes less potent as the years go on, and that the younger children in the family are less affected than the older. However, in our series, there are a number of instances in which this hypothesis is not substantiated.

3. What is the share of syphilis in the production of feeble-mindedness? The percentage of syphilitic cases found in institutions is not high. A variety of cases have been proved to be congenitally syphilitic in the absence of a positive serum W. R.

Fernald* has charted a comparison of cases diagnosticated "moron" (that is, feeblemindedness proper, in the narrower English sense) and "imbecile." Fernald says that the morons have, as a group, many more bad family histories than have the imbeciles, to quote — "Only 70% of the [imbecile] group have bad family histories. This at first seems surprising, but when we consider that more of our syphilitic, traumatic, and sporadic cases tend toward the lower end of the feebleminded group, and when we remember that with such cases there is often a seemingly normal family tree, the drop in the curve appears logical."

The situation with the idiots, of whom only 38 came into Fernald's study, was similar; 12 out of 38, or 32%, of idiots, had good family histories. On these figures, how unfortunate it would be to dub feeblemindedness hereditary! It is true, however, that 68–70.% of the idiots and imbeciles, judging by W. E. Fernald's intensive study, do have bad family histories.

Goddard† states that of all the causes of feeblemindedness,

---

* Fernald, W. E. Standardized Fields of Inquiry for Clinical Studies of Borderline Defectives. Mental Hygiene, Vol. 1, No. 2, April, 1917.
† Goddard, H. H., Feeblemindedness, its Causes and Consequences, 1914.

there is perhaps none for which there is less evidence than syphilis. Goddard found syphilis in 27 of his intensively charted cases of feeblemindedness, that is, in 9% of all his charts. He finds the majority of the syphilis cases occurring in relatives of the feebleminded to be in the hereditary group; for example, of 164 charts in the hereditary group, 17, or 10%, showed syphilis. In 34 charts in a group termed "probably hereditary" 3, or 9%, showed syphilis. Of 37 charts in the group termed "neuropathic" 4, or 11%, showed syphilis, whereas in 57 "accident" and 8 "no cause" groups, there were but 2 (4%), and one, or 13%, showing syphilis. However, Goddard concedes that much more careful studies are necessary if we are to give an exact evaluation of syphilogenic feeblemindedness.

The first ten of the Waverley Anatomical Series are shortly to be described in a forthcoming publication.* Of these ten cases, four showed some slight evidence of chronic inflammatory changes, indicating the possibility of a syphilitic or similar infectious condition. These cases, be it remembered, were not cases of juvenile paresis, but cases of what, for the lack of a better name, may be called "ordinary" feeblemindedness.

If all or any of these processes are syphilitic, the syphilis is virtually extinct. The cases had not been treated for syphilis and were not regarded as syphilitic, though several of them showed a few stigmata somewhat suggestive of syphilis. The anatomical conclusion at this time is still doubtful.

As in the text case, the hypothesis of syphilis as a direct cause for simple feeblemindedness must be entertained for a few cases. In any event, it would not seem logical to let any institution for the feebleminded run without a Wassermann analysis of the population. In addition to the Wassermann data from the blood serum, osteological data from the X-ray have proved of occasional value for syphilis diagnosis in this as in other groups.

---

* W. E. Fernald and E. E. Southard. Waverley Research Series in the Pathology of the Feebleminded. Proceedings of the American Academy of Arts and Sciences, 1917.

" Within the gates of Hell sat Sin and Death."

Paradise Lost, Book X, Line 230.

VI. NEUROSYPHILIS AND THE WAR.

Although the American toll of war syphilis has not yet begun and although the crop of neurosyphilis due to war infections may not arrive until the mid or late twenties of the century (witness German experience in the eighties of the last century), it seems proper here to give a number of abstracts *re* neurosyphilis as it has developed in the war. Available reports from English, French, and German sources have been levied upon for the years 1914–16.

It is clear that all the armies have had their share of neurosyphilitics, some clearly diseased before enlistment, some developing symptoms as a result of training, stress, or shock, others hastened or made worse by war conditions.

There are important questions of pension, retirement, and compensation for neurosyphilitics. No previous war has had the benefit of the Wassermann reaction and other exact tests bearing upon the nature, progress, and curability of neurosyphilis.

That we shall have our fill of pension and other problems can already be seen from continental reports. Thibierge,* for example, states that syphilis has become a real epidemic among the French soldiers and mobilized munition workers.

Hecht† of Austria claims that no less than an equivalent of 60 army divisions have been temporarily withdrawn from fighting on the Teutonic side for venereal diseases. He commends Neisser's idea that salvarsan and mercury should be given in the trenches. While hundreds or thousands of Austrians are sick with syphilis, sound and healthy men are being shot down in their stead. The diagnosis of syphilis, according to Hecht, ought to be a signal for sending the men to the front. He makes even the somewhat bizarre sugges-

---

* Thibierge. La Syphilis dans l'armée, 1917.
† Hecht. Wien. klin. Woch., xxix, 51.

tion that special companies of syphilitics should be formed, for convenience of treatment, on the firing line.

Not only is the syphilis problem in the army of importance to the military authorities, but also to the civil population, and perhaps to them a greater problem. With the great increase of venereal disease that is the result of the conditions of army life in war time, there will be a considerable percentage of cases developing neurosyphilis a number of years after discharge from the army, but caused by the infection acquired during service. In addition many men will bring the disease back to America in an infectious stage and spread it. We would advocate that the names of all soldiers who had acquired syphilis and were not considered cured at time of discharge should be given to health organizations in their home states that they may be given further care.

These practical and several theoretical questions are raised by the following fourteen cases which we have condensed from their sources.

A tabetic lieutenant "shell-shocked" into paresis?
Case from Donath of Vienna.

Case A.* An apparently competent German professor in an intermediate school, a lieutenant of infantry reserves, 33 years old, on the 17th August, 1914, was stunned for a while by the shock of a cannon-firing 25 feet away. Urination became difficult. Headaches and limb pains ensued, with paralysis of fingers, gastric troubles, forgetfulness especially for names, insomnia, and general scattering of mental faculties.

Neurologically, the pupils were irregular, left larger than right; Argyll-Robertson reaction. Right knee-jerk livelier than left. Achilles reactions absent. Slow and dissociated pain reactions in feet, lower thighs and lower quarter of upper thighs, with hypalgesia or analgesia. Station good; gait steady. Mentally depressed, slow of thought. Speech poor and of indistinct construction (mild dementia). Calculation ability poor. No pleasure in work.

Wassermann reaction of serum weakly positive.

It seems that for a year the patient had been subject to spells of anger. He was irritated by his wife who had been nervous since an earthquake.

On the occasion of the earthquake, 1911, the patient himself had had a spell of *difficulty with urination.* The spell had lasted two or three months. The patient had had a chancre in 1902, "cured" in four or five weeks with xeroform. In 1908, when about to marry, he had had six mercurial inunctions.

1. Is this a case of traumatic paresis? From the somewhat meagre account it would appear that Donath's lieutenant should rather be termed "shell-shock paresis," in the sense of a paretic neurosyphilis liberated by

---

* Donath. Beiträge zu den Kriegsverletzungen und -erkrankungen des Nervensystems. Wiener klin. Wchnschr., No. 27–8, 1915.

shell-shock (using shell-shock in the sense of a shock *without* direct brain injury).

2. What compensation is due such a man as Donath's lieutenant? The ordinary principles applicable to traumatic paresis are not here in point, since no symptoms pointing to trauma of brain ever supervened. See discussion under Case G.

3. How frequent is paresis in armies? R. L. Richards in White and Jelliffe's Treatment of Nervous and Mental Diseases writes as follows (of course concerning peace times):

"The French estimate that paresis cases are 7 per cent of all their military cases. The German estimate is 6.6 per cent. In our own army at the Government Hospital for the Insane, of 490 cases of mental diseases among officers and enlisted men, 37, or 7 per cent, were paresis. During the Russo-Japanese War, in the Russian Psychiatric Hospital at Harbin, the percentage of paresis was 5.6 per cent among the cases developing at the front."

> A French soldier "shell-shocked" (also burial) into incipient tabes dorsalis? Case from Duco and Blum of Paris.

Case B.* A French soldier was buried by effects of shell explosion September 8th, 1914. He sustained no wound or fracture.

Incontinence of urine developed. Anesthesia of penis and scrotum. Reflexes absent; pupils sluggish. Wassermann reactions suspicious.

The diagnosis **tabes dorsalis incipiens** was made (hematomyelia of conus terminalis eliminated).

The patient was estimated to be "40% incapacitated," according to the French "*échelle de gravité*" of conditions. A full pension would not be justified in the opinion of the French authors.

1. Is there evidence of an increase or exacerbation of tabes dorsalis in the war? Birnbaum,† reviewing German war neurology, quotes Weygandt as believing that the war has probably had to do with the production of both tabes and paresis in many instances. Other cases, however, have merely been made worse by the war stress. Thirdly, there are cases in which the war stress has done no harm whatever. Westphal has seen both tabes and paresis develop in men who had never before shown any mental or physical symptoms whatever, and accordingly, Westphal must be counted among those who regard war stress as a liberating factor for these diseases. Redlich and Donath are cited in the same connection. (The case of Donath is the case presented above as Case A.)

   A very interesting claim was made by Cimbal to the effect that he found many examples of paresis developing in the early period of the war, particularly in November and December, 1914. Later, according to Cimbal, cerebrospinal syphilis and tabes became more prevalent.

---

* Duco et Blum. Guide pratique du Médecin dans les Expertises médicolégales militaires. Paris, 1917.

† Birnbaum. Kriegsneurosen und -psychosen auf Grund der gegenwärtigen Kriegsbeobachtungen: Sammelbericht. Z. f. d. ges. Neurol. u. Psychiat., Bd. XII, H. 1, 1915.

> Neurosyphilis in a German recruit, possibly AG-
> GRAVATED ON military SERVICE. Pension not
> allowable. Case from Weygandt.

Case C.* A German, long alcoholic and thought to be
weakminded, volunteered, but shortly had to be released from
service. He began to be forgetful and obstinate, cried, and
even appeared to be subject to hallucinations. The pupils
were unequal and sluggish. The uvula hung to the right.
The left knee-jerk was lively, right weak. Fine tremors of
hands. Hypalgesia of backs of hands. Stumbling speech.
Attention poor.

It appeared that he had been infected with syphilis in 1881
and in 1903 had had an ulcer of the left leg.

The military commission denied that his service had
brought about the disease. In the phrase of the Canadian
Pension Board the German commission would probably have
rendered a report "aggravated on service," not "by service."
(See Canadian cases D, E, and F.)

1. Has paresis increased in the war? Both French and
German figures controvert the claim. Marie, for
example, found not a single paretic amongst the skull
injury cases at the Salpétrière. Most authors are
found demonstrating cases which they clearly regard as
in some way produced or unfavorably influenced by
the war. There seems, therefore, to be a little incon-
sistency between the general statement that paresis has
not increased in the war and the somewhat frequent cases
described as occurring in and modified by the war.
However, Bonhoeffer, on the basis of nine months' war
experience, also holds it to be probable that paresis is
no more frequent in the field than in the home population.

2. Is the old syphilitic especially liable to break down under
war conditions? According to Richards, Shaikewicz
says that in the Russo-Japanese war paresis was noted

* Weygandt. Kriegseinflüsse und Psychiatrie. Jahres-
kurse f. ärztl. Fortbildung, Maiheft, 1915.

especially among the officers and non-commissioned officers, and that it was undoubtedly hastened in its development by war conditions.   Steida says that while ordinarily we find paresis developing twelve to twenty years after the primary sore of syphilis, in these cases it developed in five to ten years after the primary sore. Some of the cases progressed with unusual rapidity.   It was also noticed that among soldiers from the front, under treatment, evidences of syphilis were present in 20%, while among the other soldiers under treatment, evidences of syphilis were present in 1.6%.   Undoubtedly the old syphilitic is especially liable to break down under war conditions.

But, on the whole, the German authors in this war find no evidence favoring Steida's claim of the hastened post-infective outbreak.

3. How did it come about that the efficient German system permitted this alcoholic and weakminded syphilitic to enter the army?   As will be seen, he was a volunteer. In general, the German system has been supplied with army surgeons who have been trained, not by brief and "brush-up" courses, but by longer periods, sometimes two years in duration.

Syphilis contracted before enlistment, "AGGRA-
VATED BY SERVICE." Canadian case, courtesy
of Dr. J. L. Todd, Canadian Board of Pension
Commissioners.

Case D. A laboring man, 42, who always strenuously
denied syphilitic infection, proceeded to France eight months
after enlistment. He had not been in France three weeks
when he dropped unconscious. He regained consciousness,
but remained stupid, dull in expression, and with memory
impaired. His speech was also impaired. There was dizziness and a right-sided hemiplegia.

He was confined to bed four months and was then
"boarded" for discharge.

Physically, his heart was slightly enlarged both right and
left; sounds irregular; extra systoles; aortic systolic murmur
transmitted to neck; blood pressure 140:40. Precordial
pain, dyspnoea.

Neurologically, there was a partial spastic paralysis of the
right thigh which could be abducted, could be flexed to 120°,
and showed some power in the quadriceps. There was also
a spastic paralysis of the right arm, but the shoulder girdle
movements were not impaired. There was a slight weakness
on the right side of the face. There was no anesthesia
anywhere.

The deep reflexes were increased on the right side, Babinski
on right, flexor contractures of right hand, extensor contractures of right leg, abdominal and epigastric reflexes absent,
pupils active, tongue protruded in straight line.

Fluid: slight increase in protein. W. R.+++

The Board of Pension Commissioners ruled that the condition had been aggravated *by* service. (See Case E, "aggravated *on* service.")

1. In view of the fact that the majority of the cases here
abstracted happen to be in common soldiers, is there
any evidence bearing on relative incidence in officers
and men? Quoting R. L. Richards:

"The percentage of paresis cases among officers alone is variously estimated from 50 per cent in the German army (Stier) to 58.9 per cent in the Austrian army (Drastich). Since paresis is a disease of more advanced life, it is but natural that the percentage of paresis among officers, non-commissioned officers, and older soldiers should be higher than among the whole military body, where the average age is, as we have seen, well below thirty years. Hence the above figures do not mean a greater prevalence of syphilis among those classes, but that we have no means of knowing how many of the others develop paresis. If anything it shows that these 'soldiers by calling,' have a more stable mental make-up, since they succumb chiefly to an exogenous toxin."

Rayneau at the 19th Congress of French Alienists and Neurologists at Nantes in 1909, discussing the insane of the army from a medico-legal point of view, states that the most frequent mental disease amongst officers and soldiers is general paresis. At least, this disease is the most frequent basis of invaliding, retirement, or placing in the inactive list. He states that French and foreign statistics are at one upon this matter, quoting Christian as finding 32% among the soldiers interned at Charenton; Garnier at Dijon, 59%; Meilhon at Quimper, 42% and Talon at Marseilles, 33.8%. Grilli found 31 of 40 officers interned in Florence, Sienna and Milan victims of general paresis. Stier's German statistics indicate about 50%. Rayneau himself found 16 of 20 officers paretic and 17 out of 27 subalterns and *gendarmes*.

The Neurological Society of Paris held a conference December 15, 1916, with the chiefs of the neurological and psychiatric military centres of France, and discussed a variety of questions concerning invaliding, incapacity, and compensation in neuroses and psychoses of war. Dupré dealt especially with the psychoses of war as caused by trauma, strain, infection, and intoxication. General paresis is regarded by Dupré as the most important of the dementias found in the army. The medico-legal point of view is, of course, that general paresis is necessarily related to an old syphilis, but its late development leads to misinterpretations as to its probable cause, both by the family and friends and even by magistrates. The war acts in the French nomenclature as an *agent revélateur* or as an

agent accélérateur. Although its cause is prior and
exterior to the war, general paresis in a majority of
cases is brought out (*revélé*) by the lack of adaptability
of the general paretic to the novelty and difficulties of
his surroundings and duties in war. Trauma, strain,
and alcohol in a certain number of cases accelerate the
progress of a general paresis. The aggravation of
paresis is produced by these same factors, but especially
by violent cerebral trauma. According to Dupré, the
Val-de-Grace statistics show that the number of paretics has not been increased by the war. Medico-
legally, the victim of general paresis, like the victim of
traumatic or infectious chronic mental disorder, may
be assigned an incapacity of from 50 to 100%, and
these patients are invalided under *Réforme No. 1*, — a
permanent invaliding.

Lépine of Lyons also discusses the compensation
question in general paresis. Lépine thinks that, although syphilis is indispensable in paresis, yet the truth
is that syphilis plus something else unknown to us is
responsible for general paresis. This something else is
neither a special kind of virus nor is it a particular kind
of prepared soil alone. Trauma, physical, intellectual,
and moral strain, and insomnia are the factors to which
he calls special attention as adjuncts in the production
of general paresis. As to the responsibility of the State
for the production of general paresis, according to
Lépine, the maximal responsibility should be 40% on
account of the very considerable predisposition to paresis
created by pre-existent syphilis.

Marie remarked that, although there had been
thousands of head cases at the Salpêtrière, there had
not been a single case of general paresis. Dupré agreed
with Marie that trauma was not a frequent etiological
factor; strain and alcohol were more important. The
Society agreed that in exceptional cases, where an
encephalic trauma could be regarded as accelerating
or aggravating the disease, the degree of incapacity
might be set at from 10 to 30 per cent.

Syphilis contracted before enlistment, "AGGRA-
VATED ON SERVICE." Canadian case, courtesy
of Dr. J. L. Todd, Canadian Board of Pension
Commissioners.

Case E. A laboring man, 44, acquired syphilis at a time
unknown. Ten months after enlistment this man developed
symptoms on the firing-line. He was inattentive, irrational,
incoherent. The diagnosis was then "mania."

There were, however, scars at angle of mouth and on lower
lip. Occipital glands were palpable, fine tremor of hands.
The W. R. was $+++$.

Later the patient became violent, destructive, untidy,
disoriented. Auditory hallucinations are recorded.

He was "boarded" for discharge five months after the first
symptoms. The board agreed that these symptoms would
have appeared in civil life. In view of a difference of opinion
as to the part played by stress of service, his condition was
set down as "*aggravated on service*" (not, it will be noted, *by*
service, see Case D).

1. Under what conditions should pensions be awarded for
    disability resulting from venereal diseases? According
    to a personal communication from Dr. J. L. Todd,
    Chairman of the Board of Pension Commissioners for
    Canada, pensions are awarded for all disabilities appear-
    ing *during* service, unless they can be shown certainly
    to be due to the men's own fault and negligence. It
    would appear that *during* service covers both aggra-
    vations *by* and *on* service. There remains some doubt
    as to whether contraction of venereal disease constitutes
    negligence.

2. What have been conditions in the small inactive American
    army of the past? Richards has made a study of
    statistics at the Government Hospital for the Insane,
    Washington.

    "The leading features of this mental disease were
    well exemplified in our cases the past year. They
    formed 7.5 per cent of the total number. They aver-
    aged forty years of age, and Ziehen says 80 per cent of

all cases are in the fourth or fifth decade of life. They averaged ten and a half years' service, which would indicate that the military life was their calling. Only one had any serious hereditary defect. Stigmata of degeneration were infrequent, averaging only two for each case. 66 per cent had good schooling, considering their opportunities. Physical signs were frequent in each case. Only one showed normal light reaction. Ziehen says the light reaction is retained in only 20 per cent of the cases. Patellar reflex was absent in one case and normal or exaggerated in five. The speech defect was slight in four cases. Other physical signs were present in the usual proportions. Memory defects existed in all the cases. In four the onset was with excitement. One began with a character change as the most marked feature. In only two were the transfer diagnoses correct. One, beginning as a quiet dementia, was diagnosticated paralysis agitans, because of a marked tremor. One was excited and euphoric and was called a manic-depressive psychosis. One with an obscure onset was diagnosticated as a neurasthenic. The other one was first observed in this hospital. The physical signs should have led to a correct diagnosis in each of these cases."

Duration of neurosyphilitic process important *re* compensation. Canadian case, courtesy of Dr. C. B. Farrar, Psychiatrist, Military Hospitals Commission.

Case F. A Canadian of 36 enlisted in 1915, served in England, and was returned to Canada in February, 1917, clearly suffering from some form of neurosyphilis (W. R. positive in serum and fluid, globulin, pleocytosis 108).

There is no record of any disability or symptom of nervous or mental disease at enlistment. The first symptoms were noted by the patient in May, 1916, six months or more after enlistment. The case was reviewed at a Canadian Special Hospital, October 11, 1916, by a board of examiners. This board reported that:

"The condition could only come from syphilitic infection of three years' standing" (a decision bearing on compensation); but the general diagnosis remained:

"Cerebrospinal lues, **aggravated by service.**"

The picture which the medical board regarded as of at least three years' standing was as follows:

History of incontinence, shooting pains, attacks of syncope, general weakness, facial tremor, exaggerated knee-jerks, pupils react with small excursion. Speech and writing disorder, perception dull, lapses of attention, memory defect, defective insight into nature of disorder, emotional apathy.

1. Was the conclusion "aggravated by service" sound? On humanitarian grounds the victim is naturally conceded the benefit of the doubt. But it is questionable how scientifically sound the conclusion really was.
2. Could the condition come only from syphilitic infection of at least three years' standing? Hardly any single symptom in this case need be of so long a standing; yet the combination of symptoms seems by very weight of numbers to justify the conclusion of the medical board.

Can PARETIC NEUROSYPHILIS ("general paresis") be lighted up by the stress of military service without injury or disease? A possible example from P. Marie, Chatelin and Patrikios of Paris.

Case G. In apparently good health a French soldier repaired to the colors, in August, 1914, being then 23 years old.

Two years later, August, 1916, symptoms appeared: speech disorder with stammering, change of character (had become easily excitable), stumbling gait. He became more and more preoccupied with his own affairs, grew worse, and was sent to hospital in October, 1916.

He was then foolish and overhappy, especially when interviewed. There was marked rapid tremor of face and tongue. Speech hesitant, monotonous, and stammering to the point of unintelligibility. His memory, at first preserved, became impaired so that half of a test phrase was forgotten. Simple addition was impossible and fantastic sums would be given instead of right answers; handwriting tremulous, letters often missed, others irregular, unequal, and misshapen.

Excitable from onset, the patient now became at times suddenly violent, striking his wife without provocation. After visit at home, he would forget to return to hospital. Often he would leave hospital without permission (of course the more surprising in a disciplined soldier).

No delusions were found.

The serum and fluid W. R. were positive, albumin in fluid, lymphocytosis.

Neurological examination. Unequal pupils, slight right-side mydriasis, pupils stiff to light, weakly responsive in accommodation, reflexes lively, fingers tremulous on extension of arms.

The patient had, December 5, 1916, an epileptiform attack with head rotation, limb-contractions and clonic movements.

1. Should this soldier recover for disability obtained in service? Marie was inclined to think military service in part responsible for the development of the paresis. Laignel-Lavastine thought so also, but that the amount assigned should be 5%–10% of the maximum assignable.

2. What is the duty of the military authorities relative to socalled traumatic paresis? Medico-legally speaking, Froissart, quoted by Rayneau, states that a victim of traumatic paresis *may or may not* have presented mental disorders before the accident, that is, that the paretic symptoms may develop out of a clear sky as a result of the accident. The accident itself must be of a serious nature. The accident must be followed by phenomena pointing to brain injury of traumatic nature. These phenomena need not be characteristic symptoms of general paresis at the outset. The period elapsing between the trauma and the supervening condition of paresis must be occupied without notable interruption, at first by phenomena of a purely traumatic nature, later by signs indicating the onset and evolution of general paresis.

   The French invaliding process called *Réforme No. 1* with pension is granted according to the governmental instructions only to officers, subalterns, and soldiers whose disease is due to trauma. In view of this governmental regulation, the military surgeon must write out certificates describing every cranial trauma, however slight, which might have a bearing on the development of paresis. However, he should not too readily admit trauma as a cause of paresis. If a long period of quietude, a period in which the trauma itself seems to have undergone a complete recovery, supervenes, then general paresis should not be reported by the surgeon.

   Lépine has recently noted the following features as desirable in board reports concerning paretics: nature of trauma, length of service, fatigue endured, insomnia, date of infection, treatment, W. R.

Can " gassing " light up a paresis?   Example from
de Massary of Issy-les-Moulineaux.

Case H.   A soldier, 35, was sent to the *Centre Neurologique*
with a hospital ticket reading:

"Neurasthenia, general weakness following intoxication
by gas."

The soldier was thought at first to be a neurasthenic.   But
he soon showed signs of more pronounced mental trouble.
The voice was suspicious.   There was a slight irregularity of
pupils.

An epileptiform attack occurred, followed by aggravation
of symptoms.

Lumbar puncture showed pleocytosis.   The W. R. of the
serum proved positive.

Yet the evident **neurosyphilis,** possibly **paretic** (de Massary's diagnosis), was preceded by a neurasthenia and the
neurasthenia was preceded by "gassing."

De Massary believes the patient *and his family* would
perhaps be justified in believing the condition produced by the
injury.   De Massary is not clear as to the financial deserts of
the patient.   It is not a manifest case of aggravation of ante-
bellum symptoms, even if it be neuropathologically an instance of acquired loss of resistance to pre-existent spirochetes
in body or brain.

1.   What adjuvant factors have been recognized in military
     paresis?   Aside from syphilis, Rayneau finds that alco-
     holism, malaria, sunstroke and various intoxications
     serve as causes for paresis.   Rayneau points out that the
     apparent integrity of the mind in general paresis may
     be such that they last in the army some time and have
     their oddities ascribed to misconduct or breaches of
     discipline.   In fact the Legrande du Saulle called this
     early period in general paresis the *medico-legal period*,
     showing, as it so often does, thefts, outrages against
     decency, frauds, assaults, exhibitionism and the like.
     To be sure these acts are absurd and infantile and not
     difficult to recognize as of psychotic origin.

Syphilis may bring out epilepsy in a subject having
taint.   Case from Bonhoeffer, 1915.

Case I.*   A man of 35 in the *Landwehr* acquired syphilis
some time in the summer of 1914.   He was a good soldier,
passed through several clashes, and was promoted to *Unteroffizier*.

To understand what followed it must be stated that he had
been a bed-wetter to 11, had been practically a teetotaler
(Bonhoeffer's point is perhaps that otherwise epilepsy might
have developed sooner?), and, when he did drink, vomited
almost at once, and had amnesia for the period of drunkenness.   His father had been somewhat of a drinker.   His
sister had suffered from convulsions as a child.

February, 1915, the *Unteroffizier* lost appetite, got headaches, and went to hospital for a time.   Upon getting better,
he was sent on service to Berlin.   In a Berlin hotel he had
his first convulsions and unconsciousness, biting his tongue.
He was confused for several days, and, when he had become
clear, had a pronounced retrograde amnesia together with a
tendency to fabricate a filling for the lost period.

This retrograde amnesia is uncommon in epilepsy and
suggests organic disease.   No sign of organic disease was
found on neurological examination.   The patient had no
signs of the epileptic make-up.   The serum W. R. was
negative.   On the whole, Bonhoeffer regards the epilepsy as
"reactive " to the syphilis, as a syphilogenic epilepsy.

As to the amnesia, it is of interest that alcohol should long
before have been able to cause amnesia in this man in the
same way as does now the syphilitic epilepsy.

1.   In view of the fact that this *Landwehr* man appears to
      have acquired syphilis while on campaign, what is the
      responsibility of the government for treatment?   The

---

* Bonhoeffer.   Erfahrungen über Epilepsie und Ver-
wandtes im Feldzuge.   Monatschr. f. Psychiat u. Neurol.,
Bd. 38, H. 1–2, 1915.

Canadian authorities, as stated under Case E, are in doubt whether contraction of venereal disease constitutes negligence on the part of the soldier. It would appear to us that where a government does not take suitable steps to prevent the acquisition of syphilis by the soldiers, the government must assume a measure of responsibility for the syphilis incurred. The government's responsibility would be still greater in equity, it would appear, if commercial opportunities for the acquisition of syphilis are maintained under more or less close government supervision or (even as has been claimed for certain encampments on our own Mexican border) if shelter for illicit sex relations is afforded within the limits of a military camp. In a certain community, "E," for example, it is claimed by Exner,* the district for prostitutes was "situated within the lines of military camps and protected and 'regulated' by the military authorities."

But even if the government has no legal responsibility in this regard, it would be well to consider the ultimate results of the syphilis that will probably be acquired by great numbers of soldiers under campaign conditions. Aside from the ravages of syphilis outside the nervous system, it is well known, as Weygandt intimates for German conditions, that the aftermath of war will be a high proportion of cases of neurosyphilis.

Weygandt remarks in his review of the influence of the war upon psychiatry, that the opportunity for syphilitic infection in the campaign is considerable. In the war of 1870, the conditions in this regard were extremely unfavorable, and writing in 1915, Weygandt remarks that at present there should be a prophylaxis against syphilitic infection by the soldiers, which prophylaxis should be the most energetic possible. Continence on the part of the soldiers and the isolation of infected women, with examination by specialists, have been advocated by Neisser and by Mendel. In the '80's a great number of cases of locomotor ataxia developed in Germany, which were due to syphilis acquired by the soldiers and officers in the war of 1870.

---

* Exner, M. J., Prostitution in its relation to the army on the Mexican Border, *Social Hygiene*, Vol. 3, 2, April, 1917.

> **Syphilis in a psychopathic subject. Convulsions 5 days after Dixmude. Case from Bonhoeffer, 1915.**

Case J.* A soldier in the reserves, 23, was, subsequently to his being brought to hospital, described by his wife as a rather over-sensitive fellow, who could hardly look at blood and was meticulous about the household. He had always been subject to headaches, especially after hard work. However, he had passed through his military training well in 1910, not even having been *bestraft*.

He began service in October and fought at Dixmude on the 19th. On the 24th in the trench and while being carried back, he had several spells of pallor, falling stiff, and then having convulsions. Brought finally to the Charité in Berlin, he had more spells of sudden pallor, collapse with brief convulsions, tossings in bed, and absences, post-convulsive headaches, and mild bad humor.

There were numerous attacks several days apart in the first seven weeks. The patient was not of an "epileptic" disposition, though he was rather readily dissatisfied. Headaches also occurred without relation to convulsions.

The serum W. R. was positive. Treatment by mercurial inunctions. No further convulsions. Prognosis as to the possibility of a constitutional epilepsy unknown.

---

* Bonhoeffer, *loc. cit.*

SYPHILITIC ROOT-SCIATICA (lumbrosacral radiculitis) in a fireworks man with a French artillery regiment. Case presented from Dejerine's clinic by Long.

Case K. No direct relation of this example of root-sciatica to the war is claimed nor was there a question of financial reparation.

There was no prior injury. At the end of March, 1915, the workman was taken with acute pains in lumbar region and thighs, and with urgent but retarded micturition.

Unfit for work, he remained, however, five months with the regiment, and was then retired for two months to a hospital behind the lines. He reached the Salpêtrière October 12, 1915, with "double sciatica, intractable."

There was no demonstrable paralysis but the legs seemed to have "melted away," *fondu*, as the patient said. Pains were spontaneously felt in the lumbar plexus and sciatic nerve regions, not passing, however, beyond the thighs. These pains were more intense with movements of legs; but coughing did not intensify the pains. Neuralgic points could be demonstrated by the finger in lumbar and gluteal regions and above and below the iliac crests (corresponding with rami of first lumbar nerves). The inguinal region was involved and the painful zone reached the sciatic notch and the upper part of the posterior surface of the thigh.

The sensory disorder had another distribution objectively tested. The sacral and perineal regions were free. Anesthesia of inner surfaces of thighs, hypesthesia of the anterior surfaces of thighs and lower legs. The anesthesia grew more and more marked lower down and was maximal in the feet, which were practically insensible to all tests, including those for bone sensation. There was a longitudinal strip of skin of lower leg which retained sensation.

Position sense of toes, except great toes, was poor. There was a slight ataxia attributable to the sensory disorder —

reflexes of upper extremities, abdominal, and cremasteric preserved, knee-jerks, Achilles and plantar reactions absent.

The vesical sphincter shortly regained its function, though its disorder had been an initial symptom.

Pupils normal.

The "sciatica" here affects the lumbosacral plexus. Signs of disorder at one time or other affected the first lumbar distribution of the third lumbar and first and second sacral nerves.

As to the syphilitic nature of this affection, there had been at eighteen (22 years before) a colorless small induration of the penis, lasting about three weeks. There was now evident a small oval pigmented scar. The patient had married at 20 and has had three healthy children.

The lumbar puncture fluid yielded pleocytosis (120 per cmm.). Mercurial treatment was instituted.

The treatment has not reduced the pains. Long thinks it was undertaken too long (six months) after onset. The warning for early diagnosis is manifest. There was somehow a delay under the medical conditions of the army.

Can the "lighting-up" of NEUROSYPHILIS IN
CIVIL LIFE be induced by the domestic stress of
war?   A possible example from Dr. R. Percy Smith,
London.

Case L. A German Jew in London passed into the
PARETIC form of NEUROSYPHILIS shortly after the outbreak
of war under conditions suggesting that the stress of emotions
directly or indirectly lighted up the neural process.

The man was a bank-officer, 52 years old, and married.
He had lived many years in England and was in fact a
naturalized citizen. He had been under treatment for
syphilis by Sir Jonathan Hutchinson, 29 years before, namely,
at the age of 23. Subsequently, Sir John had given him permission to marry.

It proved that for years the man had had fixed pupils,
absent knee-jerks, and a perforated ulcer of the foot. However, there had been no other mental or nervous symptoms
preventing bank-officer's work.

At the outbreak of war the man was discharged from the
bank. He grew worried and sleepless. He began to charge
himself with sex irregularity. He went down to the city and
burned trust documents belonging to others.

From worry and self-accusation he passed into depression
and agitation. He developed a belief that not only he but
also his German wife were to be executed. He thought he
was a criminal and was to be hanged.

The depression then altered to a condition of hilarity and
loquacity.

In addition to the fixed pupils and absent knee-jerks, a
speech disorder shortly developed.

The patient was placed under care, but quickly (a few
months?) passed into an advanced stage of paretic neurosyphilis and died.

> SHELL-SHOCK PSEUDOPARESIS (non-syphili-
> tic). Recovery. Case from Pitres and Marchand
> of Bordeaux.

Case M. June 19, 1915, a shell exploded some distance
from Lieutenant R. He remembers the gaseous smell, the
bursting of several shells nearby and a sensation of being
lifted into the air. When he recovered consciousness, he was
in hospital at Paris-Plage, covered with bruises and scratches.
They told him he had been delirious and had vomited and
spat blood.

June 24, his wife came to see him, but this visit he could
not remember. Nor could his wife at first recognize him, he
was so thin. He roused a few moments and recognized his
wife, but relapsed into torpor again. Speech was difficult
and ideas confused.

A few days later he was able to rise; but his mental status
grew worse, especially as to speech and writing; the latter quite
illegible. There was insomnia, or, if he slept, war dreams.

August 7, he began a period of five months' convalescence
passed with his family, depressed, given to spells of weeping,
confined to bed or couch, unable to "find words," conscious
of his state and troubled about it, speaking of nothing but
the war, and afraid to go out for fear of ambuscade. There
was at first a slight lameness of the right leg. Although he
could walk, he felt pain in the knee on flexing the right leg
on the thigh. He walked holding this leg in extension.

On going back to the colors, he was immediately evacuated
to the *Centre Neurologique* at Bordeaux, January 20, 1916.

Examination found a bored, impatient, irritated man, vexed
that a man who was not sick should be sent up "*comme fou.*"

Omitting negative details, **neurological examination** showed
slight lameness as above, body stiff and movements jerky;
difficult, unsteady gait. The lieutenant could stand for some
time on either leg, tongue and face tremulous during speech.
Limbs moderately tremulous, especially in the performance
of test movements.

Knee-jerks and Achilles jerks absent. Other reflexes, including pupillary, normal. Segmentary hypalgesia of right leg, especially about knee. Tremulous speech and writing. Patient would stop short in speaking for lack of words.

Malnutrition. Appetite good, but a bursting feeling after meals.

Skin dry, scaly on legs, fissured on fingers.

Serum W. R. negative. Fluid not examined.

Mental examination. Conscious and complaining of his troubles, Lieutenant R. claimed persistently that he was not sick. Memory for recent events was in general poor. Errands easily forgotten. Lost in the street. Complaint of corpse odors round him. Everybody is looking at him and making fun of him. He was apt to insult bystanders. He was afraid of German spies. Things in shops angered him as they seemed to him to be of German manufacture.

There were frequent periods of depression, with pallor and no spontaneous speech for some hours to a half-day. Headaches coming on and stopping suddenly.

As to diagnosis, the first impression, say Pitres and Marchand, was that of general paresis. The progress of symptoms after the shock was consistent with this diagnosis. The mental state and the physical findings seemed consistent, although the pupils were normal. His partial insight into his symptoms was not inconsistent with the diagnosis. He had a characteristic self-confidence. There had been four stillbirths (two twins); two children are alive, 11 and 13. Typhoid fever at 30. Syphilis denied. No mental disease in the family.

The patient had never done military duty, having been invalided for "right apex." But he had volunteered and been accepted in September, 1914.

1. Was this diagnosis, general paresis, at any time justified? The spinal fluid should of course have been examined. The peculiar lameness of the right leg was certainly not characteristic of general paresis, and was perhaps hysterical. (There was no limitation of visual fields or any other definite sign of hysteria.) Presumably some quality of speech defect, the amnesia, and the euphoria,

together with absent knee-jerks, led to the diagnosis general paresis. By the 20th of March, 1916, the knee-jerks had become lively; the Achilles jerks normal. At this time the patient had gained in weight, could walk though stiffly, had headache (especially right frontal) and a feeling of lead in head, less tremor, lack of desire to undertake anything. He still wanted to go back into service. He still saw spies about. Dreams terrible; devoured by spiders, leggins instruments of torture. Skin still atrophic. June 4 there was no more tremor of speech or face. Symptoms largely disappeared except a few ideas of persecution. Recovery October, 1916.

2. How was Lieutenant R. cured? Apparently by rest in the *Centre Neurologique*. Pitres and Marchand do not speak of the subtle relation between mental state and the idea of non-return to military service. This motive might still work even if Lieutenant R. kept protesting quite sincerely that he wanted to go back into military service.

SHELL-SHOCK PSEUDOTABES (non-syphilitic, serum W. R. positive). Improvement. Case from Pitres and Marchand of Bordeaux.

Case N. Innkeeper B., 36, a shell-shock and burial victim June 20, 1915, was looked on by a number of physicians as a case of genuine tabes.

Even eight months after the episode, he still showed (when observed by Pitres and Marchand, February 3, 1916) absence of knee-jerks and Achilles jerks, a slight swaying in the Romberg position, pupils sluggish to light, incoordination, delayed sensations. There was also a history of pains in the legs, compared by the patient to those of sciatica. These pains came in crises, the longest of which had lasted 30 hours.

It seems that this soldier's troubles began the day after his shock with a feeling of swollen feet and of cotton wool under them. He stayed on service, however, walking with increasing difficulty.

At the time of his evacuation, July 10, he could walk with great difficulty. "Strips of lead were between his legs." He could hardly control movements in the dark, or descend stairs. Often his legs would bend under him. Vesical function sluggish.

After a few months the patient could walk better. On February, 1916, he walked thrusting his legs forward trembling, and dragging toes a little. He could not support himself on either leg. Jerkiness and incoordination in extension or flexion of leg on thigh.

The muscular weakness was decidedly against tabes or at all events a pure tabes. The incoordination proved to be due, not to loss of position sense (which was intact) but to unsteady muscular contractions. Deep sensibility was intact.

There were no mental symptoms. There was a slight hesitation in speech and doubling of syllables, but nothing demonstrable with test phrases.

The serum W. R. was positive. Syphilis denied.

1. What is the cause of these phenomena? Pitres and Marchand lean to the hypothesis of slight internal traumatism. They believe that there is either (a) slight internal hemorrhage in the nervous system, or possibly (b) what they call "nerve cell contusion," or perhaps (c) caisson-disease-like phenomena from aerial decompression. Some authors incriminate (d) the gases. It has been reported by certain French authors that shortly after shell shock injury or burial there is a pleocytosis in the spinal fluid as well as evidence of hemorrhage. The pleocytosis is said to last only a short time; hence when patient arrives at a base hospital lumbar puncture usually discloses nothing.

Baalim and Ashtaroth

Paradise Lost, Book I, line 422.

VII. SUMMARY AND KEY

No more important human problem now exists than syphilis. Syphilis of the nervous system or, briefly, neurosyphilis is a highly important fraction of the total problem. The few outstanding dates and items which we present on the following page give but a faint idea of the amount of observation and thinking which the medical aspects of neurosyphilis alone have required. The present work deals with but a small fraction of the results of this work, nor can we more than glance at the scientific history of syphilis and neurosyphilis — a history that would form an epoch in itself.

It is only in the most recent years that syphilology and the narrower science of neurosyphilology have threatened to become separate disciplines boasting full time specialized workers. Up to recent years the contributions to the theory of syphilis have been largely by-products of work in larger sciences and arts. Thus, the cellular pathology of syphilis as worked out by Virchow and the more special vascular features as worked out by Heubner were incidental in the progress of pathological anatomy and histology. The bold procedure of Quincke in proposing lumbar puncture also had its more general ground in the extension of clinical medicine, — an interpretation likewise true of the French achievements in the cyto-diagnosis and chemical diagnosis of the lumbar puncture fluids. The careful histological definitions of the Nissl-Alzheimer group were incidental to the application of approved and classical pathological methods to neurological and psychiatric material.

Again, the work of Schaudinn, as well as that of Metchnikoff and Roux, was ingenious work with the methods of parasitology and experimental pathology. The great work of Schaudinn in establishing the constancy of the spirocheta pallida in syphilis may be said to have started syphilology as something approaching a special discipline. The ideas of one of the greatest of immunologists, Bordet, were almost

DATES, NEUROSYPHILIS

VIRCHOW	PATHOLOGY	1858
HEUBNER	ENDARTERITIS	1874
QUINCKE	LUMBAR PUNCTURE	1891
RAVAUT, SICARD, NAGEOTTI, WIDAL	CYTODIAGNOSIS, C.S.F.	1901
WIDAL, SICARD, RAVAUT	ALBUMIN, C.S.F.	1903
METCHNIKOFF AND ROUX	TRANSMISSION TO APES	1903
ALZHEIMER	HISTOPATHOLOGY, BRAIN SYPHILIS	1904
SCHAUDINN AND HOFFMANN	SPIROCHETA PALLIDA	1905
WASSERMANN, NEISSER AND BRUCK	SERUM DIAGNOSIS	1906
PLAUT	WASSERMANN REACTION, C.S.F.	1908
EHRLICH	SALVARSAN	1909
SWIFT AND ELLIS	SALVARSANIZED SERUM	1912
NOGUCHI AND MOORE	SPIROCHETES, BRAIN TISSUE, PARESIS	1913
LANGE	GOLD SOL TEST	1913

CHART 28

immediately applied to the serum diagnosis of syphilis by Wassermann and the further application of this method to the problems of neurosyphilis was almost immediate, with the spirocheta pallida as an object of attack. The commanding intelligence of Ehrlich could at once seek application of long incubated ideas of chemotherapy with the startling outcome, salvarsan.

The history of syphilis and neurosyphilis was now to be thickly sown with ideas and results growing from the achievements of Schaudinn and Ehrlich. The positive reactions in the blood and spinal fluid in the most striking of mental diseases, general paresis, led to the impression that general paresis itself might at last be proved to be what Moebius had suspected, namely, 100% syphilitic. We know how difficult is the technical proof of spirochetosis in the brains of general paretics both post mortem and ante mortem, but no one doubts the certainty of the syphilitic hypothesis concerning the origin of general paresis.

The data of the gold sol reaction ultimately obtained from the ideas of Thomas Graham concerning colloids, as developed by Szigmondi and effectively applied by Lange, have broadened and solidified the whole plane of attack.

The ingenious suggestions of Swift and Ellis (salvarsanized serum) and the notable work of Noguchi and Moore (spirochetosis in paretic brains) indicate to us as Americans what the establishment of scientific institutes may do to permit the rapid application of new ideas to branches of inquiry that are opened out. Scientific institutes do not manufacture a Virchow, a Metchnikoff, a Schaudinn, a Bordet or an Ehrlich but they directly permit such men to work and indirectly stimulate the development of more.

The series of 137 cases here at least presented does not touch systematically the problems of the neuropathology of syphilis, which would themselves require a textbook of respectable size. We have, however, presented in Part I, cases 1 to 8, some indication of the protean nature of the material and from time to time in the remainder of the book somewhat fuller accounts of the pathological anatomy and histology have been presented than are strictly necessary in the demonstration of the principles of modern systematic diagnosis and treatment.

Our work may be said to represent psychopathic hospital practice as available to us in our official capacities at the Psychopathic Department of the Boston State Hospital. A word is necessary concerning the nature of this practice. The dispensary and ward practice of a modern state psychopathic hospital, such as the Boston institution (founded in 1912) and the Ann Arbor institution (founded in 1906), is to be sharply distinguished from asylum practice. Those who have not followed the evolution of the modern psychopathic hospital with the lowering of bars to the admission of patients and the extension of its benefits to a group of sick persons far removed from the medicolegal concept " insanity ", may not soon grasp the general nature of psychopathic hospital material. Psychopathic hospital practice stands, in fact, almost midway between asylum practice in the classical sense and private practice. This has come about through the great extension of the so-called voluntary relation under which hundreds of patients now resort to the beds and outpatient rooms of a psychopathic hospital, who would formerly have remained untreated or inadequately treated. Moreover, the broadening of the concept of mental diseases as a whole has permitted in some parts of the world the establishment of laws under which psychopathic and psychotic patients may be brought to psychopathic hospitals and even to asylums under the easiest possible conditions and restrictions, omitting court procedure altogether. The operation of the voluntary and temporary care provisions of law has accordingly yielded us, in the Boston institution, a great group of cases formerly not at all accessible to hospital diagnosis and treatment. Needless to say, as always under such conditions, we have been able to show not merely that hospital diagnosis or treatment is of importance to a new group of cases, but also that home treatment, especially home treatment under supervision, is possible and even ideal for a large group of cases about which utter darkness or profound misgivings ruled in the not very distant past.

Accordingly, we are fain to insist that our material is of

importance in new programs of community organization for the stamping out of disease. The work in psychopathic hospitals upon neurosyphilis in particular is essentially a part of the public health program, although our special work will not soon be taken over by the public health officers, so complicated are the ramifications of medical and social diagnosis and treatment in the neurosyphilis group.

We have tried in Part IV (medicolegal and social cases) to give a few examples to illustrate the part played by neurosyphilis in society; but we regard this part of our work as the least satisfactory and the least representative in the total work. Our colleagues in social service, in mental hygiene, in psychopathology and in criminology will easily in the next few years provide a far more adequate basis for a full account of the public and social aspects of neurosyphilis. One point we should emphasize here. The psychopathic hospital worker, whether physician or social worker, must shortly decide upon and consolidate a program with relation to the families of neurosyphilitics.

The syphilographers of the dermatological and special syphilis clinics have their identical problems with the families of syphilitics; but the dispensaries for mental cases and in particular the psychopathic hospital and asylum out-patient departments tap another reservoir of syphilitic families at a stage when the memory of the initial horrors of syphilitic infection is dimmed or erased. Any program for the diagnosis and treatment of syphilis of the innocent must take into account not only the skin, syphilis, and internal medicine clinics but also the clinics for mental and nervous diseases wherein neurosyphilitics are not infrequent. Whether the ultimate percentage will stand at 10, 15 or 20% for the neurosyphilitics in mental clinics, is of no importance to the principle. There are enough neurosyphilitics having economical importance and humanly precious families to warrant definite steps.

The Massachusetts Commission for Mental Diseases has in the last few years employed the services of two medical workers whose time has been largely devoted to the applications of our recent knowledge in neurosyphilis and has gone so far as to establish a neurosyphilis ward in one of the district state institutions (Summer Street, Worcester, under the Grafton Hospital Board). Special social workers in the field of neurosyphilis have also been available from time to time. These social workers are enabled with the support of the medical profession to do a great deal of good, for example, with the slogan THE CHILD OF A PARETIC IS THE CHILD OF A SYPHILITIC.

The nature of the intake of patients into psychopathic hospital wards and out-patient clinics is such that great numbers of non-mental syphilitics arrive for diagnosis and possible treatment. Moreover, the existence of syphilis in non-suspects is a fact picked up by the way in routine Wassermann serum diagnosis.

The mental clinic in the modern sense with the medicolegal bars lowered or well nigh removed, turns rapidly into a clinic for neurological cases as well. The German models for mental and nerve clinics are rapidly being imitated. The result of this administrative novelty in our hospital procedure has incidentally yielded us many representative cases of entirely non-psychotic and even non-psychopathic neurosyphilis. Our impression grows and deepens that *the neurosyphilitic is seldom merely a spinal syphilitic.* The neurosyphilitic is nearly always the victim not merely of spinal disease but also of intracranial disease. Per contra, the victim of intracranial neurosyphilis is almost always more or less importantly affected by spinal neurosyphilis.

The net result of the modern work on neurosyphilis has been to bring the neurologist and the psychiatrist together upon one platform in diagnosis and more and more upon one platform in treatment. But aside from the clinical evidence that the neurosyphilitic is apt to be a victim of both brain syphilis and cord syphilis, the autopsy evidence is stronger still. Even the victim of tabetic neurosyphilis (" tabes dorsalis ") himself is rarely found at autopsy without more or less evidence of significant encephalic disease of a chronic inflammatory or degenerative nature. Aside from tabes dorsalis and Erb's paraplegia, the rule is almost universal that neurosyphilis is a matter of the entire nervous system.

In view of the generalization of neurosyphilitic process, one might question the advantage of any topical grouping of neurosyphilitic disease. Practically speaking, however, as we have shown in Chart 5, it seems advisable to separate the neurosyphilitic diseases into six roughly distinguishable groups. First, there is the great group that we have chosen to term **diffuse neurosyphilis,** including many of the cases of so-called cerebral or cerebrospinal syphilis of the neurological clinics and the group of cases that have been treated in private practice by internists and neurologists without recourse to institutions. These cases have lived at home and have not been socially hard to manage until the late phases of their disease when the victims, if poor, are sent to almshouses and infirmaries under municipal or state care. These are the cases which have been in the past regarded as most amenable to the classical iodid and mercurial treatment. Indeed there is record of numerous therapeutic successes in the group.

Whereas the lesions in diffuse neurosyphilis are chiefly chronic inflammatory and degenerative changes of a diffuse nature (with vascular changes incidental or subordinate to the inflammation and the degeneration), there is an important and large group of cases that we have termed **vascular neurosyphilis** in which the factors of inflammation and degeneration are subordinate to vascular insults. These are cases of syphilitic arteriosclerosis and the best examples are victims of cerebral thrombosis. The clinical symptoms of the immediate attacks (of apoplectiform, epileptiform or other acute nature) are not in themselves distinguishable from the immediate effects of non-syphilitic vascular disease; nevertheless the establishment of their syphilitic etiology is of the utmost importance on account of the possibilities of treatment of the underlying syphilis. For, as the neuropathologist must always insist, the immediate effects of vascular insults whether syphilitic or non-syphilitic are much more extensive than the ultimate paralytic or residual irritative effects; and by consequence a greater optimism is justifiable in the confronting of these cases than the nihilistic observer is likely to entertain.

Physicians dealing with chronic disease in general are apt to be somewhat nihilistic, but this nihilism is increased a hundred fold in disease of the nervous system. How important then is any work which shall demonstrate partial or even complete recovery from serious looking apoplectic and other seizures, besides all of which the point of syphilitic treatment naturally lies in the prevention of future insults of the same sort. Therapeutic experience in this vascular group has almost as good a toll of successes as in the diffuse neurosyphilis group above mentioned, that is to say, the modern systematic treatment and even the old pre-salvarsan treatments have succeeded fairly well in removing the products of inflammation from the membranes of the nervous system and in abolishing vascular disease.

The old principle that the dead neurone in the central nervous system cannot be regenerated remains a perfectly firm principle; but there are any number of neurones and even neurone systems that are not essential to life or to the pursuit of happiness. We accordingly have just as good a theoretical therapeutic outlook in many instances of chronic neurosyphilis as we have in chronic diseases of many other organs. Add to this the fact that a great number of the most sharply defined and grave symptoms are probably not due to destruction of neurones but to irritation and functional disability of neurones, and the conclusion is compelled that, as hinted above, an entirely unjustifiable pessimism and nihilism have prevailed in some quarters. Of course, the recoil from such pessimism with the onset of salvarsan treatment led various enthusiasts to an undue optimism.

Another great group distinguished by the existence of spinal cord disease is the group we have termed **tabetic neurosyphilis,** which group contains the classical tabes dorsalis or locomotor ataxia and its congeners.

The question of therapeutic optimism comes up most forcibly in the field of tabes. It is hard, however, at this time to give a proper and scientifically founded estimate of the therapeutic outcome in tabetic neurosyphilis with modern methods. So much can be said: namely, that the alleviation of pain and the palliation of other symptoms can be successfully claimed as a result of the renewed interest in the treatment of this affection. What was said above concerning the finality of the death process in a dead neurone is very strikingly true, of course, of some of the neurones of the posterior columns in tabes dorsalis. Still only portions of these neurones (namely, those which run an intradural course) are strikingly altered in a great many cases. Now and again one is greatly astonished to observe the restoration of the lost knee-jerk in cases of neurosyphilis (see for instance the case of Alice Morton (1), with discussion). In short, the relation of several tabetic symptoms to irritative conditions and functional disability of neurones may be considered established. Naturally, moreover, if therapy can stop the upward course of the affection as it passes from lower to higher nerve roots (according to reasonably well-established ideas of the genesis and progress of this affection), we are entitled to a further degree of optimism.

The question of therapeutic optimism *versus* pessimism is forced upon attention in the fourth great group of neurosyphilitic diseases which we have chosen to distinguish, namely, the group of **paretic neurosyphilis** including the disease formerly known as general paresis, paralytic dementia, softening of the brain and the like.

Of course, no one can gainsay there is a group of cases having in the natural course of events a prognosis of fatality within a term of years, say three to five years, and we have cases in our series which go to show that even with the modern intensive treatment the characteristic down-grade symptomatic progress and ultimate fatality occur. Still, we have other cases diagnostically on all fours with the fatal cases that have seemed to get either entirely well with the laboratory tests returning to normal and without further mental symptoms, or else lose mental symptoms on the one hand or laboratory signs on the other. We should strongly object to any account of paretic neurosyphilis which should insist that its necessary outcome is fatality within a term of years. Of course, viewing our knowledge of the affection in the past, we should be compelled to object to the generalization " *paresis fatal* " on the evidences of the universally recognized remissions. If nature can stop a paretic process, why cannot man do as much? Can it be alleged that our own apparent therapeutic successes and those of others are merely curious examples of coincidences, namely, that remissions have chosen to occur precisely when therapy was systematically applied? The percentage of therapeutic successes with modern intensive treatment, wherever it may ultimately stand, is already too high for this hypothesis of fortuitous remissions.*

Moreover, we believe that the details of the clinical progress of some of the reported cases are convincing on this point. What, however, is the distinguishing feature of paretic neurosyphilis? It is in one sense a particular kind of diffuse neurosyphilis. The tissues are apt to show not only encephalic but also spinal changes. There is apt to be a more or less well-defined meningitis, but the characteristic feature, without which the diagnosis of paretic neurosyphilis would hardly be rendered, is the existence of disease of the cerebral cortex. This disease is parenchymatous in the sense of showing nerve cell destruction. There is also an interstitial reaction in the shape of a neuroglia overgrowth, but the striking and pathognomonic feature is the infiltration of the sheaths of the small vessels in the cortex, giving evidence of an inflammation very intimately affecting the cellular mechanisms of the nervous system. It is striking how often a smaller or larger share of the cells found in the vessel sheaths are plasma cells. It does not appear, however, that the diagnosis of paretic neurosyphilis as against diffuse non-paretic neurosyphilis can be made in the stained sections with complete safety on the basis of plasmocytosis in the former and lymphocytosis in the latter. Whatever the results of careful histological differentiation by future neuropathologists may yield, it is at all events true that we cannot yet make an important differentiation clinically on the basis of the differential count of plasma cells and lymphocytes in the puncture fluids. How-

---

* We have recently reviewed the outcome in 300 *untreated* cases of paretic neurosyphilis (Psychopathic Hospital material, strictly comparable with treated cases) finding but 5 now capable of self-support and 10 more in normal-looking remission. This percentage is far lower than that in treated cases (at present, July, 1917, 50 in 200 capable of self-support).

ever this may be, there is an important distinction between diffuse neurosyphilis of the non-paretic type and paretic neurosyphilis in that paretic neurosyphilis rarely if ever fails to show important degrees of intracortical perivascular inflammation with larger or smaller numbers of plasma cells.

What has the therapeutist to face in this matter? The answer, as elsewhere, depends somewhat upon what the future may decide as to the habitat and toxic or antitoxic activities of the spirocheta pallida. The early claims that the spirocheta pallida was extravascular and lay for the most part in the parenchyma and not in the vessel sheaths were perhaps overbold, since other workers have found the spirochete in the vessel sheaths also (Mott).

Aside from the spirochete and its accessibility to spirochetocidal drugs, there seems to be no reason for supposing that the perivascular sheaths cannot be cleansed of their inflammatory contents. There is, again, no reason why the phagocytic cells should not continue to perform their scavenger function until such time as the degenerative process in the parenchyma (a process not necessarily progressive in the absence of the spirochete or its products) ceases. There is every reason to suppose that a great many of the clinical phenomena are not necessarily due to permanent destruction of neurones and neuronic organs (dendrites, axis-cylinders, nets and the like) but are due to various microphysical conditions of pressure, intoxication and the like.

The inflammatory conditions in the spinal cord of poliomyelitis, which conditions are precisely as striking as those of the paretic cortex, are beyond a question cleared away in the progress of the affection. Reference to the paradigm case (1) will show the type of our argument. There is no manner of doubt that in this paradigm case almost every portion of the nervous system had been sometime swept by spirochetosis and many of its small vessel sheaths stuffed with chronic inflammatory products. As for paretic neurosyphilis itself, a great many of its most striking clinical phenomena, such as loss of memory and disorientation, as well as great degrees of apparent dementia, are found virtually as often in cases with very slight anatomical changes as in cases with marked cortical

devastation.   The inference is plain, that these phenomena
are to a degree functional rather than structural.

In brief, we conclude not only from therapeutic experience
but also on *a priori* grounds that the histological conditions in
paretic neurosyphilis are not entirely hopeless, and certainly
not more hopeless than conditions in many chronic diseases
outside the nervous system.   Accordingly, we plead for a tem-
perate optimism as to therapeutic results in general paresis.

A fifth group of neurosyphilitic cases bulking rather largely
in textbooks of pathology is the group of the **gummata.**
For a variety of reasons (therapeutic and otherwise) the
actual number of gummata of the nervous system available
for clinical or even for anatomical study is much smaller than
the books might lead one to infer.

The sixth and last of the main groups of neurosyphilitic
diseases is that of the **juvenile forms,** among which we find not
only diffuse forms without a special and well-defined course,
but also characteristic examples of paretic and tabetic neurosyphilis.   The distinction of a juvenile or congenital group
of neurosyphilitics is, on theoretical grounds, perhaps hardly
defensible.   On practical grounds, however, the juvenile
neurosyphilitics do form a group having special relations to
feeblemindedness, epilepsy and the like.

We must be clearly understood as to the rough, six-unit
classification just given.   It is practical merely.   For comparison we have given in other charts more expanded lists
of the diagnostic entities in neurosyphilis among which that
of Head and Fearnsides is of special interest, see Chart 2,
page 21.

We shall now proceed to a brief analysis of the findings in
our chosen series of 137 cases.   We shall not reproduce the case
headings of these cases, but expand their statements where
necessary and tie them together so far as possible into a
reasonable and systematic statement of the situation in neurosyphilis.   The footnotes will contain references to other cases
in which identical points are illustrated as in the leading
cases.   The leading cases will in all instances be placed first
in the footnotes.

The paradigm * shows meningeal, vascular and parenchymatous lesions and thus illustrates our definition of the term DIFFUSE which means precisely meningeal, vascular and parenchymatous. The meningeal lesions gave rise to two prominent sets of lesions, first, the marked tabetic lesions of the spinal cord (due to the spinal root neuritis incidental to the spinal meningeal inflammation), secondly, the characteristic asymmetrical and focal atrophy of cranial nerves incidental to a now largely extinct meningeal process at the base of the brain. The vascular lesions are responsible for another important and characteristic factor in the case, namely, the bilateral pyramidal tract sclerosis; the bilateral cysts of softening of the corpora striata are characteristic effects of old syphilitic cerebral thromboses. The parenchymatous disease in our paradigm is everywhere obvious, less so perhaps in the cortex itself than elsewhere, although here also evident in the shape of lesions suggesting an early phase of tissue atrophy.

The paradigm is of interest in demonstrating what in broad lines must be taken as an ascending disease proceeding not only from spinal cord to encephalon but also traceable as proceeding from lower parts of the spinal cord to upper parts thereof and from the lower encephalon to the higher structures of the cerebral cortex itself.

The paradigm insistently calls attention to the advantage of persistent therapy not only in its display of remarkable successive recoveries from permanent looking symptoms but also histologically from the remnants of inflammatory process to be found in an otherwise almost wholly dismantled nervous system with extinct lesions.

TABETIC NEUROSYPHILIS † ("tabes dorsalis"), of course, often proceeds to death without special complications of syphilitic nature. We have chosen a case, however, to demonstrate a terminal complication with vascular insult. Incidentally the case shows another complication inasmuch as the cause of death was rupture of aortic aneurysm. It is important to bear in mind these complications in tabes dorsalis which go

---

* Alice Morton (1).   † Francis Garfield (2).

to prove that the spirochetosis of tabetic neurosyphilis is not limited to the region of the spinal roots or to the spinal region in general. Tabetic neurosyphilis is apt to be only a part of a total picture of neurosyphilis just as neurosyphilis itself is only a part of the general syphilitic process.

Our case of PARETIC NEUROSYPHILIS * ("general paresis") is a characteristic one in duration (three years and three months). The aortic sclerosis almost constantly found in neurosyphilis and especially in paretic neurosyphilis is here also shown. The spinal cord showed lesions which are also almost always found in paretic neurosyphilis. The characteristic frontal emphasis of the atrophic and indurative lesions is shown. There is also a display of gross changes in the pia mater. The characteristic so-called granular ependymitis or sanding of the ventricular surface is shown. The case is distinguishable from the paradigm in not showing the effects of vascular insults in the shape of cysts of softening. The cerebellar sclerosis of the case is fairly characteristic of paretic cases. There is even a suggestion of atrophy in the temporal region suggesting the so-called Lissauer's paresis. Clinically the case belongs in the classical grandiose group of paretics (" O. K. No. 1 superfine ").

VASCULAR NEUROSYPHILIS † is illustrated in a fourth autopsied case. It may be noted that the pia mater in this case is practically normal. The tissues outside the area of softening due to the syphilitic thrombosis of nutrient vessels are practically normal. The case was one of almost complete sensory aphasia with word-deafness. The clinical picture is accordingly quite distinct from those of the paradigm (1) and of the case of general paresis (3) just discussed.

JUVENILE PARESIS ‡ is illustrated by a case with exceedingly extensive lesions, largely meningeal and parenchymatous. The cerebral lesions are atypical since in places they suggest the tuberous sclerosis of Bourneville. The brain atrophy is extreme (965 grams) and it is possible that this apparent brain atrophy was in part hypoplasia, since the spirochetosis

---

* John Dixon (3). † James Pierce (4).
‡ John Lawrence (5).

of this case was doubtless congenital. However, clinically the patient was fairly normal up to the age of 18.

A case of so-called SYPHILITIC EXTRAOCULAR PALSY * demonstrates a characteristic meningeal process more extensive than the clinical symptoms would have indicated. In fact, focal clinical nerve palsies are as a rule, if not constantly, partial phenomena of a far more extensive process of neurosyphilis. They are far more limited clinically than anatomically and histologically. It seems at first sight improper to term them cases of diffuse neurosyphilis in view of their clinical focality, yet they are best described as partial cases of diffuse neurosyphilis.

A case of GUMMA † of the left HEMISPHERE is presented which appears to have led to death in about four years from onset. This case, like many others, is not an example of purely focalized syphilitic process inasmuch as cysts of softening indicating slight vascular insults are present elsewhere (pons). There is also a degree of leptomeningitis, particularly basal.

Our discussion of the nature and forms of neurosyphilis is completed by a rare case probably belonging in the so-called *cervical hypertrophic meningitis of Charcot* but actually due to a GUMMA OF THE SPINAL MENINGES.‡ The importance of therapeutic optimism is emphasized in this case as in the paradigm. Theoretically the meningeal inflammation of neurosyphilis ought to be almost entirely if not entirely removed by therapy, and these two cases, like several others in the series, seem to illustrate this possibility.

Neurosyphilis sometimes receives the clinical diagnosis neurasthenia simply through omission to apply proved diagnostic methods. An instance is given in which the PARETIC form of NEUROSYPHILIS (" general paresis ") received the diagnosis *neurasthenia* § for a period of five years, at any time during which period it would doubtless have been possible to render the correct diagnosis and apply treatment.

---

* Flora Black (6).

† Mrs. Lecompte (7).

‡ John Wyman (8).

§ Greeley Harrison (9). *Also* Albert Robinson (45), Alice Caperson (46), Abel Bachmann (74).

Neurosyphilis may imitate not only the psychoneuroses but also the psychoses themselves. We present a case of an architect, which looked almost precisely like *manic-depressive psychosis* * and had a history of attacks, but in which the positive serum W. R. led (in accordance with hospital rules) to an examination of the spinal fluid. The spinal fluid tests proved the case to be one of PARETIC NEUROSYPHILIS.

However, a positive serum W. R., even when associated with mental symptoms, and when those mental symptoms include grandiosity, does not prove the existence of neurosyphilis either in its paretic or non-paretic form. Our instance seems to be one of MANIC–DEPRESSIVE PSYCHOSIS. † The spinal fluid tests were entirely negative. The course of the disease was also that of manic-depressive psychosis. In the absence of positive spinal fluid tests, the diagnosis neurosyphilis was excluded.

Neurosyphilis and even PARETIC NEUROSYPHILIS may result in symptoms that would ordinarily lead to the diagnosis *dementia praecox*.‡

It is important not to rule out neurosyphilis on the ground of a *negative serum* W. R. The fluid W. R. may turn out positive. We present a case (of a salesman)§ in which the serum W. R. was repeatedly negative (even salvarsan did not act provocatively) yet the spinal fluid W. R. proved positive. The case was clinically one of classical PARETIC NEUROSYPHILIS ("general paresis"). It is a good rule to proceed to lumbar puncture, even when the serum W. R. is negative, if there are suspicious symptoms (e.g., speech defect and

---

* Lyman Agnew (10). *Also* Ethel Hunter (47), Bessie Vogel (52), Isaac Thompson (83), Juliette Lachine (11).

† JulietteLachine(11). *Also* Lyman Agnew (10), Ethel Hunter (47), Bessie Vogel (52), Isaac Thompson (83).

‡ Henry Philipps (12). *Also* Bridget Curley (59), Margaret O'Brien (68), Annie Martin (117).

§ William Twist (13). *Also* Lester Crane (20), Thomas Donovan (23).

memory impairment, grandiosity) or signs (e.g., marked reflex disorder, especially pupillary disorder).

DIFFUSE NEUROSYPHILIS was above defined as "meningo-vasculoparenchymatous." This disease is typically associated with six positive tests (positive serum W. R., positive fluid W. R., pleocytosis, gold sol reaction, positive globulin reaction and excess albumin). One or more and frequently several of these six tests are likely to run mild in diffuse neurosyphilis; that is to say, these tests are apt to run milder than the identical tests in paretic neurosyphilis ("general paresis"). The clinical course of the diffuse, and especially the meningovascular cases, is likely to be protracted. The prognosis as to life is good, barring fatal vascular insults. The illustrative case * was a case with slow course. There was a series of attacks followed by a paralytic stroke, a finding highly typical of the diffuse form of neurosyphilis. The spinal fluid reactions were mild, suitable to the general principle above stated.

These tests are likely to run stronger, as above stated, in paretic neurosyphilis (" general paresis "), than in the diffuse form. In particular, the gold sol reaction is likely to be shown in what is termed " paretic " form rather than in what is termed " syphilitic " form. The clinical course of PARETIC NEUROSYPHILIS is likely to be brief. A characteristic case † with very heavy globulin and albumin tests is presented.

TABO-PARETIC NEUROSYPHILIS ‡ (" taboparesis ") is clinically a combination of the symptoms of tabetic ("tabes dorsalis ") and those of paretic neurosyphilis (" general paresis "). First comes the tabes dorsalis lasting often for many years. Afterward follows a characteristic general paresis. The ultimate paretic picture is likely to retain, however, various characteristics of tabes. The laboratory tests in the paretic phase of taboparesis are characteristic

---

* John Jackson (14). *Also*
  Martha Bartlett (21),
  Paolo Marini (28),
  Margaret O'Brien (68).

† Pietro Martiro (15). *Also*
  Meyer Levenson (22),
  Achilles Akropovlos (50).

‡ Joseph Sullivan (16).

of general paresis and not of tabes dorsalis. The prognosis
after the paretic phase has arrived is that of general paresis.

The diagnosis of the neurosyphilitic forms would be easy
if these principles were always carried out to the letter.
The important fact is as follows: diffuse (that is, meningo-
vasculoparenchymatous neurosyphilis) may look like paretic
neurosyphilis (" general paresis ") * at certain periods of the
clinical and laboratory examination. This fact is of obvious
importance. The general prognosis of diffuse neurosyphilis
is regarded as good *quoad vitam*. The general prognosis of
paresis is bad. If, however, the differential diagnosis cannot
be rendered at particular phases of a given case, then no safe
prognosis can be offered in the individual case. In particular no prognosis affecting the administration or non-adminis-
tration of modern systematic treatment can or should be
offered in these doubtful phases.

It is not always safe to exclude neurosyphilis even when the
fluid W. R. is *negative*.† Particularly in vascular neurosyphilis the fluid W. R. and even all the other laboratory signs
in the spinal fluid may sometimes be negative. A positive
serum W. R. yields the correct pointer to diagnosis. Of
course, also in many cases of vascular neurosyphilis one or
more of the laboratory signs may be suggestive even when
the fluid W. R. is negative. Theoretically there may be
cases in which all the six tests are negative and yet the diagnosis neurosyphilis be the correct one.

A clinically important sign in neurosyphilis is the so-called
seizures. These occur both in DIFFUSE NON-PARETIC NEURO-
SYPHILIS ‡ and in PARETIC NEUROSYPHILIS.§

---

* Gregorian Petrcfski (17). *Also*
    Richard Lawlor (25),
    John Bennett (34),
    Julius Kantor (54),
    Albert Forest (112).

† Frederick Wescott (18). *Also*
    Martha Bartlett (21),
    James Burns (56),
    Victor Friedburg (108).

‡ Agnes O'Neil (19). *Also*
    Michael O'Donnell (24).
    John Edwards (104).
    Arthur Bright (121).

§ Lester Crane (20). *Also*
    Greeley Harrison (9).
    David Borofski (49).
    David Collins (61).

Aphasia is likewise a symptom in both these forms of neurosyphilis, namely, in the DIFFUSE non-paretic * and in the PARETIC form.†

The literature contains reference not only to seizures and aphasia as characteristically paretic but also to *remissions*. Remissions like seizures and aphasia are found in both the PARETIC ‡ and NON-PARETIC forms of neurosyphilis.§ They have important bearings on prognosis in all forms of neurosyphilis and are of especial significance in the evaluation of treatment. (Remissions coincident with apparent cure.)

So far we have been dealing with cases of neurosyphilis in which there was no doubt of the existence of mental symptoms. There are cases, however, in which although the laboratory signs of neurosyphilis exist, proving beyond doubt the existence of a chronic inflammatory reaction and allied pathological conditions in the cerebrospinal axis, there are no mental symptoms of neurosyphilis. We have called some of these cases PARESIS SINE PARESI ‖ and present examples.

To illustrate complications we give a case of PARETIC NEU-ROSYPHILIS with autopsy in which there were ante mortem signs of HERPES ZOSTER ¶ or, at all events, of a skin eruption limited to the area of a thoracic nerve.

A case of GUMMA of the brain ** in which decompression was warranted and performed is presented. The fluid W. R., as in many such cases, was negative; serum positive.

A case of CRANIAL NEUROSYPHILIS (extraocular palsy†† without mental symptoms) showed a positive Wassermann serum test and a negative spinal fluid.

---

* Martha Bartlett (21). *Also* Agnes O'Neil (19), Vivian Walker (87).

† Meyer Levenson (22). *Also* Albert Forest (112).

‡ Thomas Donovan (23). *Also* William Twist (13), Bessie Vogel (52), David Collins (61).

§ Michael O'Donnell (24). *Also* Alice Morton (1).

‖ Richard Lawlor (25). *Also* Bessie Vogel (52), ——— ——— (88).

¶ John Morrill (26).

** David Tannenbaum (27). *Also* Mrs. LeCompte (7), Annie Rivers (109).

†† Paolo Marini (28). *Also* Flora Black (6).

The laboratory reactions in TABETIC NEUROSYPHILIS *
(" tabes dorsalis ") run somewhat like those of diffuse non-
paretic neurosyphilis and are accordingly milder than those
of paretic neurosyphilis. The fluid W. R. and the gold sol
reaction in particular are apt to run mild. The clinical course
of tabes dorsalis is well known to be protracted and the prognosis *quoad vitam* is good except that we must alway bear in
mind the possibility of vascular insults and complications
of a syphilitic origin in the rest of the body.

It is important to remember that TABETIC NEUROSYPHILIS
is often quite atypical † clinically and may even show no
single symptom warranting the old clinical name locomotor
ataxia.

There are even cases in which the name tabes dorsalis is
not warranted in view of the fact that the lesions are not
low in the cord but are higher up (TABES CERVICALIS‡).

A rare form of neurosyphilis is ERB'S SYPHILITIC SPASTIC
PARAPLEGIA§ against which one needs to consider a number
of non-syphilitic spinal cord diseases. Our case showed a
weakly positive serum W. R., a negative fluid W. R., and the
other tests of the spinal fluid were moderately positive.

SYPHILITIC MUSCULAR ATROPHY ‖ is classified by Head and
Fearnsides both in their meningovascular group and in their
group of the so-called syphilis centralis. Our case affecting
in large part the small muscles of the hands in a teamster,
may be due either to spinal parenchymal lesions or to root
neuritis or to both.

It is a little extraordinary and very important that the
laboratory signs are apt to be positive even in the SECONDARY
period of SYPHILIS. Perhaps a third of all cases of syphilis in
the secondaries would, if tested, yield positives precisely
like those of full-blown paretic or diffuse neurosyphilis.

---

* Mario Sanzi (29). *Also*   † Stephen Green (30). *Also*
  Stephen Green (30),   Paul Halleck (31),
  Paul Halleck (31).   Henri Lepère (105),
                                  Ivan Rokicki (111).

‡ Paul Halleck (31).
§ Margaret Neal (32).
‖ Joseph Graham (33).

Strangely enough, these signs may occur without clinical symptoms. The illustrative case,* a mechanic, yielded vari- ous mental symptoms. The cases of secondary syphilis with laboratory signs of neurosyphilis but without clinical symp- toms are of the greatest theoretical importance in relation to the problem above mentioned of *paresis sine paresi*. It may well be inquired whether in some instances the neuro- syphilis of the secondaries does not persist until the ex- hibition of mental or physical symptoms of neurosyphilis years later. It must be remembered that this conception is hardly more than a hypothesis at the present time. That such signs of chronic inflammation could exist without symptoms is not so surprising when one thinks of the startling immediate improvement seen after treatment or even in remissions without treatment. One is reminded of the crisis in pneumonia wherein clinical improvement takes place en- tirely independent of the mechanical conditions in the lung which just after the crisis remain as suppurative as before.

The diagnosis of JUVENILE NEUROSYPHILIS is made upon the same lines as that of neurosyphilis in the adult. We pre- sent two cases, one with optic atrophy† and the other with signs of congenital syphilis antedating the symptoms of paresis.‡

Congenital syphilis is also apparently capable of producing a simple form of FEEBLEMINDEDNESS,§ that is to say, a form of disease non-paretic, non-tabetic, and without special tend- ency to vascular insults.

We present a case of JUVENILE TABETIC NEUROSYPHILIS ("juvenile tabes").‖ The tests were all positive.

The line of separation between typical and atypical cases of neurosyphilis is vague and indistinct and some of the

---

* John Bennett (34). *Also*   ‡ Theresa Mullen (36). *Also*
  Alice Caperson (46),   John Lawrence (5),
  Florence Fitzgerald (81),   John Friedreich (77),
  Vivian Walker (87),   Gridley Ringer (78),
  Arthur Bright (121).   James Arnold (80).

† Mary Coughlin (35).   § Isaac Goldstein (37).

‖ Archibald Sherry (38).

cases classified by us amongst puzzles perhaps belong under
systematic diagnosis and vice versa. The section on PUZ-
ZLES AND ERRORS in the diagnosis of neurosyphilis is
introduced by six cases of error in the diagnosis of the paretic
form of neurosyphilis.* These errors were made known by
autopsy. Aside from the sixth case, whose etiology must remain in doubt and which was a unique case of PERIVASCULAR
GLIOSIS, there is ground for the belief that the other five cases
in this Danvers Hospital study of diagnostic errors were perhaps actually syphilitic though not of the paretic form of
neurosyphilis. At all events, the brain tissues in these cases
failed to show the plasma cell deposits which are characteristic
in the sheaths of the intracortical vessels in paretic neurosyphilis.

A case illustrates the complication of TABES by *arteriosclerotic symptoms*, in which case the arteriosclerosis may
naturally have been of syphilitic origin. Two cases especially
illustrate the possibility of confusing the ataxia of general
paresis with CEREBELLAR ATAXIA. These cases showed
lesions of the cerebellar structures, notably of the dentate
nucleus. No one can read these cases or any of the autopsied cases in our series, without perceiving how fundamental
and even critical is the demand for autopsies in fatal cases
of neurosyphilis. The practitioner who can secure an autopsy
in a fatal case of neurosyphilis and have the tissues worked
up by approved neuropathological methods is almost bound
to add his bit to neurological theory. Even cases of classical
tabes dorsalis are often signally important to the theorist on
account of the relations of the neural to the non-neural complications.

We then proceed to a group of cases without special order
in which a variety of diagnostic questions arose.

A case of questionable neurosyphilis in the secondary stage
of syphilis brings up the problems of syphilitic *neurasthenia*.†

---

* Caroline Davis (39).   Elizabeth Brown (42).
  H. F. (40).   Robert Allen (43).
  Samuel North (41).   John Hughes (44).

          † Albert Robinson (45). *Also*
          Greeley Harrison (9).

Syphilis may act as *agent provocateur* of HYSTERIA as Charcot insisted.*

A case illustrative of difficulties in diagnosis between neuro-syphilis and manic-depressive psychosis follows.†

A case for diagnosis is given which shows that errors in the diagnosis of neurosyphilis are entirely possible even when abundant clinical and laboratory data are available. A case with a weakly positive Wassermann reaction in the spinal fluid finally turned out to be one of BRAIN TUMOR.‡

Some questions as to the diagnosis of NEUROSYPHILIS *versus Idiopathic Epilepsy* are brought up by a case in which phe-nomena of paresis seemed to have occurred very early, about two years after the initial syphilitic infection.§

A case of PARETIC NEUROSYPHILIS is offered in which *hemiplegia* and *hemitremor* strongly suggested *vascular* lesions; but the autopsy showed no coarse lesions and merely con-firmed the diagnosis paresis microscopically.‖

An autopsied case of PARETIC NEUROSYPHILIS is given, in which the pupils persisted in reacting normally. Herpes zoster-like lesions in life yielded no special signs at autopsy (all root-ganglia looked alike above and below zone of "shingles.")¶

An example of NEUROSYPHILIS, probably PARETIC, yielded symptoms highly suggestive of *manic-depressive psychosis.*** An interesting feature in this case was the birth of a healthy child nine months after the onset of the psychotic attack.

An example of *exophthalmic goitre* †† following the ac-quisition of SYPHILIS showed at autopsy a heavy scarring of the optic thalamus and unilaterally atrophic process in the cerebral cortex.

---

* Alice Caperson (46). *Also* Florence Fitzgerald (81).

† Ethel Hunter (47). *Also* Lyman Agnew (10), Bessie Vogel (52), Juliette Lachine (11).

‡ Milton Safsky (48). *Also* Daniel Falvey (55).

§ David Borosfski (49). *Also* Lester Crane (20).

‖ Achilles Akropovlos (50).
¶ Daniel Wheelwright (51).

** Bessie Vogel (52). *Also* Lyman Agnew (10), Juliette Lachine (11), Ethel Hunter (47).

†† Carrie Pearson (53).

We come to some questions concerning the *Argyll-Robertson pupil*. It is agreed on all hands that the Argyll-Robertson pupil is characteristic of the paretic and tabetic forms, but the sign occurs also in other neurosyphilitic conditions;* in fact the sign does not necessarily indicate neurosyphilis as an instance of PINEAL TUMOR demonstrates.†

The question raised above as to the possibility that neurosyphilis may exist in the absence of positive findings in the spinal fluid is illustrated in a man, a mechanic, who claimed syphilitic infection and showed an *Argyll-Robertson pupil* on one side.‡   The serum W. R. was positive; the *fluid tests* were *negative*.

An extraordinary case is given in some detail in which NEUROSYPHILIS in the form termed DISSEMINATED ENCEPHALITIS§ proved fatal within seven months of the initial infection.

We have frequently mentioned the classical assumption that paretic neurosyphilis ("general paresis") is a fatal disease. Some have suggested that there is another form clinically almost identical with general paresis except that it pursues a long course and the suggestion has been made that these cases be termed *pseudoparesis*.|| We are of the opinion that this term should be dropped and advocate the use of the word pseudoparesis only for non-syphilitic disease looking like paresis, such as alcoholic pseudoparesis and the like.

The question whether there is a form of mental disease SYPHILITIC PARANOIA¶ is raised by a case with auditory hallucinations, ideas of persecution and attacks of excitement. The diagnosis of alcoholic hallucinosis was actually made although there is no proof that the patient ever drank alcohol. Alcohol may cause symptoms identical with those of

---

* Julius Kantor (54).   *Cf.*   ‡ James Burns (56).   *Also*
  James Burns (56).   Frederick Wescott (18),
  Henri Lepère (105).   Martha Bartlett (21),
  Frederick Stone (106).   Victor Friedburg (108).

† Daniel Falvey (55).   *Cf.*   § John Summers (57).
  Francis Murphy (60). || Peter Burkhardt (58).

¶ Bridget Curley (59).

paretic neurosyphilis, including seizures, Argyll-Robertson pupils, speech defect and mental symptoms. The differentation is readily made by the negative laboratory findings. An illustration is given in our case of the alcoholic teamster. Cases such as this bear the name ALCOHOLIC PSEUDO-PARESIS.*

However, when the clinical picture is the same as in the case of our teamster, the alcohol may only be a complicating factor in neurosyphilis, as shown by our next case of the *alcoholic* steamfitter who in fact was shown to have NEURO-SYPHILIS.†

Sometimes cases of apparently frank *alcoholism*, even with apparently characteristic delirium tremens and neuritis, prove to be essentially neurosyphilitic.‡ On the other hand, true combinations of ALCOHOLISM and NEUROSYPHILIS occur which it would be proper to classify under either heading and in which therapy must take serious account of both conditions.§

As above stated, we elect to use the term pseudoparesis only for non-syphilitic cases. There are other forms of pseudoparesis than alcoholic pseudoparesis. The question of *Diabetic Pseudoparesis* is raised by an exceedingly complicated case of which our best interpretation is that the patient, a proved syphilitic (with syphilitic osteomyelitis (?)), a huge doorkeeper, was perhaps suffering from an old SYPHILITIC scarring of the PITUITARY body.|| Neither this case nor a second case, one of PARETIC NEUROSYPHILIS with *glycosuria* is actually entitled to the diagnosis diabetic pseudoparesis. The second case of paretic neurosyphilis with glycosuria brings up some unanswerable questions as to the pancreatic or basal meningitic or other origin for the glycosuria.¶

Isolated symptoms are often presented by neurosyphilitics (e.g., hemianopsia);** but we tend to regard these cases as due to focal lesions that are merely part and parcel of DIFFUSE LESIONS.

---

* Francis Murphy (60).   § Albert Fielding (63).

† David Collins (61). || Calvin Hall (64).

‡ Joseph Buck (62).   ¶ Donald Barrie (65).

          ** Lawrence Washington (66)

A neurosyphilitic case (a steward) with the rather unusual complication (for our northern region) of severe MALARIA producing cerebral thrombosis is reported.*

The diagnosis *Dementia Praecox* † was actually made in the case of a young school teacher in whom the laboratory findings proved conclusively that the condition was one of NEUROSYPHILIS. The gold sol reaction in this case was mild. The chief lesion at autopsy was a fresh looking, gelatinous pial exudate over the spinal cord which turned out to contain an almost pure display of very numerous plasma cells.

The question of LUES MALIGNA ‡ is brought up in a rectifier of spirits in whom the characteristic tremendous destruction of tissue, toxemia and failure to react to antisyphilitic treatment were illustrated. Moreover, this case had a trauma (cautery) to the tonsil, as in other cases of lues maligna.

A case somewhat suggestive of *brain tumor*, of *neurosyphilis* and of *multiple sclerosis* § turned out to be MULTIPLE SCLEROSIS (the fluid showed a pleocytosis and a moderate amount of globulin with a paretic type of gold sol reaction).

As a foil to this case that we regard as multiple sclerosis, we present a second case with nystagmus, optic atrophy and spasticity in which the suspicion of *multiple sclerosis* might well be raised but which the tests demonstrated to be NEUROSYPHILITIC.||

An even stranger imitation of well-defined non-syphilitic entities was presented by a case apparently of *Huntington's chorea*¶ (except for absence of the hereditary taint) which case, however, proved to the surprise of all diagnosticians to be one of NEUROSYPHILIS.

Frequent errors of diagnosis must occur in the field of the senile psychoses. We present a case that would at first blush warrant the diagnosis of *senile arteriosclerotic psychosis***

---

* Joseph Temple (67).   ‡ Frank Mason (69).

† Margaret O'Brien (68). *Also*   § Annie Kelly (70).
Henry Phillips (12).   James Lauder (71).
Bridget Curley (59).
Annie Martin (117). || James Lauder (71).

                        ¶ Margaret Green (72).

    ** Marcus Chatterton (73).

in a sea captain of 75 years (wife dead 15 years before of general paresis) who turned out to be a characteristic case from the laboratory standpoint of NEUROSYPHILIS.

The Protean nature of the symptomatology of neurosyphilis is sufficiently established. Still, a case that might fit into textbooks concerning DISSOCIATION OF PERSONALITY * is certainly a clinical oddity, as illustrated by a fugacious musician.

A case with strong suspicions of *neurosyphilis* of *tabetic* type turned out to be more probably one of neural complications in PERNICIOUS ANEMIA.†

NEUROSYPHILIS IN JUVENILES presents puzzling conditions. One case was marked clinically by *attacks of excitement*.‡ It is impossible to place this case among the main groups of juvenile neurosyphilis.

Another case of FEEBLEMINDEDNESS, § also NEUROSYPHI-LITIC in origin, presented physical symptoms and laboratory signs of paretic neurosyphilis; yet this case had been considered one of *simple feeblemindedness*.

A case apparently of JUVENILE PARETIC NEUROSYPHILIS in a 15 year old boy presented the rather unusual complication of shocks with quadriplegia,|| a *vascular complication* not usually expected in the paretic type of neurosyphilis in adults.

Epileptic phenomena¶ are rare as the effect of JUVENILE NEUROSYPHILIS, but occur as demonstrated in a case which slipshod methods of diagnosis might well have regarded as one of *idiopathic epilepsy*.

A case of JUVENILE PARETIC NEUROSYPHILIS with the complication of ADDISON'S DISEASE ** is given (autopsy confirmation).

The puzzle in diagnosis offered by syphilis in the secondary stage †† is illustrated by a case which showed the characteristic NEUROSYPHILITIC complications of the SECONDARY STAGE of

---

* Abel Bachman (74).
† Mrs. Brown (75).
‡ James Seabrook (76).
§ John Friedreich(77). *Cf.* Isaac Goldstein (37).
|| Gridley Ringer (78).
¶ John Doran (79).

** James Arnold (80).
†† Florence Fitzgerald (81). *Also* John Bennett (34), Alice Caperson (46), Vivian Walker (87), Arthur Bright (121).

syphilis. This patient may well have been a moron at the outset and exhibited some reactions (refusal to talk) explicable on
the basis of feeblemindedness. She was a neurosyphilitic only
in the sense of the neural complication that we find in the
secondary stage of syphilis. As stated above, we do not yet
know what the fate of these neural complications of secondary
syphilis is to be. The frequency of this finding in secondary
syphilis is probably too great to warrant the hypothesis that
it must always go on to a chronic neurosyphilis; but we
certainly are warranted in regarding these cases as potential
chronic neurosyphilitics.

A case of TABOPARETIC NEUROSYPHILIS in which the heavy
exudate characteristic of paresis became a soil for a growth
of the typhoid bacillus is presented with autopsy.* This
fatality with TYPHOID MENINGITIS is merely a concrete example of the many complications which syphilitics and especially neurosyphilitics have to sustain.

The case series then goes on to illustrate, though quite
inadequately, a variety of MEDICOLEGAL AND SOCIAL
complications of neurosyphilis. It is well known that many
social complications with grave moral, economic and even
political difficulties occur.

Our series starts with a "public character"† whose eloquence and reformatory efforts led to a considerable notoriety. The autopsy in this case showed singularly few lesions
despite the fact that the case was microscopically one of
wholly characteristic PARETIC NEUROSYPHILIS. The question might arise how far we are entitled to correlate the reformatory efforts of this always eccentric character with syphilis.
The man himself a physician, was aware of the doubt which his
Argyll-Robertson pupils threw upon his medical situation.
He explained them on the basis of an old smallpox! We are
inclined to think that the whole of this man's life, from his
giving up of medical practice to live as a kind of literary and
political hack, was due to subtle changes of neurosyphilitic

---

* Frederick Estabrook (82).

† Maj. Isaac Thompson, M.D. (83).

origin. The fact that there was a certain delinquent streak in the man is not inconsistent with this idea. Interestingly enough, a fall on the ice in the man's 61st year actually started up the fatal process, a condition of affairs amply illustrated in cases of neurosyphilis, brought out by trauma that come to the attention of the Industrial Accident Board in connection with claims for compensation.

A case of sudden *grandiosity** illustrates an episode of NEUROSYPHILITIC origin. Such a person might well be regarded by the lay newspaper reader as a crank or a grafter but the neurosyphilitic possibility should always be entertained in cases of this order.

As against the social difficulties that look in the direction of the classical paretic grandeur, we present a case of apparent *suicidal attempt* by gas, which attempt was followed by a period of amnesia that, taking into account the laboratory findings, was probably NEUROSYPHILITIC.†

Vistas of extraordinary interest are opened out by studies of the relation of neurosyphilis to *delinquency*. The case of the psychopathic reformer (Case 83) above mentioned was one in which the delinquency may possibly have been related to acquired syphilis. We present also a case of juvenile neurosyphilis, a young man of reform school type ‡ in which JUVENILE PARETIC NEUROSYPHILIS was established. This patient, in fact, deteriorated very rapidly to a condition of considerable dementia a few months after the diagnosis was established.

A striking case of so-called DEFECTIVE DELINQUENCY is presented, an alcoholic prostitute of the reformatory group.§ The NEUROSYPHILIS in this case was a complication rather than an original factor in the delinquency.

One case of PARESIS SINE PARESI was that of an habitual criminal ‖ and forger who, without showing mental or physical symptoms of neurosyphilis, yielded the laboratory signs of paretic neurosyphilis. Again, as in the case of the prostitute

---

* Lester Smith (84).

† Annie Marks (85).

‡ Frank Johnson (86).

§ Vivian Walker (87).

‖ ——— ——— (88). *Cf.*
Richard Lawlor (25).
Bessie Vogel (52).

just mentioned, the CRIMINALITY seems to have antedated the neurosyphilis and even to have been hereditary.

By way of introducing the next group of Industrial Accident Board cases, we present a case of JUVENILE PARESIS with initial TRAUM.

The Industrial Board group is of note in that the signs of the traumatic form † of paretic neurosyphilis do not occur immediately upon the accident. Some time elapses in which the physical, chemical or parasitological changes have time to work themselves out in the injured tissues. Many hypotheses may be raised as to the reason why a trauma lights up a syphilitic process. Of course, **false claims ‡ may be made for compensation by neurosyphilitics** in whom the symptoms were already in existence before the accident and in whom they may not even be markedly exacerbated by the accident. The false claimants can probably not readily frame a story which the expert psychiatrist cannot discredit if he is allowed to perform laboratory tests and give the patient the benefit of thorough examination. However, some cases of established PARETIC NEUROSYPHILIS are perhaps truly subject to *exacerbations* § of the clinical process and it may well be held that such exacerbations warrant partial compensation.

The fact that a trauma may light up a syphilitic process is illustrated in a case that came to the Psychopathic Hospital, in which a SYPHILITIC LESION developed in the skull AT THE SITE OF SKULL INJURY.||

A case of OCCUPATION-NEUROSIS ¶ that might be interpreted as a *syphilitic neuritis* is presented. The case is still in doubt as to its scientific evaluation.

The workmen's compensation group of syphilitic cases is of extraordinary general interest since it indicates that

---

* Margaret Tennyson (89).
John Lawrence (5).
Mary Coughlin (35).
Theresa Mullen (36).
John Friedreich (77).
Gridley Ringer (78).
James Arnold (80).

† Joseph O'Hearn (90).

‡ Levi Sussman (91).

§ Joseph Larkin (92).

|| Richard Marshall (93).

¶ David Fitzpatrick (94).

employers may well be on the lookout not to employ known syphilitics unless fortified by special insurance arrangements. Whether in future employers may desire **to employ only W. R. negative workmen** is one of the highly complicated questions *re* workmen's compensation and health insurance.

But the problems of neurosyphilis are not merely medico-legal and broadly public or social. The most appealing difficulties lodge within the bosom of the family. Now and then a case of INCOMPATIBILITY OF TEMPERAMENT, perhaps complicated by *alcoholism*, occurs which tests prove to be NEUROSYPHILITIC.*

Special attention should be drawn to a certain NEURO-SYPHILITIC FAMILY † in which both parents and five children showed a variety of syphilitic diseases, including syphilis without apparent neural complications, paretic neurosyphilis, juvenile paresis, aortic aneurysm, achondroplasia and caries of the spine, and an as yet indefinite neurosis. There was a sixth child that died shortly after birth, as well as three still-born.

One **cannot conclude** from the normal ‡ look of a neuro-syphilitic's family **that the normal looking members are not syphilitic,** as illustrated by the family of our draughtsman.

The most **intricate social complications** may arise. We present a case of a syphilitic man (a well-to-do merchant) who was apparently being goaded into a second marriage § because he was continually being charged with having caused his first wife's death. This he had actually done in a certain sense because his wife had died of general paresis, having contracted syphilis from him.

In the fifth section on THERAPY, we have attempted to outline some of the principles and problems that arise in the treatment of neurosyphilis. Enough has probably been said

---

* Joseph Wilson (95).   ‡ Walter Heinmas (97).

† Becky Bornstein (96).   § Mr. Jacobs (98).
  Walter Heinmas (97).
  Mr. Jacobs (98).

concerning the attitude of optimism or pessimistic nihilism that may be adopted toward the whole subject. It must be borne in mind, however, that a great deal of the work on treatment of neurosyphilis is still in the experimental stage. As a rule, each case must be considered separately and individually and the prognosis can be made satisfactorily only after treatment has been given. This section contains a group of cases that have been treated rather intensively and the results of this treatment are indicated. The section is introduced by *five untreated cases*, the brains and cords of which have been studied post mortem. These illustrate the pathological conditions which we have to meet, and from these examples we can draw the theoretical conclusion that some cases are beyond the aid of therapy on account of the brain destruction. Others, in which the symptomatology bespeaks just as grave a situation, turn out on autopsy to have very little actual damage to the brain tissues and therefore should theoretically at any rate be amenable to antisyphilitic therapy.

In order to get any adequate conception of the possibilities of therapeutic results in cases of neurosyphilis, one must consider the pathological changes that occur and how far these changes are reparable. In cases in which the destruction of tissue is marked, it is, of course, out of the question to expect to get any marked clinical improvement. A case of spastic hemiplegia * in paretic neurosyphilis is given with the autopsy findings as an illustration of irreparable damage that may occur to the parenchymatous structure, thus precluding any chance of functional recovery.

On the other hand, there is a group of cases in which the symptoms may be exceedingly severe and yet the actual destruction of tissue be almost nil. This point is illustrated by a case † in which *total duration of symptoms* terminating in death was *only 22 days*. At autopsy there was very little in the way of macroscopical lesions, and microscopically there was no marked evidence of destruction in the parenchymatous

---

* James McDevitt (99).

† Jacob Methuen (100).

tissue. The lesions were represented chiefly by perivascular infiltration. According to all our modern ideas, this type of reaction is resolvable under antisyphilitic treatment. Though this case was one of very short duration, similar pathological pictures may be obtained in cases of considerably longer standing. It is also of great importance to remember that symptomatically such a case may be in no way distinguished from a case with marked atrophy.

Another autopsied case is given which shows an exceedingly **marked meningitis.*** The meningitic processes according to the literature and experience react very readily to antisyphilitic treatment in the form either of mercury and iodid or in combination with salvarsan. The lesion here present would probably have improved had intensive treatment been given. Clinically the diagnosis of general paresis was made and, as has been the rule in the past, treatment was not given on the ground that it had no value in paresis. While this is an extreme case of meningitis, it is to be remembered that the vast majority of cases of paretic neurosyphilis show some degree of meningitis. Just as in the marked meningitis of the diffuse neurosyphilis, so with the meningitis of the paretic form, improvement is expected under treatment. As a part or even the whole of the symptomatology in a given case may be due to this meningitic process, we have reason occasionally to expect marked improvement as the result of antisyphilitic treatment.

As a contrast to this case with marked meningitis, another case of **marked atrophy** † is given. Here the atrophy was very perceptible on macroscopical examination and the mere view of the brain at once indicated that in such a case important results from treatment were not to be expected.

The **topographical variation** of the lesions in neurosyphilis must be remembered when treatment is to be instituted. Thus very marked lesions may exist in portions of the brain which do not give any very definite localizing symptoms. As a result, one may be led to believe from clinical evidence that the case is a very mild one though the lesions may

---

* John Baxter (101).   † Theodosia Jewett (102).

really be very extensive. The topographical distribution must, therefore, be taken into consideration in trying to estimate the damage done. This point of topographical distribution of the lesions is illustrated by a case.*

It has been generally recognized that **clinical improvement,** if not cure, may be **readily obtained in the group of diffuse neurosyphilis,** i.e., so-called cerebral and cerebrospinal forms of syphilis. These are cases in which the parenchyma is very slightly, if at all, affected and in which the lesion is chiefly in the meninges and blood vessels, irritative rather than degenerative. A case † is given to illustrate this point. In our experience systematic intravenous salvarsan therapy associated with mercury and iodid gives remarkably good results in the vast majority of this group of cases.

It is generally conceded that antisyphilitic treatment, particularly salvarsan, has a very satisfactory result applied to diffuse neurosyphilis. But the same good results may be obtained in cases which are not so typically of the diffuse type. An illustration is given in the case of a machinist in which the diagnosis was in doubt between paretic, tabetic or diffuse neurosyphilis.‡ The result of treatment was as satisfactory as could be expected in any type of neurosyphilis and this in a case of several years' duration with Argyll-Robertson pupils.

As a rule, the Argyll-Robertson pupil is taken as a grave omen for treatment, an idea based upon a conception that the Argyll-Robertson pupil so frequently represents the old so-called " parasyphilitic " cases, which, in the past were taught as being incapable of improvement by the ordinary antisyphilitic methods.

A second case § with Argyll-Robertson pupil shows again that the **prognosis may be very good despite the Argyll-Robertson sign.**

---

* A. W. (103).

† John Edwards (104). *Cf.*
  Henri Lepère (105),
  Frederick Stone (106),
  Arthur Bright (121),

Agnes O'Neil (19),
Paulo Marini (28).

‡ Henri Lepère (105). *Cf.*
  Julius Kantor (54).

§ Frederick Stone (106).

But even in the diffuse neurosyphilis, the symptomatic results of treatment may not be entirely happy. Under treatment it may be possible to reduce the spinal fluid tests to
negative without, however, as in the case of our hemiplegic
lady,* making the physical or mental symptoms disappear.
In other words, it may be possible to stop the active progress of the disease without removing the symptoms.

One is always warned of the danger of intravenous salvarsan
therapy in hemiplegic cases due to arteriosclerotic conditions.
While this warning is well justified, it does not mean that the
most intensive treatment is contraindicated, as shown in the
case of our hemiplegic machinist.† Such may be given over
long periods of time with the most satisfactory results.

A case ‡ is given which illustrates the value of antisyphilitic
treatment in cases showing symptoms of intracranial pressure due to syphilitic disease. In the case of the woman which
we cite, we believe that the symptoms of intracranial pressure
were probably due to a gummatous new growth, although it is
possible that they were due to a marked meningitic process.
However, the results of a limited amount of antisyphilitic
treatment in this case were very brilliant. Similar results
may often be obtained in gumma of the brain. This is not
always true, however, and it may become necessary to use
surgical procedure in order rapidly to overcome the effects of
intracranial pressure.

While it has always been conceded that treatment would
greatly help cases of diffuse and vascular neurosyphilis, the
utmost pessimism has existed concerning the results to be
obtained by treatment in cases of tabetic and paretic neurosyphilis. Only in the last five or six years, due to the stimulus
of Ehrlich's discovery of salvarsan and the introduction of the
intraspinous methods of therapy, have intensive work and
study been given to the treatment of these cases. And though
it has been by no means settled in the minds of the various
workers in this field, as to what the ultimate results of such

---

* Greta Meyer (107).   *Cf.*   † Victor Friedburg (108).
  John Jackson (14).   ‡ Annie Rivers (109).

treatment will be and though some do not believe that there is any good to be expected from our present methods, still the majority of men who are treating these cases systematically feel very much encouraged.

At times very brilliant results are to be obtained by intraspinous treatment **in tabetic neurosyphilis** (" tabes dorsalis "). A very striking illustration is given of a case of this sort in which the symptoms dated only a few months but which had all the classical symptoms, signs and laboratory tests. Five intraspinous injections of mercurialized serum were sufficient to cause the disappearance of the subjective symptoms and to reduce the spinal fluid test to negative.*

It must be emphasized that the best results in cases of tabetic neurosyphilis are usually to be expected in cases in which the symptoms are of short standing. Where the process is of long duration and much destruction of spinal cord tissue has occurred, the best one can expect is that the activity and progress may be halted. This is illustrated by our case of a baker, 43 years of age, who had been suffering from the symptoms of tabes for some years. Under treatment it was possible to get an entirely negative serology of the blood and spinal fluid.† Despite this evidence that the activity of syphilis had ceased, the symptoms continued unabated. We are ready to believe, however, that much good was accomplished. For the patient should not have any further untoward developments or the appearance of any new symptoms. These, without such treatment, might well be expected. At times excellent clinical results are obtained in long standing cases.

The results of treatment in paretic neurosyphilis (" general paresis ") have been considered even less hopeful than in tabetic neurosyphilis (" tabes dorsalis "); indeed, it has often been stated that the patients are made worse by treatment. Recent work, however, supports a much more optimistic viewpoint. We feel that **intensive treatment has been of the greatest value in a number of cases of paretic**

---

* Mr. McKenzie (110). *Cf.* † Ivan Rokicki (111).
Ivan Rokicki (111).

neurosyphilis. Two cases are given which show the most satisfactory and brilliant results of intensive intravenous salvarsan therapy in cases diagnosed as general paresis. The first case, an excellent salesman, 46 years of age, with most aggravated mental symptoms, recovered symptomatically and all his tests were rendered negative.* He has now remained entirely well and economically efficient for about two years without further treatment. The other case, † a housewife, also with very marked symptoms suggestive in all ways of general paresis, also recovered rapidly under treatment and her tests became negative. Her remission has now lasted for nearly three years without further treatment.

At times it is not possible to get the spinal fluid tests to become negative in cases of paretic neurosyphilis under the most intensive salvarsan therapy. In spite of this, the clinical condition of the patient may improve so greatly that the patient can be considered **clinically recovered.** An illustration is given of an undertaker ‡ who was brought from a condition of the greatest cachexia and mental confusion to a condition of robust appearance and mental efficiency under intravenous salvarsan therapy, in spite of the fact that his tests were very slightly if at all reduced in intensity. He has been able to resume his former occupation and his former life with great satisfaction to himself and his family.

Improvement in paretic neurosyphilis under treatment is not to be expected very early. **Two or three months of active treatment** may elapse before one sees signs of improvement. Indeed, as illustrated by our case of the shipping clerk, this improvement may begin to make its appearance only after more than four months of intensive treatment consisting of two injections of salvarsan per week.§ In spite of the long delay in this case, complete clinical recovery occurred and the tests became almost negative at the end of a year of treatment.

---

* Albert Forest (112). *Cf.* Gussie Silverman (113), Walter Henry (114), William Rosetti (116), Annie Martin (117), Levi Morovitz (122), Peter Burkhardt (58).

† Gussie Silverman (113).

‡ Walter Henry (114).

§ Henry Ryan (115).

It is not only in the central nervous system that the syphilitic process may resist the most intensive treatment. In the case of the speculator, a victim of paretic neurosyphilis, which we cite, a perennially recurrent iritis appeared after several months of the most intensive salvarsan treatment which was apparently sufficient to reduce the symptoms of the paretic neurosyphilis,* but not of non-neural syphilis.

We give the case of a charwoman having the diagnosis of paretic neurosyphilis, who, under intensive treatment, made a symptomatic recovery. The interesting point in her findings is that all the tests in the spinal fluid became negative except the gold sol reaction which remained of the "paretic" type.† There is no general rule as to the reaction of the spinal fluid tests under treatment. At times one test is the first to disappear under treatment; again it is another. We have seen many cases in which the gold sol was the first test to become negative and others, as the case given, in which it is the last to show any change. As in our undertaker, symptomatic clinical improvement may be practically complete without any change in the spinal fluid tests.

One must remember that it is the condition of the patient that is of first importance; not so much the laboratory tests. Having shown the clinical recoveries with the tests remaining positive, we now have to report two cases in which there was **improvement** as shown **by the tests but no clinical improvement**. The first patient, a bank teller‡ of 39 years, with a diagnosis of paretic neurosyphilis, received intensive intravenous salvarsan for several months. Under this treatment all the tests became negative except the gold sol which remained of the paretic type. In spite of this, there was not the slightest improvement in his mental condition.

The second case, a young man of 29 years in whom the symptoms of neurosyphilis had recently appeared, under treatment showed a marked diminution in the intensity of the spinal

---

* William Rosetti (116).

† Annie Martin (117). *Cf.* William Roberts (118).

‡ William Roberts (118). John Silver (119).

fluid tests, notwithstanding which the patient became more and more demented and died after a series of convulsions.*

Of course, good results indicated above in some of our cases of paretic neurosyphilis are not to be expected in every case no matter how intensive the treatment. We give a case of paretic neurosyphilis in which the most intensive intravenous salvarsan therapy gave no satisfactory results. This was followed by several intraventricular injections of salvarsanized serum. The results of this combined treatment, however, were still not satisfactory, and the patient died.†

In order to emphasize as strongly as possible what we believe is a great **advantage of systematic intensive treatment** for neurosyphilis, we offer two cases in different time periods of neurosyphilis. The first is a printer with the symptoms of diffuse neurosyphilis six months after the appearance of his chancre.‡ These symptoms appeared despite three injections of salvarsan, injections of mercury and mercury by mouth. Under intensive treatment (meaning injections of salvarsan twice a week and continued injections of mercury), complete recovery occurred in a few weeks.

The second case is that of a waiter with signs and symptoms of neurosyphilis in whom the diagnosis lay between the diffuse and paretic forms.§ This patient developed his symptoms in spite of continuous antisyphilitic treatment during the six years since his infection. This treatment had been comparatively mild, consisting in great part of mercury by mouth. However, he had had courses of injections of mercury and several injections of salvarsan. Under a systematic course of intravenous injections of salvarsan twice a week for a number of months, all symptoms disappeared and the spinal fluid tests became negative as well as the W. R. in the blood serum.

A final case is offered which indicates that antisyphilitic treatment may occasionally be of service in improving the mentality of a FEEBLEMINDED CONGENITAL SYPHILITIC.||

---

* John Silver (119).   John Bennett (34).

† James McGinnis (120).   § Levi Morovitz (122).

‡ Arthur Bright (121). *Cf.* || Robert Matthews (23). *Cf.*
   Levi Morovitz (122),   Isaac Goldstein (37).

No attempt has been made in this section to give a per cent evaluation of the results of treatment in any one group of neurosyphilis. Two charts (charts 25 and 26), however, are appended which give an indication of some of our results. It seems to us, however, that it is too early to make any definite statements as to how far treatment will take us in the groups of neurosyphilis. We do feel decidedly, however, that many patients, in whatever group of neurosyphilis the diagnosis may place them, will respond to intensive systematic anti-syphilitic treatment. **It is unfair to give an entirely grave prognosis in any case of neurosyphilis until the effect of treatment has been tried.**

In a separate section, entitled NEUROSYPHILIS AND THE WAR, we have presented fourteen cases selected from British, French and German writers in the war literature of 1914–16. Most of these cases were naturally somewhat inadequately reported under the critical conditions of literature made in the war. We present the cases for what they are worth: at all events they draw attention to the extraordinary interest of the neurosyphilis problem in relation to the war.

Such cases as A, one of tabes dorsalis apparently developing paresis by a process akin to shell-shock, is of value in the interpretation of the development of paresis in civil life. By " shell-shock " we commonly refer to a condition in which there is no actual traumatic injury of the brain. The hypothesis must be then that the explosion in some way indirectly caused an alteration of living conditions of the spirochetes, permitting the development of paresis.

Case B similarly seems to be a case in which a latent syphilis has turned shell-shock into tabes dorsalis.

Cases C, D, E bring up the question of aggravation of neurosyphilis *by* service and *on* service, respectively.

Case F likewise shows how, in the determination of amount of pension, the probable duration of the neurosyphilitic process is important.

Case G seems to show that war stress alone, without the emotional or physical effects of shell-shock, may kindle a latent syphilis into paretic neurosyphilis.

Case H similarly suggests that, the "gassing" process may effect the same result.

Case I seems to show that the neuropathically tainted person may have latent epilepsy brought out through syphilis, the syphilis in this case having been acquired during the first summer of the war.

Case J was an interesting case of a syphilitic who, after the stress of the Battle of Dixmude, became an epileptic.

Syphilitic root-sciatica was developed in Case K at work in the war zone.

Case L is one of a civilian who apparently would not have developed paresis at precisely the moment when he did, if he had not been discharged as a German Jew from his long-held bank position in London.

Two cases, M and N, are cases of shell-shock, non-syphilitic; yet the picture of paresis in the one case and of tabes in the other was for a long time almost convincing to the examiners. They are better termed cases of pseudoparesis and pseudotabes, using the prefix "pseudo", as usual, to signify a non-syphilitic imitation of the disease in question.

To sum up in the most general way the lessons of this book, we may emphasize again (1) *the unity-in-variety of the phenomena of neurosyphilis*, (2) *the value of a hopeful approach to the therapy of all cases of neurosyphilis, even the paretic form*, and (3) *the value of applying syphilis tests to every case of neurosis or psychosis.*

(1) RE *unity-in-variety of neurosyphilitic phenomena.*

The unity of these phenomena is confirmed, theoretically, by the common factor of spirochetosis: practically, by the Wassermann reaction, positive in serum or spinal fluid! Almost at this point the unity of phenomena ceases. Neither chronicity, nor evidence of mononuclear cell-deposits, nor evidence of serious structural damage to the nervous system, nor presence of other positive tests than the W. R.,* nor

* For cases in which, without autopsy we have risked the diagnosis neurosyphilis *in the absence of W. R. in serum or fluid*, see William Twist (13), Frederick Wescott (18), Martha Bartlett (21), Thomas Donovan (23), Paolo Marini (28), Margaret Neal (32), Bridget Curley (59), Victor Friedburg (108), Ivan Rokicki (111).

existence of mental or nervous symptoms or signs, is a common feature of neurosyphilis. Sometimes the nervous system appears to harbor spirochetes in the most cordial manner as guest-friends (*paresis sine paresi.*) Again, perhaps as an expression of elaborate processes of immunity, the spirochetes take effect in relatively huge gummata. Sometimes the neurosyphilitic process rises as if by a regular process of siege from spinal nerve-root to spinal nerve-root (tabes dorsalis and diffuse neurosyphilis). Again, the nervous system is taken by storm, as it were (disseminated encephalitis). Very frequently the neurosyphilis is simply an indirect effect of blood-vessel disease, and huge masses of tissue are scooped out in necrosis with dependent secondary degenerations; and later the extinct lesions of vascular origin may or may not betray evidence of their syphilitic origin. Sometimes diffuse processes run on, apparently, with perfect fatalism to a mortal issue in a few years both with and without treatment. Again treatment appears to accomplish much (see fuller discussion under 2). The laws governing the preference of processes to lodge in membranes, vessels, and parenchyma, and in all combinations of these, have not been worked out. Hardly a case of neurosyphilis, properly studied ante mortem and post mortem, but would throw important light on our medical approach to one of the great problems of civilization, the problem of syphilis as a whole.

(2) RE *value of a hopeful approach to the therapy of neurosyphilis.*

The prognosis of neurosyphilis is not worse than that of the chronic diseases in general. In fact, the prognosis of neurosyphilis *quoad vitam* is either good or dubious, certainly not bad. The surprising reversals of form which the spirochete shows in certain remissions are always to be awaited. Treatment of neurosyphilis has certainly effected amazing results, not so much by way of Ehrlich's *therapia sterilisans magna* as by means of systematic intensive treatment. Even paretic neurosyphilis (general paresis) seems to have been cured. Preparetic phases are theoretically hopeful. Nor is it so certain that paretic neurosyphilis will ultimately prove a perfectly distinct species of neurosyphilis. General paresis seems to us at least to be more closely related to diffuse neurosyphilis than is tabes dorsalis to diffuse neurosyphilis. In any particular case, moreover, **during a good part of the early months or years, it is difficult or impossible to tell the paretic from the non-paretic forms of diffuse neurosyphilis by any combination of clinical observations and tests.** In the instance of more protracted neurosyphilis, e.g., tabetic, the outlook for vascular complications is such that antisyphilitic treatment directed at prevention of these complications is scientifically warrantable, even if the tabetic process itself proves unassailable. The old distinction of syphilis and parasyphilis, so striking and apparently satisfactory when introduced by Fournier, seems to be a false distinction which should be dropped. Therapeutically, we should approach all cases of neurosyphilis without bias or nihilistic prejudgments.

(3) RE *universal applicability of syphilis tests in nervous and mental cases.*

The importance of putting every neurosis or psychosis through syphilis tests is not based alone on the frequency of neurosyphilis, though neurosyphilis is surely frequent enough. The importance of universally applying these tests is established by the experience of lingering doubts both in the physician's mind and (nowadays increasingly) in the patient's and friends' minds, so long as these tests are not applied. Nor should the positive serum Wassermann reaction fail to be followed by lumbar puncture and appropriate tests. The general practitioner confronting neuroses or psychoses — and what practitioner does not? — must not expect valuable results from consultation with neurologists and psychiatrists when he does not carry to these specialists the results of at least the serum W. R. in his patient. Not only are practitioners, specialists, and patients subject to discomfiture on the eventual and delayed proof of syphilis or neurosyphilis, but valuable time has been lost to treatment. How often the physician of yore (and really not so long since) had to be regarded as an eccentric virtuoso if he tested urine as routine! Well, for routine use in nervous and mental diseases, the Wassermann serum reaction is at least as important as urinanalysis. Nor would we cease our homily with the general practitioner. We know neurologists and psychiatrists who use the Wassermann test *only when it is likely to be positive!* But they are dying out.

APPENDIX A

In appendix A a brief outline is given of the six tests (W. R. on blood serum and spinal fluid, cell count, globulin test, albumin test, gold sol test). This is not intended as a complete working manual but rather as indicating the methods used in diagnosis in the cases presented herein. For more complete details the reader may be referred to textbooks on the subject of serology, among which may be mentioned Kaplan: "Serology of the Nervous System"; Plaut, Rehm and Schottmüller: "Leitfaden zur Untersuchungen der Zerebrospinalflüssigkeit"; Kolmer: "Infection, Immunity and Specific Therapy," and, for the Wassermann technique, an article by Dr. W. A. Hinton in M. J. Rosenau's "Preventive Medicine and Hygiene."

Our own W. R's. have been performed at the Wassermann laboratory of the Massachusetts State Board of Health (formerly the Neuropathological Testing Laboratory, Harvard Medical School), under the supervision of Dr. W. A. Hinton. The other tests are performed at the Psychopathic Hospital. It is very important that a close relationship should exist between the clinician and the Wassermann laboratory if the most is to be obtained from the reactions. This relationship has been effectively close between the authors and the above-mentioned laboratory; and has enabled us to get very much clearer ideas about certain cases than could otherwise have been obtained.

Cell Count. In order to obtain the number of cells per cmm., the examination should be made of the fresh fluid as soon as possible after this is withdrawn. The most convenient counting chamber for this purpose is the so-called Fuchs-Rosenthal counting chamber, the ruled spaces of which contain slightly over 3 cmm. (an ordinary blood cell counting chamber may be used). According to the method used by us the cells are stained in a pipette with Unna's polychrome methylene blue. Using a white-counting pipette, stain is drawn up to the first or second marking and the remainder of the pipette filled with spinal fluid. This makes no change in the dilution for practical purposes. After two or three minutes the staining is satisfactory and the counting may be done. With this stain a differential count may be made. Plasma cells stain a lavender as contrasted to the blue of the lymphocytes. The characteristic halo surrounding the eccentric nucleus is visible. The blood cells do not assume color with this stain; hence it is unnecessary to add any acetic acid.

For permanent preparations, and more accurate differential counts of the spinal fluid, the Alzheimer method may be used. The technique is given in a paper by H. A. Cotton and J. B. Ayer as follows:*

1. Lumbar puncture in the usual manner.

2. 96% alcohol, in proportion to twice the amount of cerebrospinal fluid, is added drop by drop and well mixed.

3. Centrifuge the mixture for one hour at high speed in a glass tube with conical end. (An ordinary electric urinary centrifuge apparatus can be employed, the tube to be well stoppered to prevent evaporation.)

4. The supernatant fluid is poured off, leaving a small coagulum in the bottom of the tube.

5. Add absolute alcohol — alcohol and ether — ether, each separately for one hour, to dehydrate and harden coagulum.

6. The coagulum can now be gently loosened from the bottom of the tube by a long needle. The tube is then inverted, and the coagulum allowed to fall into the hand by a quick tap on the end of the tube. Care must be taken not to squeeze or handle the coagulum. The hand is placed over a small homeopathic vial, containing thin celloidin, and the coagulum allowed to drop into the celloidin, where it remains over night (twelve hours usually).

7. Coagulum is placed in thick celloidin which is allowed to evaporate slowly. It is then mounted on blocks and sections cut 14 μ in thickness.

* From Mallory and Wright: Manual of Laboratory Technique.

8. The sections are stained and mounted according to the following procedure:

(*a*) Remove celloidin by absolute alcohol and ether.

(*b*) 80% alcohol.

(*c*) Water.

(*d*) Sections are carried on glass or platinum needle into a dish of Pappenheim's pyronin-methyl green stain and kept in a water-bath at 40° C. five to seven minutes.

(*e*) Quickly cool dish in running water.

(*f*) Wash off superfluous stain in plain water.

(*g*) Absolute alcohol to differentiate — until no more stain comes away from section.

(*h*) Clear in Bergamot oil.

(*i*) Mount in balsam.

The normal cell count may be stated as being up to 6 cells per cmm.; from 6 to 12 cells may be considered as suggestive of pathological condition and more than 12 cells per cmm. as definitely pathological. The type of cell in syphilitic diseases is preponderantly the small lymphocyte. A low percentage, that is, very rarely over 20%, of large lymphocytes, endothelial phagocytic cells, polymorphonuclear leucocytes and plasma cells may also be found. The finding of plasma cells in any number in the spinal fluid is suggestive although not conclusive evidence for the diagnosis of paretic neurosyphilis.

Globulin is an albumin which is precipitated by half saturation with a salt. A very simple and satisfactory test is known as the Nonne-Appelt test, which has been modified by Ross-Jones. Into a test-tube of small diameter, run 1 cc. of spinal fluid. Place under this fluid with a pipette, 1 cc. of a saturated solution of ammonium sulphate $((NH_4)_2SO_4)$. If any globulin is present a white, sharply-defined ring will form at the junction of the two fluids. According to our readings, a ring that is just visible with the aid of a black background is called 1+, a ring that is just visible without the black background, 2+; a ring easily perceptible, 3+ and a relatively very heavy ring, 4+. On shaking the tube, if globulin is present, the fluid will show turbescence.

Another simple globulin test used in our laboratory as a check on the Nonne-Appelt test is the Pandy test. A few cc. of a clarified 10% solution of phenol are placed in a watch glass. One drop of spinal fluid is run into this solution. A milky turbescence indicates globulin.

The presence of globulin in the spinal fluid is always an indication of abnormality of the cerebrospinal axis. There is nothing differential in this finding as it occurs in all inflammatory processes. However, it is characteristically present in most cases of neurosyphilis (exception to the rule: the pure vascular type does not show globulin in a very high per cent).

Albumin Test. Albumin in small quantities is present in all spinal fluids. Increase over the normal amount occurs in pathological conditions such as most cases of neurosyphilis, especially in those in which globulin is found. Any albumin precipitant may be used for rough clinical calculation, comparing the amount of precipitate with that from the normal fluid. Our method is to place 1 cc. of spinal fluid in a small test tube of about 5 mm. diameter and to precipitate the albumin by the addition of 3 drops of $33\frac{1}{3}$% of trichloracetic acid. This test has its chief value as confirmatory of the globulin test, since in the vast majority of instances where globulin is found there will also be found an increase in albumin.

The **Gold Sol Reaction** is an empirical test discovered by Carl Lange in the utilization of the work of Zsigmondi with solutions of colloidal gold and albumins. Briefly the details of the test are as follows:

Ten tubes are set up in a rack. To the first tube 1.8 cc. of a 0.4% of salt solution is added and to each of the following tubes 1 cc. of this solution. Then to the first tube containing 1.8 cc. of salt solution one adds 0.2 cc. of the spinal fluid to be tested. This gives a dilution of 1 to 10. From this tube 1 cc. is pipetted into the second tube and this process continued through the ten tubes. This gives dilutions of spinal fluid of 1 to 10, 1 to 20, 1 to 40, etc., to 1 to 5120 in the last tube. Then 5 cc. of colloidal gold solution is added to each tube. A positive reaction is indicated by the precipitation or throwing down of the colloidal gold into its metallic form.

This produces a change in color. This precipitation may be partial or complete and the amount of precipitation is indicated by the color and is read as follows:

The unchanged fluid is called 0; a slight change giving a red-blue as 1; a further change giving a blue-red as 2; a straight blue as 3; a lavender or violet as 4; and the colorless fluid representing complete precipitation as 5. The numbers are placed in a row, indicating the tube in which the color occurs. The fluid from a case of paretic neurosyphilis will give a complete precipitation beginning in the first tube and running through a number of tubes and then grading off. It may be indicated 5 5 5 5 4 3 1 0 0 0. The characteristic reaction of fluids from tabetic and diffuse neurosyphilis is less strong than from the paretic. The greater part of the reaction will take place, however, in the first five tubes, but as a rule it will not begin very strongly in the first two. A characteristic reaction is 1 2 3 3 2 1 0 0 0 0. Another reaction that may be considered characteristic of the tabetic or diffuse form is 3 3 3 2 1 0 0 0 0 0. Fluids from non-syphilitic cases as a rule give a reaction having its greatest intensity beyond the fifth tube, that is, in the high dilutions.

A reaction characteristic of brain tumor or tuberculous meningitis is 0 0 0 0 1 3 3 2 1 0.

The conclusions that may be drawn from the gold sol reaction have been summarized by one of the authors as follows:

1. Fluids from cases of general paresis will give a strong and fairly characteristic reaction, especially if more than one sample is tested, in the vast majority of cases.

2. Very rarely a general paresis fluid will give a reaction weaker than the characteristic one.

3. Fluids from cases of syphilitic involvement of the central nervous system other than general paresis often give a weaker reaction than the paretic, but in a fairly high percentage of cases give the same reaction as the paretics.

4. Non-syphilitic cases may give the same reaction as the paretics; these cases are usually chronic inflammatory conditions of the central nervous system.

5. When a syphilitic fluid does not give the strong " pa-

retic reaction," it is good presumptive evidence that the case
is not general paresis; and this test offers a very valuable
differential diagnostic aid between general paresis, tabes and
cerebrospinal syphilis.

6. The term " syphilitic zone " is a misnomer, as non-
syphilitic as well as syphilitic cases give reactions in this
zone; but no fluid of a case with syphilitic central nervous
system disease has given a reaction out of this zone (test
thus valuable negatively). Any fluid giving a reaction outside of this zone may be considered non-syphilitic.

7. Light reactions may occur without any evident significance, while a reaction of no greater strength may mean
marked inflammatory reaction.

8. Tuberculous meningitis, brain tumor and purulent
meningitis fluids characteristically, though not invariably,
give reactions in higher dilutions than syphilitic fluids.

9. The unsupplemented gold sol test is insufficient evidence on which to make any diagnosis, but used in conjunction with the Wassermann reaction, chemical and cytological
examinations, it offers much information looking toward
the differential diagnosis of general paresis, cerebrospinal
syphilis, tabes dorsalis, brain tumor, tuberculous meningitis,
purulent meningitis.

10. We believe that no cerebrospinal fluid examination
is complete for clinical purposes without the gold sol test.

The **Wassermann reaction** as carried out in the Wassermann Laboratory is based on the principles of the original
method — the only essential modification consists in the employment of cholesterinized alcoholic extracts of human
hearts as antigen instead of aqueous extracts of foetal livers
from cases of congenital syphilis. Experience has shown that
properly standardized antigens made from human hearts are
much more sensitive in the detection of true cases of syphilis.

Antigens. Three antigens are used, each being an alcoholic
extract of human heart which is saturated at room temperature with cholesterin. These antigens differ slightly in their
sensitiveness. Before the test is made each antigen is diluted
with 0.85% salt solution in the proportion of four parts of

the cholesterinized antigen extract to sixteen parts of 0.85% salt solution. The amount to be used, the dosage, is carefully determined by testing each antigen against a large number of known positive and known negative specimens of blood. The dosage of the antigens employed is less than one-half the amount which inhibits hemolysis when the antigen is incubated for one hour with the hemolytic system which consists of complement, amboceptor and cells in the proper proportions. These antigens are designated as A, B, and C. Antigen A is the most sensitive. B and C are very similar to each other quantitatively and qualitatively.

Specimens to be tested. The serum which separates from the clot is withdrawn, centrifugalized if necessary, and then heated at 55 degrees for thirty minutes. 0.1 cc. of serum is used in the test and 0.2 cc. of each specimen is used as a control to exclude the presence of anti-complementary substances. Spinal fluids are tested in two ways. As a routine 0.5 cc. of the spinal fluid is used in the test and 1.0 cc. is used in the control; or when especially requested spinal fluids are titrated by using respectively 1.0, 0.7, 0.5, 0.3, and 0.1 cc. of the spinal fluid for each test and 1.0 cc. of spinal fluid for the control. Spinal fluids are not inactivated.

Complement. The complement is obtained from the serum of guinea pig's blood. No complement is used when older than eighteen hours. A 10% solution and 0.85% salt solution is used in the test. The amount used is twice the minimum quantity necessary to hemolyze the sensitized cells.

Sheep's Corpuscles. A 5% suspension of sheep's corpuscles in 0.85% salt solution is prepared from defibrinated sheep's blood. The corpuscles are washed three times and for each washing four to five times as much 0.85% salt solution is used as the original volume of the defibrinated blood.

Amboceptor. The amboceptor is prepared by injecting sheep's corpuscles into a rabbit. The serum of this rabbit which contains amboceptor is diluted with 0.85% salt solution so that 0.25 cc. will hemolyze 0.5 cc. of a 5% suspension of sheep's corpuscles. In the test twice the quantity or 0.5 cc. of amboceptor is used.

Sensitized Cells. The sensitized cells consist of equal parts of washed sheep's corpuscles and diluted amboceptor. This mixture is incubated in a water bath at 37° C. for a half hour to effect the sensitization of the cells.

Technique of the Wassermann Test. One-tenth cubic centimeter of each inactivated specimen of serum and 0.5 cc. of each uninactivated specimen of spinal fluid is pipetted into a separate tube. A mixture is freshly prepared in salt solution, each cubic centimeter of which contains the proper amount of antigen A (the most sensitive antigen), and two units of a 10% solution of guinea pig serum (complement). One cubic centimeter of this mixture is pipetted into each test tube. These tubes are then incubated for forty minutes in a water bath at 37° C. At the end of this period, sensitized cells are added, and the tubes are again incubated in a water bath at 37° C. for one hour. Each specimen which shows any degree of inhibition of hemolysis is retested in the afternoon. For this second test antigen A is again used and in addition antigens B and C. A control is also made for each specimen retested to eliminate any possibility of the inhibition of hemolysis being due to anti-complementary substances in the serum or spinal fluid tested. The technique of the second test differs in no wise from that of the first, except for the use of a control in each retested specimen and the employment of three antigens instead of one. The degree of positiveness is noted for each retested specimen and compared with the degree of positiveness obtained for the corresponding specimen with the same antigen-complement-salt solution mixture in the morning's test. The specimen is retested on the next day when discrepancies occur between the morning reading for antigen A and the afternoon reading for antigen A. From the above description it will be noted that the negative specimens have but a single test with one antigen only, while the positive specimens are retested, thus permitting a confirmation of any positive reaction. In this way attention is focalized on the positive specimens.

Interpretation of Results. Antigen C (the weakest of the three antigens) is used entirely for diagnostic purposes and any specimen showing the slightest degree of inhibition with this antigen and stronger degrees of inhibition with the other antigens is reported as positive. The specimens which are strongly or moderately positive with antigens A and B and negative with antigen C are reported as doubtful. In testing spinal fluids by the titration method, antigen C is used and the readings are based upon the degree of inhibition of hemolysis noted. The intensity of this inhibition is indicated by Arabic numerals: " 5 " indicates complete inhibition, while " 1 " means a faint cloudiness, hence a weak reaction. Intermediate numbers show relative intensity varying between complete inhibition " 5 " (strong positive) and slight inhibition "1 " (weak positive); "—" equals no inhibition (negative).

Although it is commonly believed that the recent administration of antisyphilitic treatment will affect the reaction by making it negative, this is not our experience, and it is, therefore, not necessary that treatment be withdrawn for a short period before the specimen is submitted for examination.

The reaction as carried out in this laboratory has the following diagnostic significance: **Positive indicates syphilis,** except very rarely in acute febrile conditions such as malaria and pneumonia. **Negative does not exclude syphilis.** In obscure conditions a series of less than three negatives has little diagnostic significance. **Doubtful suggests syphilis.** It is therefore advisable to submit three or more specimens in such a case, and interpret a persistently or predominatingly doubtful reaction as indicative of syphilitic infection.

Bruck Test. A new serum test for syphilis has recently been described by C. Bruck.* Following are recent results in our laboratory with this test.†

This new test for the diagnosis of syphilis by C. Bruck has aroused much interest. The scientific standing of Bruck and the simplicity of the technique led us to overcome our prejudice, that has been the offspring of the numerous tests that have been offered of late. Bruck states that since

---

* Bruck. Münch. med. Wochen. Jan. 22, 1917.
† Smith and Solomon. Boston Medical and Surgical Jour.

the discovery of the complement fixation test for syphilis by Wassermann, Neisser and himself in 1906, he has been trying to find a simple chemical reaction that would take the place of the complicated technique of the Wassermann reaction. This method, as he has published it, was worked out and is being used at the front, in the present war, where complete laboratory equipment is not available.

Commencing our experiments with a great deal of scepticism, we were much surprised at the results obtained, which are given below. Whatever may be the final status of the test in the determination of syphilis, we feel that there is a great deal of interest in the fact that this simple chemical reaction does pick out certain differences in the composition of blood sera and that apparently a large number of syphilitic sera differ in their chemical composition percentage from the majority of non-syphilitic sera.

The technique, while exceedingly simple, offers many chances for errors and individual variations so that we have thought it well to give directions and cautions at some length.

Bruck's* technique is described as follows: "The test is made with 0.5 cc. clear serum in a test tube, to which is added 2 cc. of distilled water, and the whole shaken. Then, with a precision pipette, 0.3 cc. of the ac. nitr. purum of the German pharmacopeia is added and the whole thoroughly shaken and then set aside at room temperature for ten minutes. Then 16 cc. of distilled water at room temperature is added, and closing the tube with the finger, it is shaken up and down three times carefully, not vigorously enough to make it foam. This is repeated ten minutes later, and the tube is then set aside for half an hour. By this time the precipitate is entirely dissolved in the tube with the normal serum, while the syphilitic serum shows a distinct, flocculent turbidity. In two or three hours, or better still, in twelve hours, the gelatinous and characteristic precipitate is piled up on the floor of the test tube."

---

* Bruck: Journal of American Medical Association, Vol. lviii, No. 12, March 24, 1917, p. 944.

The acid is prepared by diluting the Acidum nitricum of the U. S. P. (Sp. gr. 1.403) with distilled water until the hydrometer shows the specific gravity 1.149, which corresponds to the nitric acid of the German pharmacopeia, but since this requires a special hydrometer, a simpler method is to make a 25 per cent solution of the Acidum nitricum, which will give about the proper specific gravity.

The serum is obtained by allowing 10 cc. of blood to stand at room temperature for an hour, and then centrifuging. Serum that has stood for some time may be used as well as the fresh, and even bloody serum does not seem to confuse the results to any great degree. The serum gives the same results with or without inactivation. Post-mortem blood gave results as constant as that obtained during life, in the few cases that we had in this series. But the reaction may be influenced markedly by the size of the test tubes. We have found that the 13 × 1.9 cm. is the most favorable size.

When one first thinks of this test it appears very simple and probably somewhat crude as a chemical reaction, but there are certain precautions that must be observed, and several hundred normal and syphilitic sera should be tried before the investigator can feel that he has a refined routine technique. There is the personal equation which must be watched, for here is probably the greatest source of error, and readily explains why two different persons get widely varying results with the same sera if they have done only a few dozen tests. We must take it for granted that the reaction is a quantitative one, where some positive reactions may differ only slightly from the normal non-syphilitic, and, furthermore, any normal serum may be made to give a positive reaction, and almost any positive serum be made to give a negative by improper manipulation at some point in the test. There are as many places for error to creep in as there are steps in the process. Bruck has omitted many details in his publication, which allow personal variations, and so we have tried to develop a routine process that will eliminate as many of these as possible.

We shall here attempt to explain the methods which we have found most satisfactory and at the same time indicate

APPENDIX A

the places where error is likely to occur. The 0.5 cc. of serum is added to 2 cc. of distilled water, and shaken thoroughly. Now add slowly exactly 0.3 cc. of acid from a precision pipette, care being taken it does not flow down the side of the tube. The tube should be shaken gently while the acid is being added, for this prevents the formation of a flocculent precipitate in normal serum which is difficult to dissolve later. After the acid is added shake each tube gently to make sure that these flakes do not persist. It is difficult to shake each tube in exactly the same manner, as must be done if we expect uniform results.

The first 250 tests of this series were made by allowing the tubes to stand for ten minutes as Bruck advocates. Then we found that practically all sera gave a positive reaction if allowed to stand 15–20 minutes, and so in the other tests of the series an attempt was made to make the reaction more sensitive by allowing the tubes to stand only 6–7 minutes. During this time the tubes should be shaken gently once or twice. The manner in which the 16 cc. of water is added also influences the reaction. If allowed to flow freely in upon the precipitate, the positive may be forced into solution as well as the negative. Both pipette and tube should be slanted and the water allowed to flow down the side of the tube without disturbing the precipitate. If all has gone well up to this point, we may see a marked difference between the normal and syphilitic precipitates, in that the normal will begin to go into solution at once, thus clouding the water, while a positive precipitate will be composed of large flakes which show little or no tendency to go into solution or cloud the water above. It must be remembered that the most flocculent positive precipitate will go into solution if the fluid is splashed or shaken too hard while the tube is being inverted. If any doubt as to the character of the precipitate now exists, it may be allowed to stand ten minutes longer, and again inverted as before, or even repeated several times during the next hour or two. We see no reason why the tubes should be left to stand over night, for during this time a precipitate usually settles in the normal tubes. This, however, differs from the syphilitic precipitate in that it is still finely granular and goes back into solution readily when the tubes are inverted.

In view of these possible grounds for error, it is only logical to run controls of known positive and known negative sera along with each group of unknown bloods, and even then certain tubes will seem doubtful, in which event the test should be repeated with added precaution to see if a definite positive or negative reaction may be obtained.

In the last tests of this series we seemed to aid the reaction by rendering the serum-water solution alkaline by one or two drops of 10 per cent potassium hydroxide before the acid was added. The positive sera have a larger precipitate, while the normal seem to dissolve more readily.

TABLE I

Syphilis: nervous system involved.

General Paresis
{ Wassermann and Bruck agree positively....... 47
       "   "   negatively....... 7
       "   "   at variance......... 10

Tabes Dorsalis { Wassermann and Bruck agree positively....... 3

Cerebrospinal
{ Wassermann and Bruck agree positively....... 8
       "   "   negatively....... 3

Juvenile Paresis { Wassermann and Bruck agree positively....... 1

Summary
      Wassermann and Bruck agree positively....... 59
       "   "   negatively....... 10
       "   "   at variance......... 10

TABLE II

Syphilis: nervous system not involved.

Syphilis
{ Wassermann and Bruck agree positively....... 12
       "   "   at variance......... 5

Congenital Syph.
{ Wassermann and Bruck agree positively....... 3
       "   "   negatively....... 2

Summary:
      Wassermann and Bruck agree positively....... 15
       "   "   negatively....... 2
       "   "   at variance......... 5

TABLE III

Non-syphilitic: Wassermann reaction negative.
      Doubtful or positive Bruck.............. 86
      Bruck test negative.................... 216

Total for three groups:
      Wassermann and Bruck agree positively.......... 74
       "   "   negatively.......... 230
       "   "   at variance......... 101

The tests here reported were made on blood sera obtained from patients admitted to the Psychopathic Hospital and its Out-Patient Department. As a routine Wassermann test is made on each patient who enters the hospital, it was only necessary to take another tube of blood from each patient, and check the results in each instance with the Wassermann reaction. As it takes several days to get the report from the Wassermann laboratory of the State Board of Health, there was no chance of being prejudiced by a previous knowledge of the Wassermann reaction. The cases for the most part were those of mental disease; the majority in good general physical health.

A comparison of the total number with the Wassermann reaction shows that there was a general agreement of 304 of the 405 cases tested, or a percentage agreement of practically 75%. In considering the cases of syphilis of the central nervous system in a group by themselves, we find that the agreement is closer, since 69 of the 79 cases tested, or 87% agreed without any question of doubt. It will be noted that in several cases of general paresis, the Wassermann reaction, which was repeated at intervals, was negative, and in most of these cases the Bruck test was negative also. Our few cases of congenital and latent syphilis also checked very closely with the Wassermann test. In the various groups of mental cases in this series, no factor of interference was discovered. It is also of interest that in the cases where the blood was obtained post mortem, the Bruck test agreed with the Wassermann result obtained on ante-mortem blood serum. Further work on post-mortem sera will be reported. Some of the patients not included in the syphilitic groups that have a negative Wassermann and no clinical signs of syphilis, give a history of previous infection at some time, which might partly account for the variations in the two tests.

CONCLUSIONS

1. We present results of the Bruck sero-chemical test in 405 cases. In 101 of these cases there were definite clinical manifestations of syphilis, in which the Wassermann and Bruck tests agreed positively in 74 or 75%. The

two tests agreed negatively in 12 instances, and were at variance in 15.

2. In the group which showed syphilis of the nervous system we had 64 cases of clinically certain general paresis, of which the Wassermann and Bruck tests agreed in 54 instances, or practically 85%. In other forms of central nervous system involvement the agreement was 100% in the 15 cases tested.

3. In the cases with no apparent involvement of the nervous system the agreement was somewhat less, being 76%. This may be in keeping with the fact that the Wassermann test was not so strongly positive in these cases.

4. The advantages of the test are: (1) the short time required to do the test; (2) the limited amount of apparatus necessary, and (3) the simplicity of the technique.

5. The disadvantages of the test seem, for the most part, to be bound up in the personal variations that are apt to occur.

6. We are here dealing, most probably, with a quantitative chemical difference in the protein content of syphilitic and non-syphilitic sera, the nature of which is not understood by us. It is our hope that this may be brought to light in the near future in the field of chemistry.

APPENDIX B

COMMON METHODS OF TREATMENT USED IN CASES OF NEUROSYPHILIS

The **treatment for neurosyphilis** according to the viewpoint of the authors **is treatment for syphilis.** It is necessary in order to cure a case of neurosyphilis to cure the syphilis in the patient. Accordingly, the methods of treatment best adapted for the cure of syphilis are indicated in the treatment of neurosyphilis. As experience shows that it is often more difficult to cure the neurosyphilitic cases, treatment will have to be pushed with greater intensity than in some non-nervous system syphilis. In general, then, the methods that have been applied by the syphilologist will be used in the treatment of cases of neurosyphilis. In addition, methods attempting to bring the drug into local contact with the central nervous system have been devised. The methods of treatment have been in part indicated in Chart 27.

The method chiefly used in treatment of the cases of this book is what we have called **intensive systematic intravenous treatment.** The treatment consists of intravenous injections of salvarsan (or a substitute for salvarsan, as arsenobenzol and diarsenol) given in a dose of about 0.6 gram and repeated twice a week over a period of a number of months. In addition, injections of mercury salicylate averaging 0.065 gram once a week are given and potassium iodid by mouth. As indicated, the important point is to keep up treatment for a long period of time. This method has produced practically no untoward results, certainly no more untoward results than are to be expected with salvarsan in smaller quantities and it has seemed to us that the therapeutic results have been as satisfactory as in any other form of treatment.

Specialized forms of treatment intended to place the drug in contact with the central nervous system may be described

486

under the headings of **spinal intradural treatment** and **cerebral subdural** and **intraventricular treatment.**

Three main therapeutic agents have been largely used. These are (1) salvarsanized serum according to the **method of Swift-Ellis (in vivo).** The serum according to this method is prepared as follows: An intravenous injection of salvarsan is given to a patient and blood withdrawn at the end of one-half hour. This is allowed to clot. The serum is removed and after inactivation at 56° C. for one-half hour it is ready for use. The average dose is 15 to 30 cc. of serum. As a matter of fact, it is not necessary to use the blood serum from the same patient to whom the intraspinous injection is to be given. (2) The salvarsanized serum according to the **method of Ogilvie (in vitro).** Blood serum is prepared from any patient and to it is added salvarsan in such a strength that the amount to be injected, 10 to 30 cc. of serum, will contain 0.0001 to 0.001 gm. (3) Mercurialized serum according to the **method of Byrnes.** Mercury bichloride is added to blood serum in such proportion that the amount of serum to be injected will contain from 0.00065 gram to 0.0026 gram.

The method of intraspinous injection is to perform lumbar puncture, withdraw an amount of fluid approximately equivalent to the amount to be injected; then allow the serum to be injected to run in by gravity.

For the **cerebral, subdural and intraventricular** injections, the same sera may be used as for the intraspinous. Five or six times as much salvarsan may be given, but a smaller amount of serum may be advisable, that is, 10 to 15 cc. To perform injections a trephine opening is made in the calvarium about the size of a dime. The location of choice for the opening is slightly back of the longitudinal prominence just to the right of the median line, to avoid the frontal sinus. For subdural injections a curved needle is thrust between the dura and the brain and the serum allowed to flow in slowly by gravity. For the intraventricular injections a blunted spinal puncture needle is thrust through the brain substance into the 3rd ventricle. When the 3rd ventricle is reached the clear cerebral fluid will flow out; then after withdrawing a sufficient amount, the serum may be introduced by gravity. The trephining may be done under local anesthesia but as a rule it is better to induce general anesthesia. The subsequent injections can be made without recourse to any anesthesia whatsoever, as they are practically painless.

All procedures both in the injections and in the preparation of sera are naturally to be performed under aseptic conditions.

INDEX

Abscess, tonsillar, associated with neurosyphilis, 250.
Addison's disease in juvenile paretic, 279.
Agraphia, 101.
Albumin test, 474.
Allbutt, Clifford, 257.
Alcoholism, chronic, 227.
Alcoholic dementia, 237.
  epilepsy, 229.
  hallucinosis, 225.
  pseudoparesis, 222, 223, 451.
Allergie, 129, 204.
Alzheimer, 428.
  method, 472.
Amboceptor, 477.
Amnesia, 195.
Anaphylaxis, 129.
Anatomical formulæ, 25.
Antigens, 476.
Aortic aneurysm, 35, 439.
  " sclerosis, 41, 46, 135.
Aphasia, 31, 43, 101, 262, 445.
Apoplexy, 197.
Argyll-Robertson pupil, 209, 212, 217, 291, 450.
  as isolated symptom, 217.
  in alcoholism, 214, 229.
Arndt, Junius and, 249.
Arsenobenzol, 375, 377, 389, 486.
Arteriosclerosis, cerebral, 101.
  not a contraindication to intensive salvarsan therapy, 359.
  radial, 68.
Ascending lesion, 23.
Asymmetrical lesions, 19.
Ataxia, 31, 223.
Atheromatous degeneration, 35.
Atrophy, cerebellar, 39.
  cerebral, 47, 134, 205.
  parenchymal, 41.
  pontine, 39.

Atypical case congenital neurosyphilis, 270.
Ayer, J. B., 472.

Ballet, 72.
Barrett, A. M., 54, 175, 187, 212, 218, 219.
Bechterew, 219.
Binet and Simon, 304.
Binet scale, 277.
Birnbaum, 403.
Blood pressure, high, 70, 262, 124.
Bly, 252.
Bonhoeffer, 404, 415, 417.
Bordet, 427.
Bratz, 278.
Bruck test, 479.
Bruck, C., 479.
Bumke, 214.

Canavan, 256.
  and Southard, 70.
Cell count, 471.
Cerebral syphilis, see diffuse neurosyphilis.
Cerebrospinal syphilis, see diffuse neurosyphilis.
Cervical hypertrophic meningitis of Charcot, 56, 441.
Chancre, extragenital, 75, 342.
Character change, neurosyphilis, 314.
Charcot, 60, 186.
Choroiditis, 242.
Christian, 407.
Cimbal, 403.
Civilization and syphilis, 76.
Clinical evidences of syphilis, 131.
Clouston, 158.
Collins, Joseph, 145.
Compensation in neurosyphilis, 309, 402, 456.
Complement, 477.

Conduct disorder, 38.
Congenital syphilis, absence of stigmata, 318.
  as cause of feeblemindedness, 159, 447.
  involvement of nervous system in, 274.
Congenital neurosyphilis, 270, 395.
  resembling feeblemindedness, 272.
Conjugal neurosyphilis, 263.
Convulsions, 43, 101, 248, 362.
  cause of in paretic neurosyphilis, 232.
  in psychopathic subject with syphilis, 417.
Corneal opacity, syphilitic, 234.
Cotard, 73.
Cotton, H. A., 472.
Craig, C. B., 152, 196.
Cramer, 125.
Cranial neurosyphilis, 140.
  tenderness, 139.
Crises, gastric, 367.
Cysts, ependymal, 59.
  of softening, 27, 36, 54.
Cytorrhyctes luis, 381.

Dana, Charles L., 65, 77, 78.
Dazed states, 264.
Deafness, 63.
Decompression, 138.
Defective delinquent — diffuse neurosyphilis, 300, 455.
Dejerine-Tinel, 61.
Delinquency and juvenile neurosyphilis, 298.
Delirium tremens, 332.
Dementia, 137.
Dementia paralytica, see paretic neurosyphilis.
Dementia praecox, 74, 185, 247.
Depression, 95, 126.
Depressive drugs, 189.
Diabetes, and neurosyphilis, 240.
  insipidus, 190.
Diabetic pseudoparesis, 238.
Diarsenol, 377, 389, 391, 486.
Differential diagnosis, alcoholism and neurosyphilis, 227, 231, 234, 236.
  brain tumor, diabetic pseudoparesis and neurosyphilis, 238.
  diffuse and paretic neurosyphilis, 165, 193, 247.

Differential diagnosis, manic-depressive psychosis and neurosyphilis, 69.
  multiple sclerosis and neurosyphilis, 253, 255.
  neurasthenia and neurosyphilis, 65, 183.
  senile arteriosclerotic psychosis and neurosyphilis, 262.
Diffuse neurosyphilis, cerebrospinal syphilis, cerebral syphilis, spinal syphilis, 17, 80, 85, 97, 103, 122, 140, 183, 193, 300, 331, 342, 359, 433, 439, 443.
  premonitory symptoms, 342.
  prognosis, 80, 103, 124, 433, 443.
  spinal fluid findings in, 348.
  symptoms, 99.
  treatment, 98, 103, 184, 302, 390.
  treatment, results, 343.
Diplopia, 50, 184, 253, 356.
  causes, 140.
Donath, 401, 403.
Drastich, 407.
Duco and Blum, 403.
Dupré, 407.
Dysdiadochokinesis, 231.

Ehrlich, 184, 428, 429.
Encephalitis, 27, 248.
  disseminated, 218.
Endarteritis, 220.
Ependymal cysts, 59.
Ependymitis, 40, 47, 49, 134.
Epilepsy, 192.
  alcoholic, 229.
  brought out by syphilis, 415.
  Jacksonian, 103.
  parasyphilitic, 194.
  relation to juvenile neurosyphilis, 277.
  syphilitic, 103, 194.
  syphilogenic, 415.
Epileptic neurosis, 195.
Erb's syphilitic spastic paraplegia, 147.
  treatment of, 148.
Euphoria, 73.
Excited states, 95.
Exner, M. J., 416.
Exophthalmic goitre, syphilitic (?), 205.
Extraocular palsy, 140, 441.
Eye changes in neurosyphilis, 257.
Eye muscles, paresis of, 17, 50.

Facial paralysis, 53.
Families of neurosyphilitics, 275, 316, 318, 320, 373, 431, 457.
Family of neurosyphilitic, normal looking, but syphilitic, 318.
Familial syphilis, 299, 306.
Farrar, C. B., 411.
Fearnsides, Head and, 21, 140, 150, 193, 217, 374, 378.
Feeblemindedness, 395.
and congenital syphilis, 159.
Fernald, W. E., 159, 273, 396.
Fildes, McIntosh and, 129, 329.
Focal changes, 221.
meningitis, 50.
softenings, pontine, 54.
Fournier, 142, 222, 186, 194, 381.
Franz, 357.
Froissart, 413.
Fugue, hysterical, 264.

Garnier, 407.
General paresis, see paretic neurosyphilis.
Glands, 270.
Gliosis, 39, 47, 49, 136, 180.
Globulin, 229.
tests, 473.
Glycosuria, 238, 241.
Goddard, 397.
Gold sol reaction, 247, 474.
in brain tumor, 100.
paretic, 85, 98.
paretic, other tests negative, 383, 385.
in purulent meningitis, 100.
syphilitic, 85, 98, 345.
Graham, Thomas, 429.
Grandiosity, 72, 295, 455.
Graves, W. W., 157.
Grille, 407.
Gross, 257.
Gumma, see gummatous neurosyphilis.
Gumma of tonsil, 250.
Gummatous neurosyphilis, 53, 56, 137, 138, 140, 221, 362, 438.

Hallucinations, 53.
in paretic neurosyphilis, 249.
Hauptmann, 348.
Head and Fearnsides, 21, 140, 150, 193, 210, 217, 374, 387.

Headache, 53, 63, 122, 247, 352.
causes of, 209.
Hecht, 399.
Hemianopsia in neurosyphilis, 242.
Hemiplegia, 31, 45, 80, 122, 262, 360.
causes of, 389.
Hemitremor, 197.
Heredity, neuropathic, 84.
Herxheimer reaction, 152.
Heubner, 427, 428.
Hinton, W. A., 471.
Huntington's chorea, 258.
Hutchinsonian teeth, 45.
Hydrocephalus, 134, 306.
Hyperreflexia, explanation of, 233.
Hypochondriacal ideas, 133.
Hysteria, 815, 301.
Hysterical symptoms, 18.

Incontinence, vesical in tabetic neurosyphilis, 144.
rectal, 56.
Incubation period of neurosyphilis, 152.
Infectiousness of neurosyphilis, 95.
Insight, 95.
Insomnia, 63.
Intracranial pressure, 139, 362.
Intraspinal lesions, 95.
Intraspinous therapy, 122, 366, 486.
unpleasant results of, 366.
Intraventricular injections, 389, 487.
Involution melancholia, 187.
Iodine, untoward results, of, 363.
Iritis, 17.

Järisch-Herxheimer reaction, 72.
Joffroy, 214.
and Mignot, 64.
Junius and Arndt, 249.
Juvenile neurosyphilis, 438, 447.
relation to epilepsy, 277.
Juvenile paresis, see juvenile paretic neurosyphilis.
Juvenile paretic neurosyphilis, juvenile paresis, 45, 154, 157, 272, 275, 298, 306, 440.
age of onset, 158.
and Addison's disease, 279.
and delinquency, 298.
prognosis, 156, 158, 162, 273, 275.
treatment, 154, 161, 278, 299.

Juvenile paretic neurosyphilis, with initial trauma, 306.
congenital amputation of toes in, 158.
Juvenile tabetic neurosyphilis, 161, 447.

Kaplan, 255, 471.
Kéraval, 257.
Key, 427.
Knee-jerks, absence of, 223.
lively, 75.
return of, 24.
Koefod, Solomon and, 243.
Kolmer, 471.
Kraepelin, 65, 66, 69, 88, 91, 95, 187, 225, 249.
Krafft-Ebing, 84.

Laignel-Lavastine, 413.
Lange, C., 428, 429, 474.
Lancinating pains, 92, 141.
Lépine, 408, 413.
Leptomeningitis, 47, 54, 135.
Lewandowski, 210.
Liability of paretic, 295.
Lissauer's paralysis, 38.
Locomotor ataxia, see tabetic neurosyphilis.
Long, 418.
Lucke, Baldwin, 93, 144.
Lues maligna, 250, 452.
Lumbar puncture, untoward effects, 352.
treatment of, 354.
Lüth, 278.
Lymphocytosis, 23, 30, 40, 49.

McDonagh, 381.
McIntosh, Fildes and, 129, 329.
Malaria, cerebral, simulation of paretic neurosyphilis, 245.
Mallory and Wright, 472.
Manic-depressive psychosis, 68, 71, 77, 187, 202, 291, 384, 442.
Marie, Chatelin and Patrikios, 412.
Marie, 408, 414.
Martin, E. G., 313.
Massary, de, 414.
Mattauschek and Pilcz, 347.
Medicolegal and Social, 454.
period of paretic neurosyphilis, 414.

Meilhon, 407.
Memory, failing, 63.
Meningitis hypertrophica cervicalis of Charcot, 56.
sympathica, 19.
syphilitic, 103.
Mercurialization, 98.
Mercury, 58, 83, 85, 98, 148, 193, 235, 376, 377, 389, 391, 395, 486.
untoward results of, 363.
Metasyphilis, 89.
Metchnikoff and Roux, 427, 428.
Microgyria, occipital, 47.
Mignot, Joffroy and, 64, 66.
Migraine, 19.
Mitchell, H. W., 218.
Moebius, 429.
Mott, F. W., 158, 257, 308, 396, 437.
Multiple sclerosis, 253, 256.
relation of syphilis to, 254.
spinal fluid findings in, 254.
Muscular atrophy, 149, 446.
syphilitic relation to amyotrophic lateral sclerosis, 150.
Muscular weakness, 279.
Myerson, A., 196.

Nageotti, 428.
Nausea, 63.
Neisser, 399.
Nerve trunk tenderness, 148, 234.
Nervousness, 63.
Nervous indigestion, 63.
Neurasthenia, 63, 183.
Neuritis, cranial, 51.
optic, 365.
root, 235.
syphilitic, 235.
Neurorecidive, 152, 153, 184, 196, 235.
Neuroses, relation of syphilis to, 186.
Neurosyphilis, 187, 238, 240, 242.
aggravated on military service, 404.
atypical, 258, 346.
atypical case resembling hysterical fugue, 264.
dates, 428.
forms of, 20, 21, 28, 29, 95.
galloping, 328.
history cf, 427.
incubation period, 152.
infectiousness of, 95.

Neurosyphilis, laboratory findings in, 82.
latent, 142, 203.
lesions, 303.
lighted up by stress of military service, 412.
and marriage, 319.
prevention, 320.
onset, 64.
in primary stage, 186.
in secondary stage, 185, 283, 390.
in secondary stage, prognosis, 390.
in secondary stage, treatment, 153.
spinal, 23.
and the war, 399, 466.
Nissl-Alzheimer method, 427.
Noguchi, 381.
and Moore, 428, 429.
Nonne, 82, 125, 152, 186, 195, 196, 214, 216, 235, 254, 265.
-Apelt test, 473.
Numbness, 56.
Nystagmus, 45, 253, 256, 279.

Obersteiner, 249.
Occupation neurosis, 312.
Ogilvie method, 487.
Operation for gumma, 139.
Optic atrophy, 256.
in juvenile paretic neurosyphilis, 154.
Optic thalamus, syphilitic lesion of, 205.
Osteitis, syphilitic, 311.
Ozena, 350.

Pains, 31.
Pandy test, 474.
Paralysis, 123.
recovery from, 342.
of respiration, 248.
Paranoia, syphilitic, 225.
Paraphasia, 19, 43.
Paraplegia, 26, 30.
Parasyphilis, 89.
Paresis sine paresi, 126, 186, 204, 303, 445.
Paresis, see paretic neurosyphilis.
Paretic neurosyphilis, dementia paralytica, general paresis, softening of the brain, 37, 63, 68, 74, 78, 80, 85, 97, 131, 188, 192, 197, 199, 202, 227, 241, 262, 289, 295, 309, 314, 323, 338, 372, 375, 377, 382, 384, 386, 388, 392, 435, 440, 442.
adjuvant causes of, 414.
causing social complications, 289.
causes of death in, 197.
course, 85.
duration, 88.
forms, 95.
improvement, 377.
incidence among officers, 407.
incidence among soldiers, 402.
lesions of, 131.
"lighted up" by domestic stress in civil life, 420.
"lighted up" by "gassing," 414.
mortality from, 89.
nomenclature, 88.
onset, 192.
pathology of, 436.
prognosis, 435, 444.
symptoms, 90, 131.
symptoms, mental, 87.
symptoms, physical, 86.
versus diffuse neurosyphilis, 165.
versus vascular neurosyphilis, 169, 172.
with very marked meningitis, 332.
with very marked brain atrophy, 335.
without mental symptoms, 315.
traumatic exacerbation, 310.
traumatic form, 308, 413.
traumatic, shell shock, 401.
treatment of, 85, 370, 372, 377, 382, 384, 386, 388, 392.
treatment, results of, 351.
Pensions for disabilities resulting from venereal disease, 409.
Pensions for neurosyphilis, 411.
Peripheral neurosyphilis, 19.
Perivascular infiltration, 41.
Pernicious anemia with spinal symptoms, 267.
Petit mal attacks, 195.
Pförringer, 61.
Phobia, 67.
Pilcz, Mattauschek and, 347.
Pitres and Marchand, 421, 424.
Plaut, 249, 348, 428.
Plaut, Rehm and Schottmüller, 471.
Plasmocytosis, 40, 49, 55.

Pleocytosis, 23, 220, 247, 344.
effect of antisyphilitic treatment on, 244, 376.
in remissions, 243.
significance of, 243.
spinal fluid otherwise negative, 270.
Polydipsia, 190.
Polyuria, 190.
Pontine hemorrhage, 219.
softening, 54.
Posey and Spiller, 257.
Potassium iodid, 58, 85, 98, 193, 222, 376, 377, 389, 486.
Preparesis, 65, 77, 78.
Prince, Morton, 195.
Psammoma, 213.
Pseudoneurasthenia, 66.
Pseudoparesis, 449.
alcoholic, 222, 229, 451.
diabetic, 238.
senile, 263.
shell shock, 421.
syphilitic, 223, 371.
Pseudoparetic neurosyphilis, 222.
Pseudotabes, shell-shock, 424.
Psychogenic neurosyphilis, 189.
Psychographic disturbance, 228.
Psychopathic personality, 302.
Ptosis, 350.
Pupillary reaction, changes in, 261.
signs, 69.
Pupils, Argyll-Robertson, see Argyll-Robertson pupils.
irregular, 79, 201.
normally reacting in paretic neurosyphilis, 199.
sluggish reaction to light, 188.
stiff as isolated symptom, 265.
Purkinje cells, binucleate, 48.
Putnam, James J., 19, 56.
Pyramidal tract lesion, bilateral, 326.
sclerosis, 44.

Quadriplegia in juvenile paretic neurosyphilis, 275.
Quincke, 427, 428.

Randsklerose, 24.
Ravaut, 428.
Ravaut, Sicard, Nageotti, Widal, 428.
Rayneau, 407, 413, 414.

Recovery, 77.
Recurrences, 70.
Redlich, 403.
Régis, 73.
Remissions, 122, 435, 445.
Retardation, 187.
Retention of urine, 56.
Retinitis, hemorrhages, 365.
Richards, R. L., 402, 404, 406, 409.
Robertson, A. R., 59.
Rod cells, 226, 297.
Romberg sign, 141, 216, 279.
Root sciatica, syphilitic, 418.
Rosenau, 471.
Ross-Jones test, 473.
" Rum fit," 229.
Ryder, Charles T., 42.

Saddle-shaped nose, 210.
Salivation, 98.
Salmon, Thomas W., 89.
Salvarsan, 75, 83, 85, 193, 222, 377, 389, 486.
provocative, 78, 79.
untoward results of, 363.
Salvarsanized serum, 75.
Schaudinn, 427, 429.
Sciatic pain in neurosyphilis, 149.
Seizures, 31, 64, 83, 103, 444.
causes of in paretic neurosyphilis, 194.
Jacksonian, 392.
minor, 392.
Senile arteriosclerotic psychosis, 262.
Sensitized cells, 478.
Sérieux and Ducaste, 96.
Shaikewicz, 404.
Shanahan, 278.
Sheep's corpuscles, 477.
Shock, 42, 81.
Sicard, 428.
Six tests, 80, 85.
in tabetic neurosyphilis, 141.
Smith and Solomon, 479.
Social cases, 454.
service, 232.
Solomon, 142, 255.
and Koefod, 243.
Smith and, 479.
Southard and, 202, 303.
Somnolence, 45.

Southard, E. E., 48, 134, 212.
  and Canavan, 70.
  and Solomon, 202, 303.
  and Taft, 397.
Spasms, clonic, 326.
Spastic hemiplegia in paretic neuro-
    syphilis, 323.
Spastic paraplegia, Erb's, 147, 306.
Spasticity, 18, 256.
Speech defect, 69, 133.
Spiller, 150.
  Posey and, 257.
Spinal fluid findings in secondary stage
    of syphilis, 151, 185, 283.
  in juvenile paretic neurosyphilis, 275.
  negative in diffuse neurosyphilis, 140.
  negative in gummatous neuro-
    syphilis, 138.
  negative in neurosyphilis, 216.
  negative in tabetic neurosyphilis,
    269.
  in tabetic neurosyphilis, 141.
Spinal fluid, withdrawal for therapeutic
    purposes, 377, 379.
Spinal syphilis, see diffuse neuro-
    syphilis.
Spirochetes, "drug fastness," 381, 394.
  strains, 76, 263, 276, 381, 394.
Steida, 405.
Sterility in tabetic neurosyphilis, 144.
Stier, 407.
Stokes, Wile and, 186.
Suicide, 92, 126, 240, 296, 301.
Summary, 427.
Syphilis aggravated by service, 406,
    411.
  on service, 409.
Syphilis as cause of diabetes, 241.
  as cause of feeblemindedness, 396.
  hereditaria tarda, 160, 318.
  history of, 427.
  lesions in, 329.
  of lung, 211.
  from Mongolian, 76.
  primary, 65.
  secondary, 65.
  tertiary, lesions in, 329.
Syphilitic feeblemindedness, pathology
    of, 160.
  neuritis, 312.
  psychosis, 91.

Syphilophobia, 67, 361.
Syphilotoxins, 72.
Swift, 129, 212.
Swift and Ellis, 428, 429.
  method, 428, 487.

Tabes dorsalis, see tabetic neuro-
    syphilis.
Tabetic neurosyphilis, tabes dorsalis,
    locomotor ataxia, 30, 31, 141, 146,
    366, 367, 434, 446.
  associated with cerebral symptoms,
    177.
  atypical, 143.
  cervical, 146.
  course, 141.
  with negative spinal fluid findings,
    269.
  prognosis, 94.
  shell shock, 403.
  "shell shocked" into paretic neuro-
    syphilis, 401.
  symptoms, 93.
  symptoms in order of frequency, 145.
  treatment, 145, 366, 367.
  plus vascular neurosyphilis, 175.
  with vascular insult, 30, 439.
  versus pernicious anemia, 267.
Taboparesis, see Taboparetic neuro-
    syphilis.
Taboparetic neurosyphilis, taboparesis,
    92, 135, 195, 284, 443.
  course, 92.
  nomenclature, 94.
  prognosis, 92, 443.
  and typhoid meningitis, 284.
Taft, A. E., Southard, E. E., and,
Talon, 407.
Taylor, E. W., 50.
Temperature, paretic, 376.
Tests, changes under treatment, 102.
  changed to negative in paretic neuro-
    syphilis without clinical improve-
    ment, 385.
  changed to less strongly positive in
    paretic neurosyphilis without clini-
    cal improvement, 386.
Therapeutic conception, 324.
Thibierge, 399.
Thierry, 158.
Throbbing in head, 63.

Thrombosis, cerebral, 36, 42, 342, 357, 360, 124.
Thymus, persistent, 282.
Tibial exostoses, 100.
Tigges' formula, 248.
Todd, J. L., 406, 409.
Transient deafness, 18.
  blindness, 18.
  paralysis, 124.
  paralysis, condition in which occurs, 123.
Trauma and juvenile neurosyphilis, 278, 306.
  neurosyphilis, 456.
  paretic neurosyphilis, 199, 308, 310.
  syphilitic osteitis, 311.
Treatment of neurosyphilis, 67, 75, 83, 124, 148, 184, 222, 235, 299, 328, 332, 335, 342, 346, 350, 351, 355, 359, 365, 366, 370, 372, 375, 382, 384, 390, 392, 395, 419, 439, 457.
  case in which theoretically of no avail, 323.
  methods, 356, 486.
Treatment of syphilis, effect on development of neurosyphilis, 142, 347.
Tremor, 197.
  intention, 256.
Tubercle, 80.
Tuberous sclerosis of Bourneville, 47.
Tumor, cerebral, 53, 191, 238, 253.
  pineal, 213.

Unconsciousness, 53.
  causes of, 389.

Vascular changes, 220.
Vascular neurosyphilis, 31, 42, 72, 296, 359, 433, 440.

Vascular neurosyphilis, plus tabetic neurosyphilis, 175.
  prognosis, 433.
  versus paretic neurosyphilis, 169, 172.
Veeder, B. S., 274.
Vertigo, 122.
Viet, 278.
Virchow, 427, 428.
Vomiting, 53, 63.

Warthin, 241.
Wassermann reaction, 191.
  and alcoholism, 230.
  in congenital syphilis, 160, 271.
  meaning of "doubtful," 360.
  negative in diffuse neurosyphilis, 184.
  negative in juvenile paretic neurosyphilis, 298.
  negative in spinal fluid in spinal syphilis, 148.
  negative in spinal fluid in neurosyphilis, 101.
  negative in neurosyphilis, 252.
  negative in paretic neurosyphilis, 77.
  technique, 476.
  titrations in spinal fluid, 348.
Wassermann, Neisser and Bruck, 428.
Weiler, 214.
Weygandt, 403, 404.
Widal, Sicard, Ravaut, 428.
Wiles and Stokes, 186.
Word deafness, 35, 43.

X-ray diagnosis of bone conditions, 136.

Yerkes-Bridges, 304.

Ziehen, 409.
Zsigmondi, 429, 474.

MENTAL ILLNESS AND SOCIAL POLICY
THE AMERICAN EXPERIENCE

AN ARNO PRESS COLLECTION

Barr, Martin W. Mental Defectives: Their History, Treatment and Training. 1904.

The Beginnings of American Psychiatric Thought and Practice: Five Accounts, 1811-1830. 1973

The Beginnings of Mental Hygiene in America: Three Selected Essays, 1833-1850. 1973

Briggs, L. Vernon, et al. History of the Psychopathic Hospital, Boston, Massachusetts. 1922

Briggs, L. Vernon. Occupation as a Substitute for Restraint in the Treatment of the Mentally Ill. 1923

Brigham, Amariah. An Inquiry Concerning the Diseases and Functions of the Brain, the Spinal Cord, and the Nerves. 1840

Brigham, Amariah. Observations on the Influence of Religion upon the Health and Physical Welfare of Mankind. 1835

Brill, A. A. Fundamental Conceptions of Psychoanalysis. 1921

Bucknill, John Charles. Notes on Asylums for the Insane in America. 1876

Conolly, John. The Treatment of the Insane Without Mechanical Restraints. 1856

Coriat, Isador H. What is Psychoanalysis? 1917

Deutsch, Albert. The Shame of the States. 1948

Dewey, Richard. Recollections of Richard Dewey: Pioneer in American Psychiatry. 1936

Earle, Pliny. Memoirs of Pliny Earle, M. D. with Extracts from his Diary and Letters (1830-1892) and Selections from his Professional Writings (1839-1891). 1898

Galt, John M. The Treatment of Insanity. 1846

Goddard, Henry Herbert. Feeble-mindedness: Its Causes and Consequences. 1926

Hammond, William A. A Treatise on Insanity in Its Medical Relations. 1883

Hazard, Thomas R. Report on the Poor and Insane in Rhode-Island. 1851

Hurd, Henry M., editor. The Institutional Care of the Insane in the United States and Canada. 1916/1917. Four volumes.

Kirkbride, Thomas S. On the Construction, Organization, and General Arrangements of Hospitals for the Insane. 1880

Meyer, Adolf. The Commonsense Psychiatry of Dr. Adolf Meyer: Fifty-two Selected Papers. 1948

Mitchell, S. Weir. Wear and Tear, or Hints for the Overworked. 1887

Morton, Thomas G. The History of the Pennsylvania Hospital, 1751-1895. 1895

Ordronaux, John. Jurisprudence in Medicine in Relation to the Law. 1869

The Origins of the State Mental Hospital in America: Six Documentary Studies, 1837-1856. 1973

Packard, Mrs. E. P. W. Modern Persecution, or Insane Asylums Unveiled, As Demonstrated by the Report of the Investigating Committee of the Legislature of Illinois. 1875. Two volumes in one

Prichard, James C. A Treatise on Insanity and Other Disorders Affecting the Mind. 1837

Prince, Morton. The Unconscious: The Fundamentals of Human Personality Normal and Abnormal. 1921

Putnam, James Jackson. Human Motives. 1915

Russell, William Logie. The New York Hospital: A History of the Psychiatric Service, 1771-1936. 1945

Sidis, Boris. The Psychology of Suggestion: A Research into the Subconscious Nature of Man and Society. 1899

Southard, Elmer E. Shell-Shock and Other Neuropsychiatric Problems Presented in Five Hundred and Eighty-Nine Case Histories from the War Literature, 1914-1918. 1919

Southard, E[lmer] E. and Mary C. Jarrett. The Kingdom of Evils. 1922

Southard, E[lmer] E. and H[arry] C. Solomon. Neurosyphilis: Modern Systematic Diagnosis and Treatment Presented in One Hundred and Thirty-seven Case Histories. 1917

Spitzka, E[dward] C. Insanity: Its Classification, Diagnosis and Treatment. 1887

Supreme Court Holding a Criminal Term, No. 14056. The United States vs. Charles J. Guiteau. 1881/1882. Two volumes

Trezevant, Daniel H. Letters to his Excellency Governor Manning on the Lunatic Asylum. 1854

Tuke, D[aniel] Hack. The Insane in the United States and Canada. 1885

Upham, Thomas C. Outlines of Imperfect and Disordered Mental Action. 1868

White, William A[lanson]. Twentieth Century Psychiatry: Its Contribution to Man's Knowledge of Himself. 1936

Willard, Sylvester D. Report on the Condition of the Insane Poor in the County Poor Houses of New York. 1865